Textbook of Caesarean Section

Digital media accompanying the book

Individual purchasers of this book are entitled to free personal access to accompanying digital media in the online edition.

These online ancillary materials, where available, are noted with iconography throughout the book.

 Video

The corresponding media can be found on *Oxford Medicine Online* at:
www.oxfordmedicine.com/textbookofcaesareansection

If you are interested in access to the complete online edition, please consult with your librarian.

Textbook of Caesarean Section

EDITED BY

Professor Eric Jauniaux

Professor in Obstetrics and Fetal Medicine, Academic Department of Obstetrics
and Gynaecology, Institute for Women's Health, University College London, UK

Professor William A. Grobman

Professor in Obstetrics and Gynaecology-Maternal Fetal Medicine,
Center for Health Care Studies, Institute for Public Health and Medicine
and Preventative Medicine, Northwestern University, Chicago, Illinois, USA

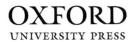

OXFORD
UNIVERSITY PRESS

OXFORD
UNIVERSITY PRESS

Great Clarendon Street, Oxford, OX2 6DP,
United Kingdom

Oxford University Press is a department of the University of Oxford.
It furthers the University's objective of excellence in research, scholarship,
and education by publishing worldwide. Oxford is a registered trade mark of
Oxford University Press in the UK and in certain other countries

First Edition published in 2016

Impression: 1

Published in the United States of America by Oxford University Press
198 Madison Avenue, New York, NY 10016, United States of America

British Library Cataloguing in Publication Data
Data available

Library of Congress Control Number: 2015950769

ISBN 978–0–19–875856–3

Printed and bound by
CPI Group (UK) Ltd, Croydon, CR0 4YY

Acknowledgements

The editors would like to thank David Bloomer and Julia Tissington (Global Library for Women Medicine) for their support in developing this project, Nicola Pritchard and Glenn Chappell for their support in filming the surgical procedures, Dan Haythorn for the editing and providing the voice-over of the videos, Olivier Jauniaux for the diagrams in Chapter 12, and Valerie Sadoun for the photography in Chapter 5. We would also like to thank all the authors and co-authors of the different chapters for giving up their time and their fees to help the distribution of this book and the training videos to low-income countries.

Contents

List of Contributors

Michael A. Belfort Department of Obstetrics and Gynecology and Center for Medical Ethics and Health Policy, Baylor College of Medicine, Houston, Texas, USA

Vincenzo Berghella Department of Obstetrics and Gynecology, Division of Maternal-Fetal Medicine, Jefferson Medical College of Thomas Jefferson University, Philadelphia, Pennsylvania, USA

Natalie Greenwold University College Hospital, London, UK

William A. Grobman Professor in Obstetrics and Gynaecology-Maternal Fetal Medicine, Center for Health Care Studies, Institute for Public Health and Medicine and Preventative Medicine, Northwestern University, Chicago, Illinois, USA

Paul Howell St Bartholomew's Hospital, Barts Health NHS Trust, West Smithfield, London, UK

Laurie Montgomery Irvine Watford General Hospital, Vicarage Road, Watford, Hertforshire, UK

Eric Jauniaux Professor in Obstetrics and Fetal Medicine, Academic Department of Obstetrics and Gynaecology, Institute for Women's Health, University College London, UK

Davor Jurkovic Department of Obstetrics and Gynaecology, University College Hospital, London, UK

Tom Lissauer Department of Paediatrics, Imperial College Healthcare Trust, London, UK

Emily S. Miller Department of Obstetrics and Gynecology, Northwestern University, Feinberg School of Medicine, Chicago, Illinois, USA

Michel Odent Primal Health Research Centre, London, UK

Daniel Pasko Department of Obstetrics and Gynecology, Division of Maternal-Fetal Medicine, University of Alabama Birmingham School of Medicine, Birmingham, Alabama, USA

Susan P. Raine Department of Obstetrics and Gynecology and Center for Medical Ethics and Health Policy, Baylor College of Medicine, Houston, Texas, USA

Desikan Rangarajan Homerton University Hospital NHS Foundation Trust, London, UK

Emily Robertson Department of Infectious Disease Epidemiology, Imperial College, London, UK

Michael Stark The New European Surgical Academy (NESA), Berlin, Germany, VEDICI-Vitalia Hospital Group, Paris, France and MIPT University, Moscow, Russia.

Philip J. Steer Academic Department of Obstetrics and Gynaecology, Chelsea and Westminster Hospital, Imperial College London, London, UK

Akila Subramaniam Department of Obstetrics and Gynecology, Division of Maternal-Fetal Medicine, University of Alabama Birmingham School of Medicine, Birmingham, Alabama, USA

Alan T. N. Tita Department of Obstetrics and Gynecology, Division of Maternal-Fetal Medicine, University of Alabama Birmingham School of Medicine, Birmingham, Alabama, USA

James Walker Department of Obstetrics and Gynaecology, University of Leeds, UK

Matthew J. West Fernville Surgery, Midland Road, Hemel Hempstead, Hertfordshire, UK

Caesarean section

INTRODUCTION TO THE 'WORLD'S NO. 1' SURGICAL PROCEDURE

Eric Jauniaux and William A. Grobman

Introduction

All around the world, women giving birth and their babies are facing the same types of basic obstetric complications: mainly, obstructed labour and post-partum haemorrhage. What varies widely is the outcome, both short term and long term, of childbirth, as these complications are more common and have more severe outcomes in low-resource settings with limited or no access to trained healthcare professionals and surgical facilities than in high-resource settings. Essential care, such as access to surgical or instrumental delivery for obstructed labour and/or non-reassuring fetal status, prophylactic uterotonics for placental delivery, prophylactic antibiotics for emergency caesarean section or prolonged rupture of the placental membranes, intravenous fluid and blood products, $MgSO_4$ for eclampsia prophlyaxis, and basic neonatal care, is often not available in many low-income countries (LICs), and this lack is a major contributor to severe maternal outcome, mainly, such as severe morbidity and death.

The caesarean section is now the most commonly performed major operation around the world, with more than 1 million procedures performed each year in the United States alone. It has become such a common procedure that it is one of the first surgical procedures performed independently by residents/trainees in obstetrics/gynaecology [1]. In most of the world, the rise in the frequency of caesarean is a relatively recent occurrence. Prior to the 1980s, rates of caesarean section were generally less than 10%. These rates, however, have risen such that they have reached over 30% in the last decade in many developed countries (see Chapter 3). This rise has been even greater in countries with rapidly industrializing economies, such as Brazil and China, where caesarean section rates are now around or over 50% [2]. The high caesarean birth rates have become a matter of concern to international public health agencies (see Chapter 13).

Nevertheless, despite the rise in the frequency of caesarean delivery in many countries, caesarean section rates in rural areas of many African and Asian countries remain lower than the 10%–15% ideal rates proposed by the World Health Organization as a target to optimize maternal and perinatal health [3]. There is no doubt that, if substantial reductions in maternal and perinatal mortality are to be achieved, universal availability of life-saving interventions needs to be matched with comprehensive emergency care and overall improvements in the quality of maternal and neonatal healthcare [4]. Progress can be made through the use of evidence-based interventions, such as oxytocin for the prevention and treatment of post-partum haemorrhage [5]. There is also increasing interest in the provision of essential surgical care such as caesarean section as part of public health policy in developing countries [6]. However, because of the lack of obstetrician/gynaecologist specialists in most LICs, the provision of emergency care for mothers and babies outside main urban areas is difficult to implement.

Increased international awareness of the need to provide accessible essential or emergency obstetric and newborn care in developing countries has resulted in the recognition of new training needs and in a number of new initiatives to meet those needs. In some cases, educational programmes have been implemented to train general practitioners and nurses in performing emergency caesarean section in rural areas of India and sub-Saharan Africa [7–11]. However, these initiatives have had limited impact, partly because of the lack of a distribution network for quality medical literature, including medical textbooks, and the lack of direct contact between trainees and their trainers, who are often based in far-away cities or abroad. Other initiatives include capacity building through academic partnership with national and international organizations [12] such as the International Federation of Gynecology and Obstetrics (FIGO), and the Tropical Health and Education Trust (THET).

The increased access to smart mobile phones and the internet in LIC provides new opportunities for web-based educational resources (e.g., http://www.glowm.com; http://www.medicalaidfilms.org) while simultaneously enhancing faculty effectiveness and efficiency. This book about caesarean delivery will make use of these web-based resources to provide information about why caesarean delivery has evolved in the manner it has, as well as how the procedure has been and is currently performed in different parts of the world.

The rise of the modern caesarean delivery

New knowledge of human anatomy in the eighteenth century led to the first modern caesarean section by Henry Thomson and John Hunter in London in 1769 (see Chapter 1). Although nineteenth-century surgeons further developed the technique, the outcome of the procedure for both a mother and her baby remained bleak. Only after the Second World War, with the development of anaesthesia, antibiotics, blood transfusion, and neonatal care, was the outcome associated with the procedure improved. Since that time, further improvements in anaesthesiology (Chapter 7) and neonatal care (Chapter 10) have made the procedure of caesarean section safer than it ever has been.

Vertical (midline) abdominal skin incision was the technique of choice to enter the abdomen from the start of modern surgery in the eighteenth and nineteenth centuries. Surgeons preferred this technique for caesarean section because it allowed a larger space to deliver the baby, better access to the pelvis and lower abdomen, and a faster operation, compared to other techniques. It also gave good visibility of both the pelvis and abdomen at a time when operating theatre equipment, in particular lighting, was rudimentary. For similar technical reasons, uterine incisions for caesarean section were vertical, which exposed the women to a very high risk of uterine rupture in subsequent pregnancies. Martin Munro Kerr (1868–1960) was the first

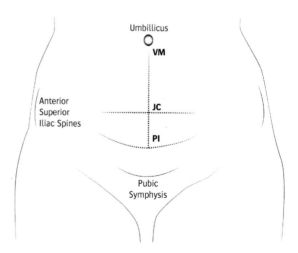

Figure E.1 Different types of skin incisions used for caesarean section; VM, vertical midline; JC, Joel-Cohen; PI, Pfannenstiel incision.

to combine the horizontal suprapubic skin incision described by Pfannenstiel (1900) and the low transverse uterine opening described by Kehrer (1881) and Sänger (1882) and is considered as the father of modern caesarean section (Chapter 1). If the low transverse uterine incision was quickly incorporated by obstetricians and gynaecologists from the beginning of the twentieth century, the suprapubic transverse skin incision remained unpopular until the 1970s. The Pfannenstiel incision was originally described for urologic surgical procedure and required more dissection and was therefore slower than the vertical skin incision. This fact explains why some surgeons continue to use the vertical skin incision for their emergency caesarean section operations, despite the higher rates of long-term post-operative complications such as wound dehiscence and abdominal incision hernia, and cosmetic issues compared to the transverse skin incision (Chapter 4). Interestingly, the same surgeons have shown little interest in using the Misgav Ladach technique described by Stark and colleagues 20 years ago (Chapter 5), although this technique, which is based on the Joel-Cohen (1972) incision, provides faster pelvic entry and access than the Pfannenstiel entry (Figure E.1).

The modern caesarean section has evolved over more than 100 years and it has led to many different technical habits and beliefs, which are sometime difficult to change within a generation of surgeons. If one considers the different options of opening the skin, opening the different layers, using an intra- or extraperitoneal approach, creating or not creating a bladder flap, closing the uterus, closing or not closing the peritoneum and the subcutaneous fat, closing the skin, and using or not using a sub-rectus sheath drain, there are thousands of ways of performing a caesarean section (Chapter 4). Only a few of these options have been evaluated by adequately powered randomized controlled trials, and overall any results and conclusions must therefore be interpreted with caution. Correspondingly, there is a need for more randomized controlled trials to reach a consensus on the safest, most efficient and most economical ways of performing a caesarean section in the twenty-first century.

The iatrogenic consequences of the caesarean section excesses

A planned (elective) caesarean section carries an overall risk of complication that is only slightly higher than that of a vaginal delivery when performed at full term by an experienced team with adequate resources. Nevertheless, caesarean section, and in particular emergency caesarean section, is associated with increased risks of haemorrhage, infection, hysterectomy, thromboembolic disease, and bladder injury (see Chapter 8). Furthermore, in subsequent pregnancies, a caesarean section can lead to placenta accreta (see Chapter 9), pelvic adhesions, and uterine scar rupture in cases of a trial of labour (see Chapters 6 and 11).

Moreover, the marked rise in the rate of caesarean section over the last decade in developed countries has taken place without an accompanying marked improvement in neonatal outcome. There is actually some evidence that caesarean section has had some adverse effects on the newborn.

In the short term, caesarean section in the absence of labour is associated with increased respiratory morbidity (see Chapter 10). In the long term, alterations of the neonatal microbiome caused by non-vaginal birth have been associated with an increased risk of asthma and type 1 diabetes mellitus (see Chapter 12).

Why, in the absence of associated improvements in maternal and perinatal health outcomes, has the caesarean section rate risen so substantially? Reasons for the increase may be differences in the maternal population (e.g. increased maternal age and BMI, an increase in the number of maternal co-morbidities) as well as the fear of litigation [13–17]. In the United Kingdom, the mean age of a mother giving birth is at an all-time high of 29.8 years, and women aged 40 and over have the fastest rising pregnancy rates [14]. Similarly maternal overweight and obesity have been rising rapidly since the 1980s, reaching 50% in many regions of the United States and Europe [15, 16, 18].

Nevertheless, these factors can only partially explain the increase in caesarean section rates. There also has been an increase in maternal request for caesarean section for both elective and medical reasons, such as breech presentation [19, 20]. However, a recent report on caesarean section on maternal request suggests that this indication is responsible for less than 3% of all deliveries in the United States [21]. Also, as less than 3% of fetuses present in the breech position at term, these factors do not represent a major contribution to the rising rates of caesarean section in the United States, South America, China, and Europe.

Regardless of the ultimate reasons for the increase in caesarean section rates, leading professional organizations in many countries and the World Health Organization now increasingly support prevention of the first caesarean section and promotion of a trial of labour after caesarean (see Chapter 11). External cephalic version for breech presentation and a trial of labour for women with twin gestations when the first twin is in cephalic presentation are examples of interventions recently highlighted by the American College of Obstetricians and Gynecologists and the UK National Institute of Clinical Excellence (NICE) that can contribute to the lowering of the primary caesarean delivery rate (see http://www.guidance.nice.org.uk/) [22]. Using a 6 cm dilatation as the cut-off for active labour, allowing adequate time for the second stage of labour, and the use of operative vaginal delivery, when appropriate, also have been suggested as important strategies to reduce the primary caesarean delivery rate in singleton term pregnancies [23].

The tide might be difficult to reverse, as an indirect effect of the rapid increase in caesarean section rates is fewer obstetricians skilled in vaginal breech delivery, external and internal version, and instrumental vaginal delivery. However, recent data showing no difference in outcome for planned vaginal birth versus caesarean section in breech presentation [24, 25] suggest that it might not be too late to control the situation. Furthermore, financial incentives and policy interventions, such as a fee changes, could be important strategies to consider in reducing the overutilization of caesarean section in developed countries [26].

Training the MD for caesarean section

Regardless of the particular surgical technique employed, there is a core set of principles that should be followed and skills that should be present at the time of a caesarean section procedure. The 2008 World Health Organization Surgical Safety Checklist (see http://www.who.int/patientsafety/safesurgery) was introduced to improve the safety of surgical procedures and has been widely accepted. A recent systematic review has evaluated the current evidence regarding the effectiveness of this checklist in reducing post-operative complications [27]. The corresponding meta-analysis showed a strong correlation between a decrease in post-operative complications and adherence to the checklist. Modified versions of the checklist for obstetrics have been recently proposed (http://www.nrls.npsa.nhs.uk/resources/type/guidance; http://www.sogc.org/wp-content/uploads/2013/04/JOGC-Jan2013-CPG286-ENG-Online.pdf). The most important modification of the checklist (Figure E.2) seems to be the adoption of a classification of the level of urgency of caesarean section (caesarean section grades). A recent retrospective study of the impact of the World Health Organization Obstetric Safe Surgery checklist in a teaching hospital in London has shown that implementation of the modified checklist improves the communication of caesarean section grade between specialist obstetricians and anaesthetists [28].

In Europe and the United States, changes in physician trainees' working patterns and hours have resulted in less exposure of trainees to surgical procedures. A recent Danish survey has highlighted the

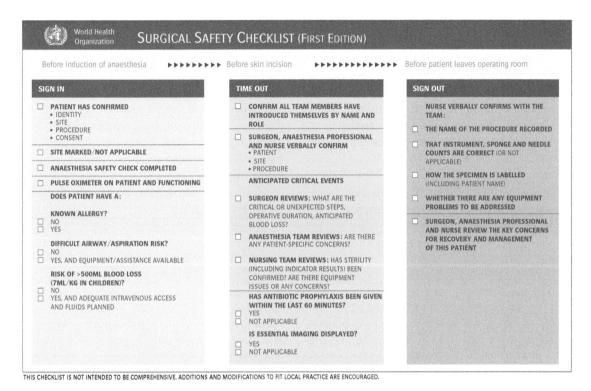

THIS CHECKLIST IS NOT INTENDED TO BE COMPREHENSIVE. ADDITIONS AND MODIFICATIONS TO FIT LOCAL PRACTICE ARE ENCOURAGED.

Figure E.2 World Health Organization Obstetric Safe Surgery checklist (http://www.who.int/patientsafety/safesurgery).
Reprinted from WORLD HEALTH ORGANIZATION – Patient safety, Safe Surgery, Copyright (2015).

need for trainees to have basic surgical proficiencies regarding instruments, sutures, and surgical technique, as well as basic anatomy (see Chapter 2), before entering a specialist training programme for caesarean section [1]. The investigators also recommended that a training programme for caesarean section skills should include theoretical instruction, video tutorials, practical experience, 40 supervised caesarean sections, and direct supervision of 10–15 caesarean sections before trainees are allowed to operate independently [1].

Validated methods of assessment are therefore required to assure the surgical competency of future obstetric specialists. One assessment of technical competence that can be used to assess the capacity of an obstetrician to carry out caesarean section is the Objective Structured Assessment of Technical Skill tool. Trainee feedback suggests that the effectiveness of the tool diminishes as the seniority of the trainee increases, with technical competence assessed less effectively in more complex procedures [29].

Recent data from the United States indicate that patients delivered by obstetricians with low delivery volume are at significantly higher risk for caesarean delivery after adjusting for patient and obstetrician characteristics [30]. These findings not only should prompt discussions regarding the role of volume in credentialing but also lead to practice models that direct patients to obstetricians with high delivery volume. In addition, these findings, in concert with the fact that it has become impossible to train a junior doctor in all aspects of modern women's healthcare, underscore the need to continue to train specialists in both obstetrics and gynaecology in the twenty-first century in high-income countries.

Simulation in medicine in general and in obstetrics in particular is gaining popularity quickly and its use may improve management of obstetric emergencies [31]. Since the first simulation manikins, then called phantoms, were fabricated in the seventeenth century, out of wicker and leather, simulators have grown increasingly more realistic. Modern simulators have been used by mainly by the military and airline industry to prepare for rare but life-threatening scenarios. Introduction of multidisciplinary teamwork training with integrated acute obstetric training interventions in a simulation setting is potentially effective in the prevention of errors [32]. Simulations can improve the performance of individuals and obstetric teams and the training of junior doctors. The evidence is also overwhelming that, with simulated practice, obstetricians improve their technical and communication skills. Shoulder dystocia has been the most widely studied complication addressed by simulation-based drills. There is limited experience of the use of simulator in operative obstetrics. Caesarean section at full dilatation can be associated with high maternal and neonatal morbidity (Chapter 4), in particular when performed by an operator with limited experience. A recent study has validated a new delivery simulator and has established expert consensus on the most effective techniques for safe delivery in full dilatation caesarean section [33].

Training the 'non-physician' for caesarean section

Many essential surgical interventions are cost-effective or very cost-effective in LICs [34]. Quantification of the economic value of surgery provides a strong argument for the expansion of surgery's role in the global health movement. A study from Burkina Faso has shown that the training of general practitioners appears to be both effective and cost-effective in the short run but that care provided by non-physician clinical officers is associated with a high newborn case fatality rate [35]. The investigators conclude that training substitutes for physicians is a viable option to increase access to life-saving operations in district hospitals, but that high newborn case fatality rate among these clinical officers would need to be addressed by a refresher course and closer supervision.

The World Health Organization recommends task shifting to improve access to key maternal and newborn interventions. Surgical task shifting is not new and, since the 1980s, non-medical clinical officers have been trained to perform selected surgical procedure, mainly in East Africa. However, access to new technologies including low-cost ultrasound machine and anaesthetic monitoring equipment is transforming rapidly the diagnosis and management of obstetric and neonatal complications. A holistic, cost-effective, and sustainable training approach including basic obstetric ultrasound, management of complicated labour, and neonatal resuscitation is essential to address supply shortages of skilled health personnel in LICs [36].

Aim of this book

The main objective of our book is to provide an overview of the caesarean section, including its history, the technical details of the procedure, and the different techniques currently in use around the world (see Chapters 4 and 5). We will present a detailed account of the worldwide epidemiology of caesarean section and the possible short-term and long-term complications of the procedure (see Chapters 3, 8, and 9).

Anaesthetic and neonatal implications also will be reviewed (see Chapters 7 and 10). In resource-limited settings, there is still a high unmet capacity for medically indicated caesarean section, as well as limited or no access to appropriate medications and equipment for comprehensive emergency obstetric care, safe and timely surgical procedures, and appropriate supervision from health professionals (see Chapters 6 and 13).

The profits from the sale of our book in the United States and Europe will be used to make a condensed version in a variety of local languages that are used in the developing world. This version will be distributed along with video material made by Medical Aid Films (http://www.medicalaidfilms.org) to local NGOs and via the Global Library of Women Medicine website (http://www.glowm.com) so that obstetric trainees as well as general practitioners and nurses in developing countries have access to the information.

References

1. Madsen K, Grønbeck L, Rifbjerg Larsen C, Østergaard J, Bergholt T, Langhoff-Roos J, et al. Educational strategies in performing cesarean section. Acta Obstet Gynecol Scand 2013; 92(3): 256–63.
2. Lumbiganon P, Laopaiboon M, Gülmezoglu AM, Souza JP, Taneepanichskul S, Ruyan P, et al. Method of delivery and pregnancy outcomes in Asia: The WHO global survey on maternal and perinatal health 2007–08. Lancet 2010; 375(9713): 490–9.
3. World Health Organization. Appropriate technology for birth. Lancet 1985; 2(8458): 436–7.
4. Souza JP, Gülmezoglu AM, Vogel J, Carroli G, Lumbiganon P, Qureshi Z, et al. Moving beyond essential interventions for reduction of maternal mortality (the WHO Multicountry Survey on Maternal and Newborn Health): A cross-sectional study. Lancet 2013; 381(9879): 1747–55.
5. Nelissen EJ, Mduma E, Ersdal HL, Evjen-Olsen B, Van Roosmalen JJ, Stekelenburg J. Maternal near miss and mortality in a rural referral hospital in northern Tanzania: A cross-sectional study. BMC Pregnancy Childbirth 2013; 13:141.
6. Grimes CE, Henry JA, Maraka J, Mkandawire NC, Cotton M. Cost-effectiveness of surgery in low- and middle-income countries: A systematic review. World J Surg 2014; 38(1): 252–63.
7. Hounton SH, Newlands D, Meda N, De Brouwere V. A cost-effectiveness study of caesarean-section deliveries by clinical officers, general practitioners and obstetricians in Burkina Faso. Hum Resour Health 2009; 7: 34.
8. Evans CL, Maine D, McCloskey L, Feeley FG, Sanghvi H. Where there is no obstetrician-increasing capacity for emergency obstetric care in rural India: An evaluation of a pilot program to train general doctors. Int J Gynaecol Obstet 2009; 107(3): 277–82.
9. Wilson A, Lissauer D, Thangaratinam S, Khan KS, MacArthur C, Coomarasamy A. A comparison of clinical officers with medical doctors on outcomes of caesarean section in the developing world: Meta-analysis of controlled studies. BMJ 2011; 342: d2600.
10. Nyamtema AS, Pemba SK, Mbaruku G, Rutasha FD, Van Roosmalen J. Tanzanian lessons in using nonphysician clinicians to scale up comprehensive emergency obstetric care in remote and rural areas. Hum Resour Health 2011; 9: 28.
11. Milland M, Bolkan H. Surgical task shifting in Sierra Leone: A controversial attempt to reduce maternal mortality. BJOG 2015; 122(2): 155.
12. Anderson FWJ, Johnson TRB. Capacity building in obstetrics and gynaecology through academic partnership to improve global women's health beyond 2015. BJOG 2015; 122(2): 170–3.
13. Moore EK, Irvine LM. The impact of maternal age over forty years on the caesarean section rate: Six year experience at a busy District General Hospital. J Obstet Gynaecol 2014; 34(3): 238–40.
14. Khalil A, Syngelaki A, Maiz N, Zinevich Y, Nicolaides KH. Maternal age and adverse pregnancy outcome: A cohort study. Ultrasound Obstet Gynecol 2013; 42(6): 634–43.
15. Hollowell J, Pillas D, Rowe R, Linsell L, Knight M, Brocklehurst P. The impact of maternal obesity on intrapartum outcomes in otherwise low risk women: Secondary analysis of the Birthplace national prospective cohort study. BJOG 2014; 121(3): 343–55.
16. Athukorala C, Rumbold AR, Willson KJ, Crowther CA. The risk of adverse pregnancy outcomes in women who are overweight or obese. BMC Pregnancy Childbirth 2010; 10: 56.
17. Groves T. The pressure of pregnancy. BMJ 2014; 348: g2789.
18. Zeal C, Remington P, Ndiaye M, Stewart K, Stattelman-Scanlan D. The epidemiology of maternal overweight in Dane County, Wisconsin. WMJ 2014; 113(1): 24–7.
19. Lawson GW, Keirse MJ. Reflections on the maternal mortality millennium goal. Birth 2013; 40(2): 96–102.
20. Hannah ME, Hannah WJ, Hewson SA, Hodnett ED, Saigal S, Willan AR. Planned caesarean section versus planned vaginal birth for breech presentation at term: A randomised multicentre trial. Term Breech Trial Collaborative Group . Lancet 2000; 356(9239): 1375–83.
21. Ecker J. Elective cesarean delivery on maternal request. JAMA 2013; 309(18): 1930–6.
22. American College of Obstetricians and Gynecologists; Society for Maternal-Fetal Medicine. Obstetric care consensus no. 1: Safe prevention of the primary cesarean delivery. Obstet Gynecol 2014; 123(3): 693–711.
23. Boyle A, Reddy UM, Landy HJ, Huang CC, Driggers RW, Laughon SK. Primary cesarean delivery in the United States. Obstet Gynecol 2013; 122(1): 33–40.

24. Vistad I, Cvancarova M, Hustad BL, Henriksen T. Vaginal breech delivery: Results of a prospective registration study. BMC Pregnancy Childbirth 2013; 13: 153.

25. Borbolla Foster A, Bagust A, Bisits A, Holland M, Welsh A. Lessons to be learnt in managing the breech presentation at term: An 11-year single-centre retrospective study. Aust N Z J Obstet Gynaecol 2014; 54(4): 333–9.

26. Chen CS, Liu TC, Chen B, Lin CL. The failure of financial incentive? The seemingly inexorable rise of cesarean section. Soc Sci Med 2014; 101: 47–51.

27. Bergs J, Hellings J, Cleemput I, Zurel Ö, De Troyer V, Van Hiel M, et al. Systematic review and meta-analysis of the effect of the World Health Organization surgical safety checklist on postoperative complications. Br J Surg 2014; 101(3): 150–8.

28. Mohammed A, Wu J, Biggs T, Ofili-Yebovi D, Cox M, Pacquette S, et al. Does use of a World Health Organization obstetric safe surgery checklist improve communication between obstetricians and anaesthetists? A retrospective study of 389 caesarean sections. BJOG 2013; 120(5): 644–8.

29. Landau A, Reid W, Watson A, McKenzie C. Objective Structured Assessment of Technical Skill in assessing technical competence to carry out caesarean section with increasing seniority. Best Pract Res Clin Obstet Gynaecol 2013; 27(2): 197–207.

30. Clapp MA, Melamed A, Robinson JN, Shah N, Little SE. Obstetrician volume as a potentially modifiable risk factor for cesarean delivery. Obstet Gynecol 2014; 124(4): 697–703.

31. Argani CH, Eichelberger M, Deering S, Satin AJ. The case for simulation as part of a comprehensive patient safety program. Am J Obstet Gynecol 2012; 206(6): 451–5.

32. Merién AE, Van de Ven J, Mol BW, Houterman S, Oei SG. Multidisciplinary team training in a simulation setting for acute obstetric emergencies: A systematic review. Obstet Gynecol 2010; 115(5): 1021–31.

33. Vousden N, Hamakarim Z, Briley A, Girling J, Seed PT, Tydeman G, et al. Assessment of a full dilatation cesarean delivery simulator. Obstet Gynecol 2015; 125(2): 369–74.

34. Chao TE, Sharma K, Mandigo, M et al. Cost-effectiveness of surgery and its policy implications for global health: A systematic review and analysis. Lancet Glob Health 2014; 2(6): e334–345.

35. Hounton SH, Newlands D, Meda N, De Brouwere V. A cost-effectiveness study of caesarean-section deliveries by clinical officers, general practitioners and obstetricians in Burkina Faso. Hum Resour Health 2009; 7: 34.

36. Greenwold N, Wallace S, Prost A, Jauniaux E. Implementing an obstetric ultrasound training program in rural Africa. Int J Gynaecol Obstet 2014; 124(3): 274–7.

CHAPTER 1
Caesarean section

FROM ANTIQUITY TO THE TWENTY-FIRST CENTURY

Matthew J. West, Laurie Montgomery Irvine, and Eric Jauniaux

Introduction

Use of caesarean section has been recorded since ancient times, with accounts in both Western and non-Western cultures; yet, the origins of this procedure remain surrounded by myth, complicated further by the fact that the procedure has changed over time and culture in both its meaning and indication.

Historically performed to save the infant, despite occasional references to operations on living mothers, it was almost invariably used to retrieve the infant from a deceased or moribund woman.

Nevertheless, it was rare for such births to survive and, rather than being motivated by the vain hope of saving the infant's life, state law or religious edicts likely required the procedure be done so the infant might be buried separately from the mother. As a measure of last resort, the operation was rarely intended to preserve the mother's life. The maternal death rate following caesarean section showed little improvement until the nineteenth century, when surgeons started to remove or suture the uterus after delivery of the baby [1, 2].

Origins of the caesarean section

Julius Caesar and the origin of the term 'caesarean'

One of the most prevailing myths associated with caesarean section concerns the birth of Gaius Julius Caesar (13 July 100 BC–15 March 44 BC), the Roman general and statesman (Figure 1.1). Legend holds that Caesar was delivered abdominally, and references to this legend have persisted in popular culture as the origin of the term caesarean. Such a delivery is almost certainly unlikely at this time

in history, and all the more given that his mother, Aurelia Cotta, lived to hear of, and congratulate, her son's invasion of Britain [3, 4].

The renowned biographer of Roman emperors, Suetonius (famous also for his witness to the historicity of Jesus Christ, and the impact of Christendom in the Roman capital just 17 years after the crucifixion) quotes Pliny the Elder as the source for this belief [5]. However, Pliny was referring to an ancestor of Julius Caesar—Sextus Julius Caesar, Praetor of Sicily in 208 BC, *a caeso matris utero* ('born

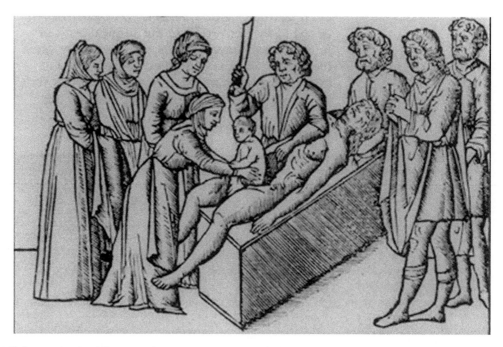

Figure 1.1 An early printed illustration of a caesarean section. Purportedly the birth of Julius Caesar. A live infant being surgically removed from a dead woman. From Suetonius' *Lives of the Twelve Caesars*, 1506 woodcut.

(Reproduced from the National Library of Medicine's History of Medicine Division)

by caesarean section'). Yet, within the dynasty, there were Gaius Julius Caesar, Sextus Julius Caesar, Lucius Julius Caesar, and Numerius Julius Caesar, all complicating identification of the individual from whom the myth arose [6].

'Caesarean delivery' may not be the only tradition cited for the additional of Caesar to the family name; others include a family member who was born with a shock of hair and thus called *caesaries* ('hairy'), or those with bluish-grey eyes (*oculi caesii*; although Julius Caesar's eyes were reputedly black). Caesar himself seemingly favoured the tradition that the familial name was derived from a word meaning 'elephant', reputedly *caesai* in the Moorish Punic or Gaul language, with claims of an ancestor being killed by an elephant. Indeed, Caesar was familiar with the creatures, using them during his European conquests, displaying 40 elephants on the first day of 'Caesar's Gallic Triumph' in Rome, and even placing an elephant above the name 'Caesar' on his first denarius. The fact that Caesar issued coins featuring elephants suggests that he favoured this interpretation of his name [7, 8].

Etymology of the term 'caesarean section'

The etymological derivation of caesarean section is from the Roman legal code, the *Lex Caesarea*, which began as the *Lex Regia* during the reign of Numa Pompilius (715–673 BC). It specified that a baby should be cut from the mother's womb if she died before giving birth, forbidding the mother's burial prior to excision: *Negat lex regia mulierem quae pregnans mortua sit, humari, antequam partus ei excidatur: qui contra feceret, spem animantis cum gravida, peremisse videtur.* ('The lex regia forbids the burial of a pregnant woman before the young has been excised: who does otherwise clearly causes the promise of life to perish with the mother.') [9] When the Roman Empire was formed, this law Lex Regia became part of the *Lex Caesaris, or Lex Caesarea*, under the rule of the emperors, and the term 'caesarean' may have derived from the law Lex Regia decreeing this procedure, from a description of infants born under the law (*caesone*), not simply from the Latin verb *caedere* ('to cut') [3, 4]. Until the sixteenth century, the procedure was known as caesarean birth, which gradually became known as caesarean operation. The term 'caesarean section' (la section césarienne) was first used by the French obstetrician Jacques Guillimeau in his 1609 book on midwifery, *De l'heureux accouchement des femmes*. Interestingly, caesarean section is one of the few operations that has similar terminology in almost all other languages; for example, *Kaiserschnitt* ('Emperor's cut') in German, *keisersnit, kejsersnit*, and *keizersnede* in Norwegian, Danish, and Dutch, respectively, *sezaryen* in Turkish, *wilaada qaySaríyya* in Arabic, and *cesariana* in Portuguese.

Legendary abdominal births

Numerous legendary references to the surgical delivery of infants appear in ancient Hindu, Egyptian, Chinese, Greek, and Roman folklore. Perhaps one of the earliest and most well known is the Greek myth about the birth of Asklepios, the god of medicine and healing, who was cut from the abdomen of his dead mother Coronis by his father, the god Apollo (Figure 1.2); his name is derived from the circumstances surrounding his birth, as it means 'to cut

open' in ancient Greek. Similarly, in Roman mythology Bacchus, the god of the grape harvest, winemaking, and wine, was delivered from his mortal mother Semele by his father, the chief god Jupiter [10]. In another version of the same story, Bacchus, known as Dionysus in Greek mythology, was rescued by his father Zeus from his dying mother and sewn into Zeus' thigh to be reborn a few months later.

There is no mention of the operation in the Bible. Discussion of the surgical birth is found within the Mishnah (AD 200), the Gemara (AD 450), and the Talmud, where rabbinical writers were familiar with the procedure. Children who survived were to be called *yotse dofan* ('go out of the body wall'). The fact that the rituals a woman should observe after the operation are also described may suggest that survival for mother and child was anticipated; but these rituals may equally have been written 'in the event' of successful surgery [1]. There are early reports of caesarean section within Islamic writings, including the birth of the Persian warrior Rostam as described in the *Shahnameh*, which was written between 940 and 1020 [11–13]. Other antique mythological surgical deliveries are presented in Table 1.1.

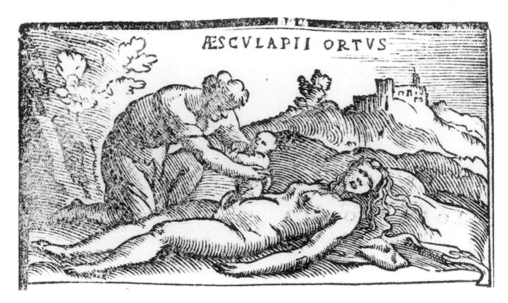

Figure 1.2 The extraction of Aesculapius from the abdomen of his mother Coronis by his father Apollo. Woodcut from the 1549 edition of Alessandro Beneditti's *De Re Medica* V.

(Reproduced from the National Library of Medicine's History of Medicine Division)

Table 1.1 Descriptions of mythical caesarean sections from antiquity to the Middle Ages

Year (source)	Location	Name	Description
1023 BC (Luzhong)	China	Jilian (1st Mi Emperor)	Mother had six sons all born by 'cutting open the body'
320 BC (Dipavanca and Mahavamsa)	India	Bindusara (Second Samrat Emperor)	Mother who was accidentally poisoned was delivered by Chanakya (teacher and adviser)
c.50 BC (Lugaid Riab)	Ireland	Furbaide Ferbend (legendary prince)	Born following the murder of his mother by her sister
AD 1000 (Shahnameh)	Persia	Rostam (Persian hero)	Rostam's mother Rudaba was having a difficult labour; his father Zal, inspired by the magical being Simurgh, performed a Rostamzad (Persian equivalent of a caesarean delivery)

Caesarean section throughout history

Caesarean section from antiquity to the fifth century

There exists an authenticated report of an infant named Gorgias, who is alleged to have survived the operation in Sicily in approximately 508 BC [3]. However, other records as far back as the fifth century BC, implying favourable outcomes for both mother and child, cannot be substantiated and as such remain dubious. It is in the second century BC when we have the first accurately recorded case in the legal adoption proceedings of a two-year-old who at birth had been 'pulled out of its mother's womb', a possible allusion to a caesarean section [1, 2].

The Greek physician Aelius Galenus, better known as Galen of Pergamon (129–200), was principally influenced by the then-current theory of humourism, as advanced by many ancient Greek physicians such as Hippocrates (460–370 BC). His theories dominated and influenced Western medical science for more than 1300 years. His anatomical reports, based mainly on dissections of monkeys and pigs, remained uncontested until the sixteenth century, his theory on the physiology of the circulatory system persisted until the seventeenth century, and medical students around the world continued to study Galen's writings until well into the nineteenth century. Interestingly, in all his writing, he only made one reference about the procedure of abdominal delivery as described by earlier authors [7]. There is also no mention of the procedure in Soranus of Ephesus' *Gynaikeia* (second century AD), the most prominent surviving ancient treatise on midwifery; this fact suggests that it was considered to be a post-mortem procedure, as at the time, common complications would have not allowed the mother to survive [8].

Caesarean section in the Middle Ages (from the fifth to the fourteenth century)

Following the fall of the Roman Empire at the end of the fifth century AD, standard medical knowledge was based mainly upon surviving Greek and Roman texts which had been preserved in monasteries. After the Crusades, the influence of Islamic medicine grew, and many medical texts both on ancient Greek medicine and on Islamic medicine were translated from Arabic during the thirteenth century. The most influential of these texts was *The Canon of Medicine*, a medical encyclopaedia written c.1030 by Ibn Sīnā (also known as Avicenna; 980–1037); it summarized the medicine practised by Greek, Indian, and Muslim physicians at that time and was used in the medical schools of the universities of Montpellier and Leuven until the seventeenth century.

The famous Jewish philosopher and physician Moses Maimonides (1135–1204) was knowledgeable about Greek and Arabic medicine and followed the principles of humourism in the tradition of Galen. In his writings, he stated that 'it was well known in Rome how to deliver an infant abdominally without killing the mother, but was seldom performed', although this statement not supported by his own experience or by the knowledge of human anatomy at the time, and therefore highly improbable [1, 7] (Figure 1.3).

Throughout the Middle Ages, there were only isolated reports of notable figures born by caesarean section. Raymond Nonnatus (1204–1240), the Catalan saint, was reportedly given his surname from the Latin *non natus* ('not born') following abdominal delivery, his mother dying in childbirth. Robert II of Scotland was allegedly born by caesarean section in 1316 after his mother, Marjorie Bruce, died following a fall from her horse at Paisley Abbey; this story possibly provided inspiration when Shakespeare wrote *Macbeth* in 1606: after having been told by witches that 'none of woman born' should harm him, Macbeth is dismayed to discover that his attacker Macduff was 'from his mother's womb untimely ripp'd' [14].

In Switzerland *c.*1500, a sow gelder is reported to have performed a caesarean delivery on his wife, who was unable to deliver her baby despite the support of 13 midwives. Not only did both mother and baby survive, but she was to subsequently give birth normally to another five children. The story was recorded 82 years later and not surprisingly has raised a few questions about its accuracy from many historians [1, 2]. Even granted the most generous acceptance, it is most unlikely that subsequent vaginal deliveries ensued without rupture, unless possibly this was an extraordinary extrauterine abdominal delivery [7, 10, 15].

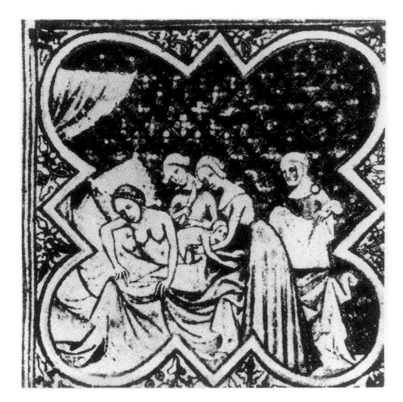

Figure 1.3 Caesarean section performed on a living woman by a female practitioner. Miniature from a fourteenth-century *Historie Ancienne*.

(Reproduced from the National Library of Medicine's History of Medicine Division)

Caesarean section from the Renaissance to the early modern period

The Renaissance brought an intense focus on scholarship and the teaching of medicine; this focus started in Bologna (1219) and Padua (1222) and then expanded rapidly to the rest of Christian Europe. A major effort to translate the Arabic and Greek scientific works into Latin emerged. Europeans scholars gradually became experts not only in the ancient writings of the Romans and Greeks but also in the contemporary writings of Islamic scientists. During the later centuries of the Renaissance came an increase in experimental investigation, particularly in the fields of human anatomy and surgery.

Andries van Wezel or Andreas Vesalius (1514–1564) was a Belgian anatomist, physician, and author of one of the most influential books on human anatomy *De Corporis Humani Fabrica*, published in 1543. Vesalius is often referred to as the founder of modern human anatomy, as his predecessors, such as Galen, were not allowed for cultural and religious reasons to perform human autopsies. His groundbreaking work contributed much through accurate anatomical depictions of the female pelvis and abdominal structures, providing theoretical foundations for the obstetric developments of the eighteenth and nineteenth centuries [1, 16] (Figure 1.4).

Another important figure in the progress of obstetrics and surgery in the mid-sixteenth century was the French barber surgeon Ambroise Paré (1510–1590). He revived the practice of podalic version, and showed how even in cases of head presentation, surgeons with this maneuver could often deliver the infant safely, instead of having to dismember the infant and extract the infant piece by piece.

In 1581, the French physician François Rousset (Franciscus Roussetus; 1535–1600) published *Hysterotomotokia*, a treatise on caesarean delivery, advocating that the operation could be performed without losing the life of mother and child and therefore being the first to advise it be done on living women. In his book, Rousset described seven cases, and Bauhin, his translator from French to Latin (1582), surreptitiously added several others. However, there

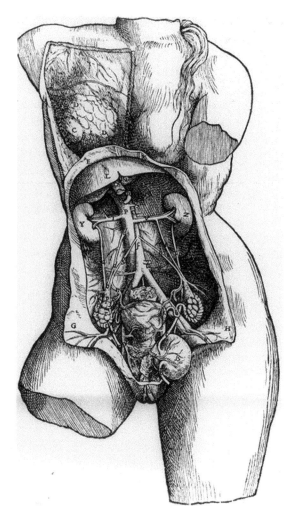

Figure 1.4 The female pelvic anatomy.

From Vesalius's *De Corporis Humani Fabrica*, 1543. (Reproduced from the National Library of Medicine's History of Medicine Division).

is no evidence that Rousset performed this procedure himself and it is very likely that he may have taken all his examples from other writers [17].

Great personal risk was associated with undertaking caesarean sections during the sixteenth and seventeenth centuries, as illustrated by the story of John Bullawanger, described as 'late of Buckden, Huntingdonshire, yeoman, self-claimed physician and surgeon' [18]. He was indicted before the justices of Assize for the Norfolk Circuit for performing an incision in the belly (*per ventris sui incisionem*) of Agnes Redborne, who was 'labouring under diverse infirmities', in Folksworth on 17 June 1573.

He opened her belly on the left side with a knife, giving her 'a blow six inches long and three inches deep, carelessly penetrating with the knife'. Agnes languished until 28 June and then died of the wound. The lapse of 10 days between the operation and the death of the patient suggests that the operation was successful and that Agnes died from sepsis rather than from intra- or post-operative bleeding. The outcome of the child is unknown, but Bullawanger was found guilty. Nonetheless, the justices recognized that he had been the first doctor to do the operation in the British Isles, and a pardon ensued [18].

By the end of the sixteenth century, a few novel surgical treatises became available to the midwifery profession. In 1596, Scipione Mercurio (1540–1615), a Roman medical physician, published a book entitled *La commare o raccoglitrice* [19], which contains the first detailed indications for the execution of caesarean sections, which he initially observed during a visit to France around 1571 (Figure 1.5). Mercurio studied medicine in Bologna under Julius Caesar Aranzi (known as Arantius; 1529–1589), a disciple of Vesalius, and his knowledge of female anatomy enabled him to improve erroneous midwifery practices that had previously contributed to infant and maternal mortality [19]. *La commare* was translated into German (*La commare: Kindermutter oder Hebammen-Buch*) and circulated in Italy and Germany for over a century, a fact which implies

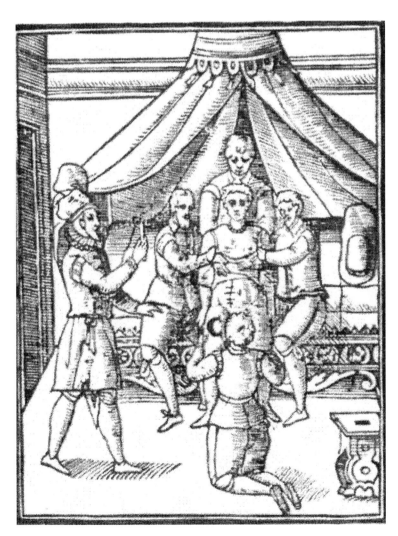

Figure 1.5 'Illustration of Birth by Caesarian Section'.

from Scipione Mercurio La Commare o Raccoglitrice. Verona, 1642.

that there was a growing demand for information on safe childbirth.

The first authenticated case of caesarean section, reported in a medical journal, was performed by Dr Jeremiah Trautmann of Wittenberg in 1610. He operated in front of a small audience, with the baby surviving but the mother succumbing to infectious complications on Post-operative day 25 [1, 4, 7]. Another European, Dr Van Roonhuyze of Amsterdam, performed a successful operation in 1663, publishing clear diagrams of his technique. Towards the end of the seventeenth century, in 1692, a post-mortem demonstrated a well-healed uterine scar from a caesarean section undertaken 14 years previously [1, 4, 7]. Important developments in caesarean section since the Renaissance are presented in Table 2 (also see Figure 1.6).

Caesarean section in the Age of Enlightenment

In the eighteenth century, anatomists and surgeons extended their knowledge of the normal and pathological aspects of the human body. The first independent clinics and hospitals opened in London (Guy's Hospital, 1721) and the colonies (Pennsylvania Hospital, 1752).

Only a few caesarean deliveries took place during the eighteenth century. In Edinburgh on 29 June 1737, the surgeon Robert Smith operated successfully in the presence of seven colleagues, with the infant stillborn and the mother dying 18 hours later. In London, on 21 October 1774, Henry Thomson, assisted by John Hunter (1728–1793), the genial anatomist and founder of modern surgery, performed a caesarean section on Martha Rhodes [20]. Having dosed her with opium, they made a six-inch-long incision in her abdomen and then opened the womb and delivered the baby. Martha died 5 hours later, probably because of internal bleeding, and her baby died 2 days later. Of nineteen operations recorded in the British Isles during the eighteenth century, only six children survived, with no mother surviving' [4]. During that period, the only doctors recorded as saving a mother were James Barlow, who was assisted by Charles White, a pupil of John Hunter, in Blackburn, in 1793. The following year, Dr Jesse Bennett of Frankford,

Table 1.2 Important technical steps in caesarean section procedures since the Renaissance

Year	Name	Country	Description
1543	A. Vesalius	Belgium	First human anatomy book *De Corporis Humani Fabrica*
1581	F. Rousset	France	Describes caesarean sections performed on living women in *Hysterotomotokia*
1596	S. Mercurio	Italy	First detailed caesarean section indications in *La commare o raccoglitrice*
1610	J. Trautmann	Germany	First authenticated caesarean section with survival of the mother
1769	J. Lebas	France	First closure of the uterus after caesarean section
1786	S. Johnson	United Kingdom	First description of lower segment uterine incision
1876	E. Porro	Italy	Caesarean section followed by supracervical partial hysterectomy and salpingo-oopherectomy
1882	F. Kehrer and M. Sänger	Germany	Transverse incision of lower uterine segment and uterine closure using sutures made of silver wire
1900	H. Pfannenstiel	Germany	Described transverse suprapubic skin incisions
1908	M. Munro Kerr	United Kingdom	First series of suprapubic skin incision and transperitoneal lower segment caesarean sections

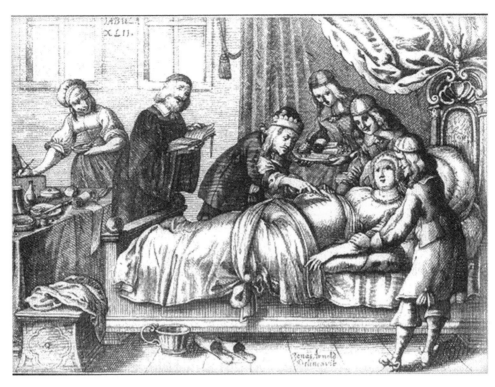

Figure 1.6 Plate XLII from Scultetus' *Armamentaerium Chirugicum Bipartum*, 1666.
(Reproduced from the National Library of Medicine's History of Medicine Division)

Pennsylvania, is credited with the first successful professional caesarean delivery in the USA. He operated on his own wife and also removed her ovaries so that neither of them would face the same experience again [4, 5].

Outside of the medical profession, the details of the first women to survive a caesarean section in the British Isles were published by surgeon Duncan Stewart, of Dungannon, in 1741. Three years prior, in 1738, in Charlemont, Co. Armagh, Alice O'Neill, a thirty-five-year-old, multiparous farmer's wife had been in labour for 12 days, with the infant believed to have died on Day 1. An illiterate woman by the name of Mary Donnelly was infamous for extracting dead infants in the traditional fashion through the birth canal following craniotomy and so was called in this instance. After failing with the traditional methodology, she proceeded to perform the caesarean section, layer by layer using a razor. Closure was with tailor's silk and needle, the wounds dressed with egg whites and herbal salve.

Complete recovery ensued, and confirmation provided from Dr Gabriel King of Armagh when he reviewed the patient and removed the silk stitches from her wound [14].

Throughout the seventeenth and eighteenth centuries, the operation was not in any way refined; yet, despite its crudeness, Samuel Johnson's 1755 definition 'cutting a child out of the womb, either dead or alive, when it cannot otherwise be delivered' was a succinct summary of a seemingly familiar procedure [1]. A significant procedural omission until 1769 was closure of the uterus itself; the use of this procedure, first performed by the French surgeon Jean Lebas, had an immediate effect as it minimized haemorrhage, while use of an incision through the lower uterine segment, rather than through the contractile segment of the myometrium, was described by Johnson in 1786, developed by Osiander in 1805, and over a century later in 1908 suggested by Selheim as responsible for significantly decreased haemorrhage and uterine dehiscence

[4, 14]. Nevertheless, traditional techniques of caesarean section persisted until the latter nineteenth century, as evidenced by the British obstetrician Fleetwood Churchill recording in 1872 that 'no sutures are required in the uterus; as it contracts, the wound will be reduced to 1–2 inches and the lips will come into opposition, if it be healthy' [7].

However, critics considered that a baby could always be delivered vaginally and that the results of an abdominal delivery did not justify its barbarity. The 1776 case of Dr Osborne illustrates the point. His patient had rickets; her height was 3 feet, 6 inches, she was unable to stand without crutches, and her greatest pelvic antero-posterior dimension was less than 2 inches. Following 72 hours in labour, she was exhausted and had haemorrhaged substantially. It was after 84 hours that four colleagues assisted in craniotomy and extraction of the infant, followed 12 hours later by a learning exercise for 30 medical students as they crowded in and examined the poor woman's unique pelvis. Osborne remarked that the woman demonstrated great fortitude and he subsequently published the episode in the medical literature [14].

The opposition to caesarean section was evidenced in 1742 when Sir Fielding Ould wrote in his *Treatise of Midwifery*, 'I have taken upon myself absolutely to explode the Caesarean operation as repugnant not only to all the rules of Theory and Practice but even of humanity itself—a detestable, barbarous, illegal piece of inhumanity.' Dr Dease, of Dublin, added in 1783, 'It is only practised by rash and ignorant men who have no reputation to lose and are anxious to acquire one.' When Dr Simmonds of Manchester in 1798 published a tract to explicitly condemn the operation, his colleague Dr Hull, the first Englishman to do two caesarean sections, took violent exception: 'A compound of unjust and malicious insinuations against a man who never gave you the least offence. Pernicious precepts, false assertions, garbled extracts, ribaldry, libel, hypocrisy, nonsense' [4, 5].

Caesarean section in the nineteenth century

Advances in medicine and a better understanding of human anatomy and physiology and of disease prevention took place in the nineteenth century and were partly responsible for rapidly accelerating population growth in the Western world. Paris and Vienna became the two leading medical centres on the Continent between 1770 and the 1850s.

During the nineteenth century, caesarean section was observed in a number of countries around the world, including an 1879 encounter by Dr R.W. Felkin with indigenous operators in Uganda. The patient's abdomen was prepared with alcohol made from bananas; some of the alcohol was then given orally with herbal mixtures as a form of analgesia and sedative to the patient, and then more of the alcohol was used to disinfect the operators' hands, prior to delivering abdominally [2, 4, 21]. From the well-developed nature of the procedures employed, European observers concluded that the procedures had been employed for some time (Figure 1.7).

It was during the nineteenth century that anaesthesia began to be developed, beginning with ether and soon followed by chloroform. Initial opposition for the use of anaesthesia in childbirth, due to moral or religious reasons, receded after Queen Victoria, despite her openly religious convictions, used chloroform during the birth of Prince Leopoldo in 1853 and of Princess Beatrice in 1857. The way was paved for a new era in obstetrics and, towards the end of the nineteenth century, caesarean section delivery became more sustainable [7] (Figure 1.8).

The terrible post-operative mortality following caesarean section was correctly attributed by Eduardo Porro (1842–1902), Professor of Obstetrics at Pavia, to the continued practice of retaining the open (unstitched) uterus in the peritoneal cavity, with associated haemorrhage and peritonitis [1, 2]. He began performing supracervical hysterectomy and bilateral salpingo-oophorectomy during caesarean section, a technique which he described and advocated in his book *Della amputazione utero-ovarica come complemento di taglio cesareo*, published in 1876. Removing the uterus and the adnexae was associated with reduced rates of infection and haemorrhage and consequently improving maternal mortality, although at the expense of future childbearing. It had been suggested and successfully performed on rabbits by Blundell of Guy's Hospital, London, in 1834 [22]. The removal of the unstitched uterus greatly improved the risks of

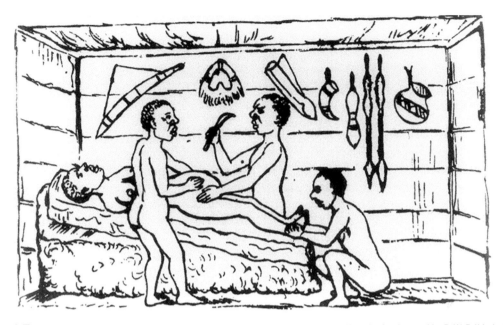

Figure 1.7 Successful caesarean section performed by indigenous operators in Kahura, Uganda. As observed by R. W. Felkin in 1879 from his article 'Notes on Labour in Central Africa'.

internal haemorrhage and sepsis, and a review of world literature undertaken 5 years later in 1881 by R. P. Harris showed that 50 cases had been delivered by the Porro method, with a maternal mortality of 58% and a fetal survival of 86% [7]. Prior to Porro, no one in Pavia had survived a caesarean section while, from 1885 to 1889, 158 such operations were performed with a 29% maternal mortality [1, 10].

However, if this was a major improvement of the caesarean section technique, it was a mutilating one-off operation, nevertheless.

Suturing the uterus after caesarean section was first advocated by Lebas in 1769 [22]. Traditionally, sutures were not used inside the abdomen or pelvis, since it was thought that they would be impossible to remove once the cavity had closed. Like many

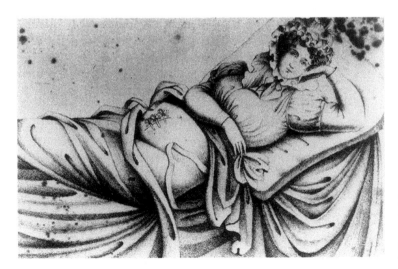

Figure 1.8 A caesarean patient prior to dressing the wound.

From Edward Siebold, *Abbildungen aus dem gesammtgebiete der theoretisch-praktischen geburtshülfe*, 1829.

advances in medicine, the procedure was opposed by the 'pundits' in obstetrics of those days. A century later, in the early 1880s, two German obstetricians, Ferdinand Adolf Kehrer (1837–1914) and Max Sänger (1853–1903), independently of each other, developed uterine closure methods using sutures made of silver wire, as utilized by the American gynaecologist James Marion Sims (1813–1883), who had seen great success in the treatment of vesico-vaginal fistulae in North America [23]. Max Sänger in 1882 challenged the ancient practice with his publication on caesarean section, advocating two-layer uterine closure (Figure 1.9), the use of antisepsis, and abdominal delivery during the early stages of labour—not simply as a means of preventing a woman dying undelivered but as a way to save the woman's life. Although Kehrer has the priority by a few months, Sänger's name was most generally associated with this revolutionary improvement in the technique caesarean section, in the early twentieth century. However, on 25 September 1881, in the town of Meckesheim, Kehrer performed the first modern caesarean section in Germany. The patient was a 26-year-old woman, and the operation proved to be a success. Kehrer's novel approach involved a transverse incision of the lower uterine segment, at the level of the internal cervical os; this procedure minimizes bleeding, and Kehrer is now recognized as the father of the 'lower segment operation' [22]. This 'conservative' (non-sterilizing) procedure, as opposed to the radical caesarean section hysterectomy used by Porro, did not become popular until the early twentieth century.

With improvements in operative technique and general safety, including developments in anaesthesia, asepsis, suturing, and non-interference early in labour, caesarean section became safer than ever before and could be used at earlier stages than had previously been possible in difficult labours. Maternal mortality decreased substantially through the nineteenth century, from 65%–75% to less than 10% [1, 7].

Caesarean section in the twentieth century and in contemporary history

Significant advances in the twentieth century included the widespread adoption of the transverse incision over the 'classical' vertical approach (shown in Figure 1.9). Several surgeons, including Kehrer, had utilized the transverse incision in the twentieth century, but the procedure only become widespread following strong support by John Martin Munro Kerr (1868–1960), Regius Professor of Midwifery at the University of Glasgow from 1927 to 1934. Fluent in German and French, Munro Kerr spent a number of years after his graduation in Germany, Austria, and Ireland, studying obstetrics and gynaecology at Berlin, Vienna, and Dublin. Appointed Visiting Surgeon at the Glasgow Royal Maternity Hospital in 1900, he published to great success Operative Midwifery in 1908, popularizing the lower segment caesarean section in preference to the classical operation [22]. The advantages of this 'Kehrer–Kerr' technique were less haemorrhage, less infection, and a reduced risk of uterine rupture during subsequent trials of vaginal delivery. Slowly the technique combining transverse incision and lower segment operation gained wide acceptance.

A major advance occurred before the availability of antibiotics when Frank (1907), Veit and Fromme (1907), and Kronig (1912) described improved healing with the extraperitoneal caesarean section operation [22]. In brief, they used a longitudinal abdominal incision together with an incision thorough the utero-vesical (visceral) peritoneum. The parietal and visceral peritoneums were then temporarily stitched together and the lower segment opened longitudinally. This procedure allowed the peritoneal cavity to be sealed before the uterus was opened with a vertical incision, thereby preventing peritoneal contamination and risk of sepsis [1, 7, 10]. Another pivotal contribution was made by Hermann Johannes Pfannenstiel (1862–1909), a German gynaecologist who in 1900 described a transverse suprapubic incision (shown in Figure 1.10), a method intended to decrease the risks of incisional hernia associated with the vertical abdominal incision [24]. The fact that he described his technique, which is now known as 'Pfannenstiel's pelvic skin incision', for genitourinary surgery may partially explain why obstetricians around the world were reluctant to use it routinely for caesarean section until the 1970s.

A.

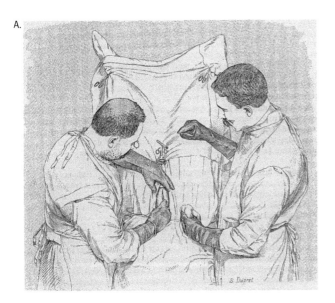

B.

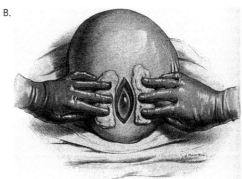

C.

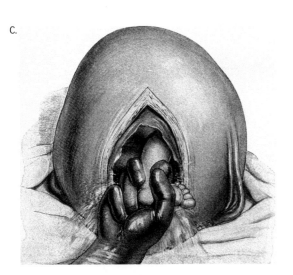

D.

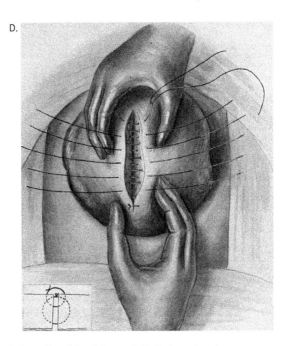

Figure 1.9 Surgeon performing a classical caesarean section. A. Vertical opening of the abdomen. B. Vertical opening of an exteriorized uterus. C. Delivery of a fetus in breech. D. Double closure of the uterus.

(From Laurent O; *Anatomie clinique et technique operatoire*; 1906 and JM Muro-Kerr *Operative Midwifery*, 1908)

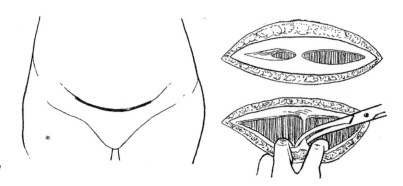

Figure 1.10 The Pfannenstiel incision, in curvilinear fashion approximately 2 cm above the pubic symphysis.

(From Laurent O; *Anatomie clinique et technique operatoire*; 1906).

The 1921 September special issue of the *Journal of Obstetrics and Gynaecology of the British Empire*, dedicated to the caesarean section, provides insight on the procedure from the beginning of the twentieth century [25]. This issue followed the annual meeting of the British Medical Association at Newcastle-on-Tyne and presented the statistics of nearly 4000 caesarean sections performed in the United Kingdom since 1910. The data were collected by John M. Munro Kerr and Eardley Holland, who also reported on their personal experiences of the procedure and on their views about its use for the future in obstetrics practice [26, 27]. Among others, the meeting was attended by Lady Barrett (1867–1945), a consultant surgeon at the Royal Free Hospital in London and one of the leading gynaecologist and obstetricians of her time, who discussed at length the indications for caesarean sections and the still very high morbidity and mortality of the procedure. With regard to the method, she confessed to having used the classical procedure because of the 'bad results' that followed the low incision (Pfannenstiel incision) procedure she saw in Vienna [25]. Interestingly, some of the kinds of instruments used at the time are still in use today for caesarean section in the United Kingdom (Figure 1.11).

Although transverse abdominal incisions were increasingly used, fascial incisions continued to be longitudinal; it was Pfannenstiel who advocated that the sheath be cut transversally for more secure closure and less post-operative pain than with longitudinal incisions [24]. Currently, the Pfannenstiel incision, performed in curvilinear fashion approximately 2 cm above the pubic symphysis,

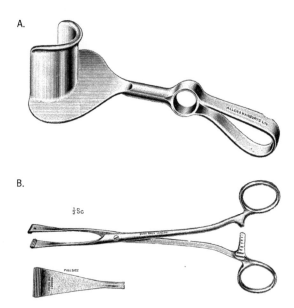

Figure 1.11 A. The DeLee universal retractor. B. Green-Armytage haemostatic forceps.

is most commonly employed; however, some evidence suggests that the linear Joel-Cohen incision (approximately 2–3 cm more superiorly) without peritonealization is equally successful but with a shorter opening and reduced operative time than the Pfannenstiel incision [25, 26]. Another method is the Misgav Ladach section described by Michael Stark 20 years ago [28, 29]; his method is based on minimalistic principles. He examined all the steps in caesarean sections in use, analysed them for their necessity and, if the steps were found to be necessary, for the optimal way of performing them. For the abdominal incision, he used the modified

Joel-Cohen incision, comparing the longitudinal abdominal structures to strings on musical instruments. As blood vessels and muscles have lateral sway, it is possible to stretch rather than cut them. The peritoneum is opened by repeat stretching, no abdominal swabs are used, the uterus is closed in one layer with a big needle to reduce the amount of foreign body as much as possible, the peritoneal layers remain unstitched, and the abdomen is closed with two layers only.

Improvements in patient care have progressively established the caesarean section as safe, both as an emergency and as an elective procedure. Blood transfusions and the introduction of antibiotics after the Second World War substantially reduced adverse outcomes. Advances in anaesthesia and improvements in post-operative care have further contributed to declining mortality rates in economically developed countries. Ergot alkaloids for uterine contraction and consequent reductions in haemorrhage have been utilized since the early nineteenth century, with Chassar Moir first isolating ergotamine from three alkaloids of crude ergot in 1932 [7, 30]. Oxytocin was synthesized in 1953, and its use in significantly reducing post-partum haemorrhage has become widespread. Such developments, together with advances in anaesthesia and improvements in post-operative care, have further contributed to declining mortality and morbidity rates over the last half century.

References

1. Gabert HA, Bey M. History and development of cesarean operation. Obstet Gynecol Clin North Am 1988; 15(4): 591–605.
2. Sewell JE. Cesarean Section: A Brief History. 1993. http://www.nlm.nih.gov/exhibition/cesarean.
3. Boley JP. The history of caesarean section. CMAJ 1991; 145(4): 319–22.
4. Harley JMG. Cesarean section. Clin Obstet Gynecol 1980; 7(3): 529–59.
5. Katz VL, Cefalo RC. History and evolution of cesarean delivery. In: Phelan JP, Clark SL, eds. Cesarean Delivery. New York, NY: Elsevier, 1988; 1–18.
6. Healey J (trans). Pliny the Elder, Natural History: A Selection. London: Penguin Books, 1991.
7. Todman D. A history of caesarean section: From ancient world to the modern era. Aust N Z J Obstet Gynaecol 2007; 47(5): 357–61.
8. Todman D. Childbirth in ancient Rome: From traditional folklore to obstetrics. Aust N Z J Obstet Gynaecol 2007; 47(2): 82–5.
9. Skinner HA. The Origin of Medical Terms. London, 1949 (s.v. 'Caesarean section').
10. Speert H. A Pictorial History of Gynecology and Obstetrics. Philadelphia, PA: Davis Press, 1973.
11. Payman B. Rostam revisited. ACOG Clin Rev 2001; 6(4): 16.
12. Khatamee MA. 'Rostam' is born: How? By cesarean section (940–1020 AD) ACOG Clin Rev 2000; 5(2): 12–16.
13. Hillan EM. Caesarean section: Historical background. Scot Med J 1991; 36(5): 150–4.
14. O'Sullivan JF. Caesarean birth. Ulster Med J 1990; 59(1): 1–10.
15. Reiss H. Abdominal delivery in the 16th century. J Royal Soc Med 2003; 96(7): 370.
16. Jackson I, Park K (eds.) Andreas Versalius de Humani Corpus Fabrica. Basel: The Warnock Library, 1998.
17. King H. Midwifery, Obstetrics and the Rise of Gynaecology: The Uses of a Sixteenth-Century Compendium. Aldershot: Ashgate Publishing, 2007.
18. Pugh RB. An early case of caesarean section in England. BJOG 1949; 56(5): 872–4.
19. Schega ML. Between imagination and observation: Reasoning monstrous births in Scipione Mercurio's La Commare. Tiresias 2013; 2: 46–54.
20. Moore W. The Knife Man. London: Bantam Press, 2005.
21. Felkin RW. Notes on labour in Central Africa. Edinb Med J 1884; 20: 922–93.
22. Chassar Moir J. Munro Kerr's Operative Obstetrics. 6th Ed. London: Bailliere, Tindall and Cox, 1956.
23. Todman D. Max Sänger (1853–1903): A historical note on uterine sutures in caesarean section. IJGO 2008; 10(1): http://print.ispub.com/api/0/ispub-article/6817.
24. Pfannenstiel HJ. Über die Vortheile des suprasymphysären Fascienquerschnitts für die gynäkologischen Koliotomien, Zugleich ein Beitrag zu der Indikatiosstellung der Operationswege. Samml Klin Vortr 1900; 268: 1735–56.
25. Lyle RPR. The indications for caesarean section. BJOG 1921; 28(3–4): 571–9.
26. Munro Kerr JM. Indications for caesarean section. BJOG 1921; 28(3–4): 338–48.
27. Holland E. Methods of performing caesarean section. BJOG 1921; 28(3–4): 349–57.
28. Stark M, Finkel AR. Comparison between the Joel-Cohen and Pfannenstiel incisions in caesarean section. Eur J Obstet Gynecol Reprod Biol 1994; 53(2): 121–2.
29. Stark M, Chavkin Y, Kupfersztain C, Guedj P, Finkel AR. Evaluation of combinations of procedures in cesarean section. Int J Gynecol Obstet 1995; 48(3): 273–6.
30. Rayburn WF, Schwartz WJ. Refinements in performing a cesarean delivery. Obstet Gynecol Surv 1996; 51(7): 445–51.

CHAPTER 2
The anatomy of the female pelvis

Natalie Greenwold

Introduction

A good knowledge of human anatomy is pivotal to the development of surgical techniques. There were very few attempts to explore human anatomy before the fifteenth century, and in particular there were very few descriptions of the pregnant uterus until the eighteenth century. John Hunter (1728–1793), the British surgeon who became arguably the greatest anatomist in medical history and was a pioneer of many different surgical specialities, was the first to describe in detail the anatomy of the pregnant woman. One of his pivotal discoveries took place in May 1754. By injecting melted wax into the main vessels of the womb of a pregnant corpse, John Hunter and Colin Mackenzie conclusively demonstrated that maternal and fetal blood circulations are separate, thus putting

to rest a debate that had engrossed anatomists, including Galen, Leonardo Da Vinci, and Vesalius, for many centuries. John Hunter's unique collection of human and animal specimens was to become a major attraction for the intellectual elite of the eighteenth century and has inspired several generations of doctors in Europe and the United States.

The present chapter reviews the basic anatomical knowledge required to perform a standard caesarean section. This approach will enable the surgeon to fully appreciate the surgical risks and to optimize all steps of the operation in order to ensure minimal tissue disturbance. More detailed information on the anatomy of the female pelvis is available from specialized textbooks [1–4].

Incision of the skin in caesarean section

The lower segment caesarean section is the most commonly employed technique. The incision may be either the lower Pfannenstiel incision or the higher Joel-Cohen incision. The anatomical landmarks of the two techniques are as follows:

The Pfannenstiel incision

This approach uses a 15 cm incision which has outer edges that curve upwards slightly and a midpoint which is 3 cm above the pubic symphysis (see Chapter 4).

The Joel-Cohen incision

This approach uses a straight incision running 15 cm in length (see Chapter 5). The midpoint of the incision lies 3 cm below the midpoint of an imaginary line joining both anterior superior iliac spines.

The nerve supply of the abdominal wall is provided by thoracic nerves T6–T12, including the subcostal nerve, and the cutaneous branches of the iliohypogastric nerve and the ilioinguinal nerve, both of which derive from the lumbar nerve L1. This nerve supply can be mapped as follows: the xiphisternum

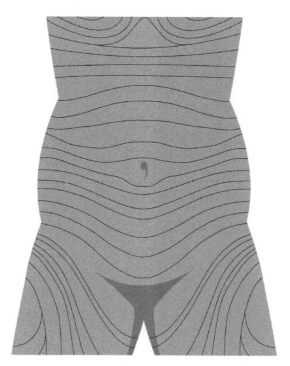

Figure 2.1 Diagram showing direction of Langer's lines on the anterior abdominal wall.
Alternative View Studios

is innervated by T6, the umbilicus by T10, and the groin by L1. As a result, regional anaesthesia for a caesarean section must extend to the T6 level.

Langer's lines—also known as cleavage lines—are natural lines of cleavage of the skin (see Figure 2.1).

They correspond to the areas where the skin is least flexible and are determined by the direction of alignment of collagen fibres. When the skin is incised along the direction of the Langer's lines, scar formation is minimized.

Abdominal entry in caesarean section

Entry into the abdomen requires knowledge of the tissue planes and vasculature in order to minimize trauma to the tissues and bleeding (see Figure 2.2). The layers of the abdominal wall below the umbilicus are as follows: the skin, the superficial (Camper's) fascia, the membranous (Scarpa's) fascia, the rectus sheath, muscle, and the parietal peritoneum [1, 2].

The skin, the fatty fascia, and the rectus sheath are all incised or divided digitally and horizontally in the lower segment caesarean section. Under the rectus sheath lies the rectus abdominis muscles.

The recti, which run in a longitudinal plane, arise from the fifth, sixth, and seventh costal cartilage and insert inferiorly into the crest of the pubis.

Tendinous intersections run across the body of the recti in a horizontal direction at the level of the xiphoid, at the level of the umbilicus, and halfway between these two landmarks. Sometimes a fourth intersection runs across the recti below the level of the umbilicus as well. These intersections fasten the rectus to the anterior rectus sheath but are not present posteriorly, where the rectus muscle lies completely free.

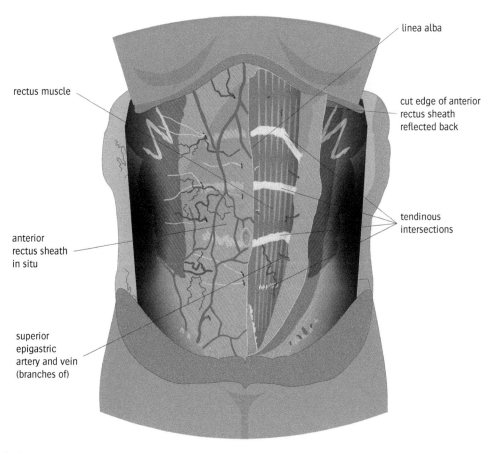

linea alba

rectus muscle

cut edge of anterior
rectus sheath
reflected back

tendinous
intersections

anterior
rectus sheath
in situ

superior
epigastric
artery and vein
(branches of)

Figure 2.2 Diagram showing the anatomy of the anterior abdominal wall.

Alternative View Studios

Superficially, the inferior part of the abdominal wall is supplied medially by the superficial epigastric artery and laterally by the superficial circumflex artery. Both are branches of the femoral artery. Below the superficial level, the inferior epigastric artery supplies the medial part of the lower abdomen, and the deep circumflex iliac artery supplies the lateral part. Both of these arteries are branches of the external iliac artery. The veins run in the plane between the superficial and the deep fascia. The superficial inferior epigastric veins are usually approximately 4 cm lateral to the midline of the Pfannenstiel incision, on either side. They are superior to the rectus sheath. The inferior epigastric arteries are posterior to the rectus muscles. Branches of the superior epigastric artery and vein pierce the rectus at each intersection. In repeat caesarean section, there are often adhesions in the plane between the anterior rectus sheath and the rectus muscle and these may require surgical division in order to free the rectus sheath sufficiently from the muscle to enable it to be lifted superiorly and thus create sufficient space for subsequent delivery of the fetal head. Awareness of the vessels in this plane and use of cautery or ligation, if the vessels are divided, is crucial to avoid the risk of rectus sheath haematoma later on.

The rectus sheath is formed from the medial aponeurotic extensions of the lateral abdominal wall muscles (from anterior to posterior, the external oblique muscle, the internal oblique muscle, and the transversus muscle). Below the midpoint between the umbilicus and the symphysis pubis, all three aponeuroses pass anterior to the rectus muscle. The line marking the level below which all three aponeuroses pass in front of the rectus is known as the arcuate line. Above the arcuate line, the internal oblique aponeurosis splits around the rectus muscle, and the transversus aponeurosis passes behind the rectus. In the midline, all three aponeuroses blend to form a white line, the 'linea alba', running vertically along the length of the recti from the xiphisternum to the symphysis pubis.

A vertical incision on the abdomen, when performed, passes through the linea alba, which is an almost bloodless line allowing rapid entry to the abdomen.

Entry to the peritoneal cavity

Access to the peritoneal cavity is made by parting the recti from the midline in a lateral direction as superiorly as the transverse incision allows. The reason for this procedure is to avoid perforating the bladder if sharp entry is used. Also for this reason, some operators use blunt digital entry into the peritoneal cavity. At sharp entry, loops of bowel which may lie beneath the peritoneum must also be avoided; therefore, the surgeon often raises a thin peritoneal layer between forceps and checks that there are no other underlying tissues before using scissors to incise the peritoneum.

The peritoneum is derived from the embryological endothelial lining of the primitive coelomic cavity. The visceral peritoneum denotes peritoneum covering the viscera or organs, and the parietal peritoneum lines the body wall (see Figures 2.3 and 2.4).

It is essential to understand the extra- and intra-peritoneal relations of the pelvic organs. Of particular interest is the vesico-uterine peritoneal fold. Once the parietal peritoneum has been breached to open the abdominal cavity, the retro- peritoneal bladder is visible as a golden-yellow globular structure in the pelvis. The visceral peritoneum covers the upper part of the bladder and passes posteriorly, onto the body of the uterus. In order to push the bladder down and out of the way of the surgical

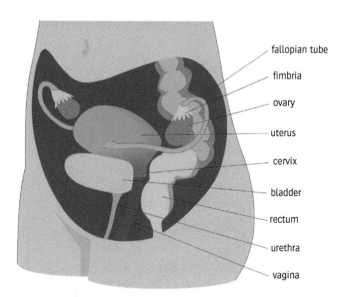

fallopian tube

fimbria

ovary

uterus

cervix

bladder

rectum

urethra

vagina

Figure 2.3 Diagram showing a side view of the non-pregnant female pelvic anatomy.

Alternative View Studios

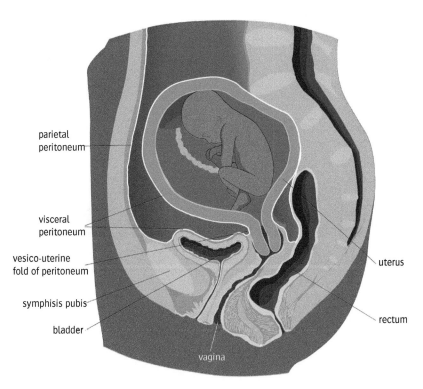

Figure 2.4 Diagram showing the anatomical relations of the pregnant uterus to the other pelvic organs (Lateral view of the pelvis).
Alternative View Studios

field, it is important to identify this fold of perito-neum and carefully incise it. The bladder can then gently be pushed inferiorly, using a sterile gauze. The lower segment of the uterus is thus revealed, with the bladder and ureters cleared from the oper-ative field. The ureters lie close to lateral fornices of the vagina at the level of the uterine cervix and pass directly under the uterine arteries at this point.

Entry to the uterine cavity in caesarean section

It is important to be mindful of the altered anatomy of the lower segment of the uterus during advanced stages of labour, as this is often the time in which caesarean section may be performed. In advanced labour, the cervix may be fully or almost fully dilat-ed and so the lower segment is drawn up cephalad. If one is not vigilant, incision of the uterine cavity is performed at a level that in advanced labour may in fact be cervix and not lower uterine segment. In these circumstances, the incision should be placed a little higher than it would be at early labour, in order to avoid incision of the cervix.

The uterus has several significant anatomical relationships that are of importance to the sur-geon (see Figure 2.4):

- The anterior wall of the uterus lies directly poste-rior to the superior part of the bladder, with the vesico-uterine fold of peritoneum coursing over the bladder and onto the anterior body of the uterus. The supravaginal cervix is also directly posterior to the bladder.

- The pouch of Douglas lies posterior to the uterus. This cavity has been used as a point of access to the pelvic intraperitoneal cavity via the posterior vaginal fornix.

- A particularly important relation is that of the ureters to the supravaginal cervix. Lying 1.5 cm lateral to the supravaginal cervix and passing directly beneath the uterine arteries, the ureters can be injured when the uterine arteries are ligated during a hysterectomy (see Figures 2.5 and 2.6).

- Lateral to the uterus is the peritoneal broad ligament. A double, peritoneal layer forms the broad ligaments, running from the sides of the uterus out to the lateral walls and floor of the pelvis. In the upper free border of each side of the broad ligament lie the fallopian tubes. The lateral border of the broad ligament is drawn superiorly over the ovarian vessels as the suspensory ligament of the ovary.

- The ovaries lie within a small mesentery called the mesovarium, which is suspended from the posterior part of the broad ligament.

- The round ligaments run in the anterior layer of the broad ligament. They pass form the lateral border of the uterus to the deep inguinal ring on each side.

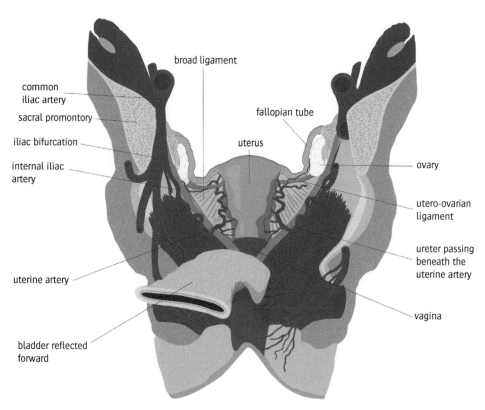

Figure 2.5 Diagram showing the arrangement of the pelvic arteries and the anatomical relationship between the uterine arteries and the ureters (anterior view).

Alternative View Studios

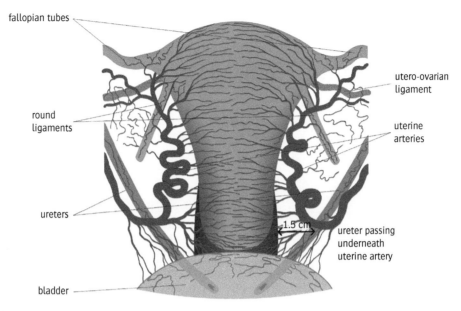

fallopian tubes

utero-ovarian ligament

round ligaments

uterine arteries

ureters

1.5 cm

ureter passing underneath uterine artery

bladder

Figure 2.6 Diagram showing the anatomical relationship between the uterine arteries and the ureters (Anterior view).
Alternative View Studios

Blood supply to the uterus and ovaries

Arterial supply to the uterus and ovaries

The uterus and fallopian tubes are supplied by the uterine arteries, with collateral supply from the ovarian arteries. The uterine arteries are branches of the internal iliac arteries. The internal iliac arteries arise from the common iliac arteries at the level of the fourth lumbar vertebra. The uterine artery passes medially from the pelvic side wall to the level of the junction between the uterus and vagina. As it passes medially, it crosses the ureter at a point 1.5 cm lateral to the lateral fornices of the vagina. The ureters pass below the uterine arteries at this point. The uterine arteries then divide into ascending and descending branches, with the former passing along the lateral margin of the uterus, and the latter forming a vaginal branch (see Figures 2.5 and 2.6).

The ovarian arteries are branches of the abdominal aorta. They descend along the posterior abdominal wall and then cross over the external iliac arteries at the pelvic brim, at which point they enter the

suspensory ligaments to supply the ovaries. Tubal branches then anastomose with tubal branches of the uterine arteries to supply the fallopian tubes. Thus, both uterus and ovaries receive collateral circulations from their respective primary arteries.

Venous supply to the uterus and ovaries

The venous drainage of the uterus, the cervix, the upper vagina, and the ovaries is via a plexus of veins running within the parametrium. The plexus forms veins that run alongside the arterial blood supply. With the exception of the left ovarian vein, which drains into the left renal vein, these veins drain into the inferior vena cava.

Internal artery ligation

In extreme cases of post-partum haemorrhage, it may be deemed useful to perform internal iliac artery ligation as a life-saving procedure. The internal iliac artery is identified at the pelvic brim. The peritoneum is incised, revealing the common iliac bifurcation. The internal iliac is gently dissected from the loose areolar connective tissue surrounding it. The ureter is identified medially and can be seen characteristically peristalsing; it is then retracted medially. At a point 4 cm distal to the bifurcation and, with the surgeon being mindful of the posterior internal iliac vein, a suture is placed beneath the artery from lateral to medial, and the artery is ligated.

Additional anatomical features of the female pelvis

The Fallopian tubes and the ovaries

The cavity of the uterus is flattened and triangular. The fallopian tubes enter the uterine cavity bilaterally in the superior-lateral portion of the cavity, an area known as the cornua. Each tube is approximately 10 cm in length and 1 cm in diameter and is situated within a portion of the broad ligament called the mesosalpinx. The distal portion of the fallopian tube ends at the ovary.

The ovary is in the shape of an almond. It is 4 cm long and is attached to the back of the broad ligament by the mesovarium. The ovaries have two further supports—the utero-ovarian ligaments, which run from the ovaries to the cornua of the uterus, and the suspensory ligaments also known as infundibulo-pelvic ligaments, which run to the pelvic side walls and contain ovarian vessels, sympathetic nerve fibres, and lymphatics from the side wall of the pelvis. The ovarian arteries originate directly from the aorta. The ovarian veins drain to the inferior vena cava on the right side and to the left renal vein on the left side. The lymphatic drainage of the ovary is to the para-aortic nodes. The ovarian nerve supply is from the thoracic nerves T10 and T11 (from the aortic plexus). These are pain-conducting sympathetic fibres; thus, pain from the ovaries is typically experienced in the groin.

Innervation of the female pelvis

Nerves of the pelvic autonomic nervous system consist of the hypogastric nerves, which are primarily sympathetic fibres and originate from the superior hypogastric plexus lying over the sacral promontory. The fibres of the pelvic splanchnic nerves, which come from the sacral roots S2–S4, are mainly parasympathetic.

Sympathetic fibres are responsible for bladder compliance, urinary continence, and small muscle contractions at orgasm.

The parasympathetic supply is responsible for vaginal lubrication and genital swelling during arousal, as well as detrusor contractility and various rectal functions. The parasympathetic pelvic splanchnic nerves also control motility in the distal third of the transverse colon, in the sigmoid colon, and in the rectum, and transmit pain sensation from the same part of the lower digestive tract and the cervix.

The inferior hypogastric plexus is formed by the fusion of the iliohypogastric and the splanchnic nerves and lies in an area extending from the antero-lateral rectum to the cervix, the vaginal wall, and the base of the bladder. It lies close to the ureter, where it is crossed over from above by the uterine artery, and it is closely related to the venous plexus of the bladder and vagina.

Uterine ligaments and support

The ligamentous supports of the cervix and upper vagina are formed from condensations of the pelvic fascia that line the pelvic floor covering the levator ani and the obturator internus muscle. The ligaments effectively sling the pelvic viscera from the pelvic side walls. The cardinal ligaments—also known as the transverse cervical or Mackenrod's ligaments—pass laterally from the cervix and the upper vagina to the pelvic side walls. The uterosacral ligaments pass backwards from the posterior aspect of the cervical isthmus and the vaginal fornices to the periosteum in front of the sacroiliac joints. The pubo-cervical fascia extends forwards from the cardinal ligaments to the pubis, forming a sling around the bladder neck. The broad ligament and the round ligaments already have been described (see 'Entry to the uterine cavity').

The pelvic floor in females

Also known as the pelvic diaphragm, the muscles forming the pelvic floor divide the pelvis superiorly from the perineum inferiorly. The levator ani and the coccygeus muscle constitute the pelvic floor. The levator ani is a V-shaped muscle that forms a sling around the rectum. It extends posteriorly from the superior surface of the pubic rami, with its fascia covering the sidewall of the pelvis over the obturator internus and the spine of the ischium, and inserts medially and behind the rectum onto the lower coccyx and the median anococcygeal raphe.

Three-dimensional anatomy of the female pelvis

A better understanding of the pelvic anatomy is essential for clinicians and surgeons involved in obstetric care. This enables a clear understanding of the common complications of caesarean (see chapter 8) and natural deliveries [5] but also the rare complications of pelvic surgery [6]. The traditional method of anatomic teaching of the last centuries, using resources such as cadavers, is progressively being replaced by methods that use views obtained with new imaging technologies such as MRI or three-dimensional ultrasound [7, 8]. State-of-the-art radiology department workstations with industry-standard software applications can provide exquisite demonstrations of anatomy, pathology, and, more recently, physiology. Similar advances in personal computers and software can allow anatomy departments and their students to build their own three-dimensional virtual models.

One of the first interactive, three-dimensional (3D), computer-based anatomical training systems, using virtual anatomical models (virtual body structures), was proposed by Temkin et al. in 2006 [9]. The model allowed a real-time, self-guided virtual tour of the entire body and was designed to provide detailed anatomical information about structures, substructures, and proximal structures. The system facilitates learning of visual-spatial relationships at a level of detail that may not be possible by any other means. The use of volumetric structures allows for repeated real-time virtual dissections, from any angle, at the convenience of the user.

The Visible Human Project (VHP) of the US National Library of Medicine is a detailed online data set of cross-sectional photographs of the human body [10, 11]. To generate this data set, one male cadaver and one female cadaver were frozen and cut into thin slices, which were then photographed. These images were then adapted to create three-dimensional, computer-generated anatomical models (see http://www.nlm.nih.gov/research/visible/visible_human.html).

The objective of the VHP was to provide both labelled and unlabelled high-quality, high-resolution sections of the human body, so that these sections could be used in both basic and continuing medical education. To provide an overview of the body, 370 axial sections were selected from both the male and the female data sets, with special regard to regions of clinical interest. Each section is accompanied by its corresponding computer tomography image and, if available, MRI images, for quick and easy comparison of morphologic and radiologic structures.

The first three-dimensional model of a female pelvis was reported in 2010 [12]. The model includes the pelvic girdle, the organs of the pelvic cavity, the surrounding musculature, the perineum, neurovascular structures, and the peritoneum. Each structure can be controlled separately (e.g. added, subtracted, made transparent) to reveal the organization and/or relationships between structures. The model can be manipulated and/or projected stereoscopically to visualize structures and relationships from different angles with excellent spatial perception.

More recently, Luo et al. have created a PDF which contains a detailed three-dimensional, interactive anatomic model of 23 pelvic structures, including the muscles, ligaments, and fascia of the pelvic floor, and the organs that the floor supports [13]. Bones, blood vessels, and the perineum are illustrated as

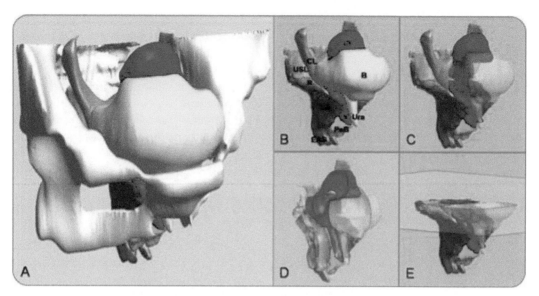

Figure 2.7 The user can manipulate the three-dimensional model of pelvic structures. A. A three-quarter right anterolateral view. B. Hiding the bones reveals selected features. C. Making the bladder and urethra transparent reveals the underlying structures. D. Sample sagittal cross-section of the remaining structures. E. Sample axial cross-section; B, bladder; CL, cardinal ligament; EAS, external anal sphincter; LA, levator ani; PeB, perineal body; R, rectum; Ura, urethra; USL, uterosacral ligament; Ut, uterus; V, vagina.

Luo. A model patient: female pelvic anatomy viewed in diverse 3-dimensional images. Am J Obstet Gynecol 2011.

well. To produce this tool, three-dimensional volumetric models were created from serial images that were 5 mm thick and were obtained with a 3-Tesla MRI scanner. Each structure was traced with the use of the most clearly visible axial and/or coronal plane images and then incorporated into a three-dimensional virtual model that was based on previous anatomic work. Models were validated against the original scans and tracings and exported as a universal three-dimensional file that would allow the user to manipulate the three-dimensional model (see Figure 2.7).

Anatomy changes of the female pelvis following delivery

The anatomical changes following caesarean delivery such as scar defects and adhesions are discussed in chapter 9. Disruption or denervation of anatomical components of pelvic floor support system, particularly levator ani muscle complex, is associated with later development of pelvic floor disorders. These disorders affect women of all ages and are associated with significant economic burden and poor quality of life and have contributed to the debate around women choices of the mode of delivery, i.e. elective caesarean versus vaginal birth.

A recent prospective study has compared pelvic floor function and anatomy between women who delivered vaginally versus those with caesarean delivery prior to the second stage of labor [14]. The authors found that vaginal birth resulted in prolapse changes and objective urinary incontinence but not in increased self reported pelvic floor dysfunction at 6 months postpartum compared with women who delivered by caesarean prior to the second stage of labour. A previous study from Australia has shown that a quarter of women continent before pregnancy reported new incontinence at 3 months postpartum [15]. Compared with women who had a spontaneous vaginal birth, women who had a caesarean section before labour or in the first stage of labour were less likely to be incontinent 3 months postpartum. At 4 years, 29.6% of women reported urinary incontinence and 7.1% reported faecal incontinence [16] but the odds of reporting incontinence at 4 years were for women experiencing symptoms in pregnancy

These data suggest that the second stage of labour has an effect on postpartum pelvic floor anatomy and function but that there are important individual variations, probably linked to anatomical differences and fetal size at birth. Overall, this effect is probably modest but the risks of persistent urinary incontinence is common after childbirth and is more likely following prolonged labour in combination with operative vaginal birth i.e. forceps and/or episiotomy [17]. Within this context, three-dimensional ultrasound is increasingly used to evaluate anatomical injuries to the pelvic floor musculature following different modes of delivery [18, 19]. This also highlights the importance of an accurate knowledge of the corresponding anatomical structures, which is pivotal to better understanding of the underlying pathophysiology of the pelvic complications following all methods of delivery.

Key learning points

1. Knowledge of the pelvic and lower abdomen anatomy is essential to perform caesarean section.
2. The relative merits of the Pfannenstiel incision and Joel-Cohen incisions are that the former lies lower on the abdominal wall, below the 'bikini-line', whereas the latter lies higher but provides less chance of incising the inferior epigastric vessels because they can 'bow string' out laterally if digitally deflected. The Joel-Cohen incision also provides greater access, which is especially useful in emergency situations.
3. When the skin is incised along the direction of the Langer's lines, scar formation is minimized.
4. Beware of damaging underlying loops of bowel when opening the parietal peritoneum.
5. Know the anatomy of the vesico-uterine peritoneal fold so as to avoid damage to the underlying bladder, particularly in repeat caesarean section, when fibrous adhesions may elevate the bladder in the operative field.
6. Be aware of the relations of the ureters in the pelvis, to avoid inadvertent damage to them. The ureters lie close to the lateral fornices of the vagina at the level of the uterine cervix and pass directly under the uterine arteries at this point.
7. The uterine arteries are branches of the internal iliac arteries. The ovarian arteries are branches of the aorta.
8. Both the uterus and the ovaries receive collateral circulations from their respective primary arteries.
9. Three-dimensional, computer-based, interactive anatomical training systems are increasingly replacing cadaveric study.

References

1. Moore KL, Dalley AF, Agur AMR. Clinically Oriented Anatomy. 7th Ed. Baltimore: Lippincott Williams & Wilkins, 2014.

2. Agur AMR, Dalley, AF. Grant's Atlas of Anatomy. 13th Ed. Baltimore: Lippincott Williams & Wilkins, 2009.

3. Ellis H, Mahadevan E. Clinical Anatomy: Applied Anatomy for Students and Junior Doctors. 12th Ed. London: Wiley-Blackwell, 2011.

4. Standring S. Gray's Anatomy: The Anatomical Basis of Clinical Practice. 40th Ed. Philadelphia: Churchill-Livingstone-Elsevier, 2008.

5. Miller JM, Low LK, Zielinski R, Smith AR, DeLancey JO, Brandon C. Evaluating maternal recovery from labor and delivery: bone and levator ani injuries. Am J Obstet Gynecol 2015;213(2):188.e1-188.e11

6. Liu S, Wen J. Ovarian Vein Thrombosis with Involvement of the Renal Vein After Cesarean Section. A Case Report. J Reprod Med 2015;60(5–6):269–72.

7. Paramasivam S, Proietto A, Puvaneswary M. Pelvic anatomy and MRI. Best Pract Res Clin Obstet Gynaecol 2006; 20(1): 3–22.

8. Wasnik AP, Mazza MB, Liu PS. Normal and variant pelvic anatomy on MRI. Magn Reson Imaging Clin N Am 2011; 19(3): 547–66.

9. Temkin B, Acosta E, Malvankar A, Vaidyanath S. An interactive three-dimensional virtual body structures system for anatomical training over the internet. Clin Anat 2006; 19(3): 267–74.

10. Jastrow H, Vollrath L. Anatomy online: Presentation of a detailed WWW atlas of human gross anatomy: Reference for medical education. Clin Anat 2002; 15(6): 402–8.

11. Jastrow H, Vollrath L. Teaching and learning gross anatomy using modern electronic media based on the visible human project. Clin Anat 2003; 16(1): 44–54.

12. Sergovich A, Johnson M, Wilson TD. Explorable three-dimensional digital model of the female pelvis, pelvic contents, and perineum for anatomical education. Anat Sci Educ 2010; 3(3): 127–33.

13. Luo J, Ashton-Miller JA, DeLancey JO. A model patient: Female pelvic anatomy can be viewed in diverse 3-dimensional images with a new interactive tool. Am J Obstet Gynecol 2011; 205(4): 391.e1–2.

14. Rogers RG, Leeman LM, Borders N, Qualls C, Fullilove AM, Teaf D, Hall RJ, Bedrick E, Albers LL. Contribution of the second stage of labour to pelvic floor dysfunction: a prospective cohort comparison of nulliparous women. BJOG 2014; 121(9): 1145–53.

15. Brown SJ, Gartland D, Donath S, MacArthur C. Effects of prolonged second stage, method of birth, timing of caesarean section and other obstetric risk factors on postnatal urinary incontinence: an Australian nulliparous cohort study. BJOG 2011; 118(8):991–1000.

16. Gartland D, MacArthur C, Woolhouse H, McDonald E, Brown SJ. Frequency, severity and risk factors for urinary and faecal incontinence at 4 years postpartum: a prospective cohort. BJOG 2015. [Epub ahead of print]

17. Gartland D, Donath S, MacArthur C, Brown SJ. The onset, recurrence and associated obstetric risk factors for urinary incontinence in the first 18 months after a first birth: an Australian nulliparous cohort study. BJOG 2012; 119(11): 1361–9.

18. Memon HU, Blomquist JL, Dietz HP, Pierce CB, Weinstein MM, Handa VL. Comparison of levator ani muscle avulsion injury after forceps-assisted and vacuum-assisted vaginal childbirth. Obstet Gynecol 2015; 125(5): 1080–7.

19. V.olløyhaug I, Mørkved S, Salvesen Ø, Salvesen KÅ Forceps delivery is associated with increased risk of pelvic organ prolapse and muscle trauma: a cross-sectional study 16–24 years after first delivery. Ultrasound Obstet Gynecol 2015; 46(4): 487–95.

CHAPTER 3
The epidemiology of caesarean delivery

Daniel Pasko, Akila Subramaniam, and Alan T. N. Tita

Introduction

Caesarean section is one of the most commonly performed major surgical procedures worldwide, with an estimated 18.5 million cases performed annually [1, 2]. Despite its common utilization, the decision to proceed with delivery via caesarean section is complex and influenced by multiple factors.

In order to facilitate an understanding of the role of caesarean section in modern obstetrics, this chapter explores the epidemiology of the procedure by highlighting its prevalence, indications, and risk factors, as well as recent efforts towards preventing its use when not necessary.

Global trends in caesarean section rates

In 1985, the World Health Organization indicated that national rates of caesarean delivery between 10% and 15% were considered optimal [3]. However, significant variation exists globally with regard to the respective rates of caesarean delivery. These variations are marked, particularly between developed and developing nations, although discrepancies also exist within these groupings. Recently, WHO reported that population-based rates above 10% are not associated with improvements in maternal or newborn deaths and proposed a 10-group (Robson) classification system to better compare rates at the facility level [4].

Caesarean section rates in developed nations

In the United States, the caesarean rate far exceeds 10%–15%. In 2012, the Consortium on Safe Labor reported on 228,668 deliveries across 19 US hospitals from 2002 to 2008 and documented a 30.5% caesarean section rate [5]. Their findings are consistent with data published for all US births by the Center for Disease Control, which has documented a rising caesarean rate among singleton deliveries from 19.7% in 1996 to 31.3% in 2011 (Figure 3.1) [6]. In response to this dramatic rise, the US Department of Health and Human Services established a 'Healthy People' target caesarean rate of 23.9% for the year 2020 [7].

The findings from the countries in the Organization for Economic Co-operation and Development (OECD) reveal significant variation in caesarean rates among developed and developing member nations, with a range of 14.7% (Iceland) to 49% (Mexico) [8]. A comparison with data from previous years also demonstrates that the overall trend in the past 10 years in most of the industrialized

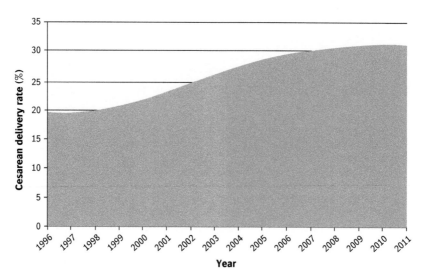

Figure 3.1 US caesarean delivery rate for singleton pregnancies, 1996–2011.

Adapted from Osterman MJ, Martin JA. Changes in Caesarean delivery rates by gestational age: United States, 1996–2011. NCHS data brief 2013 (1244). Hyattsville, MD: National Center for Health Statistics. 2013.

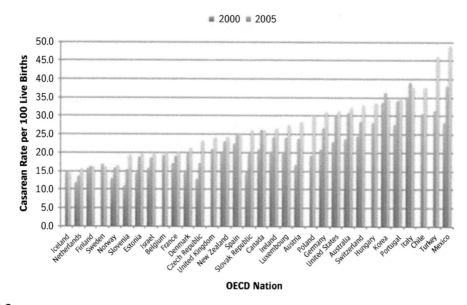

Figure 3.2 Organization for Economic Co-operation and Development caesarean delivery rate, 2000–2011.

Adapted from OECD: Health at a Glance 2013: http://www.oecd.org/health/health-systems/health-at-a-glance.htm

nations has been an increasing caesarean delivery rate (Figure 3.2). Furthermore, the majority of countries represented by the OECD currently exceed the US Healthy People target of a 23.9% or lower caesarean rate for 2020 [7].

Caesarean section rates in developing nations

In the last decade, the World Health Organization conducted a global survey on maternal and perinatal health, which examined the delivery records of 373 health facilities in 24 developing countries (see Chapter 13). The results of the global survey revealed that significant variation in the rate of caesarean delivery also exists among developing nations [9–11]. The findings from the World Health Organization have been reaffirmed by other studies. While Asian and Latin American countries consistently demonstrate caesarean rates well above 15%–20% (Figure 3.3), their counterparts largely demonstrate rates less than 10%–15% (Figure 3.4) [12–14]. Importantly, an association has been demonstrated between increasing caesarean section rates and decreasing mortality rates in developing nations in the setting of overall caesarean section

rates less than 10%–15%. Furthermore, the average caesarean rate among the world's 49 least-developed nations is 2%, and these same countries are plagued by elevated rates of maternal and neonatal mortality [12].

Causes underlying the differences in caesarean section rates between developed and developing nations

The underlying cause for the variation in caesarean delivery rates in both developed and developing nations is likely multifactorial, with the ease of availability of caesarean facilities and supplies as a major factor. This fact becomes apparent upon examination of the rates of caesarean delivery when stratified by presence of a skilled birth attendant and geographic region. Africa and South East Asia have average caesarean rates of 3.8% and 8.8%, respectively. This finding is paired with low respective rates of births attended by skilled personnel (Figure 3.5). Based on data from the World Health Organization, it also appears that income level contributes to the caesarean rate; a drastic increase in the percentage of deliveries by caesarean section occurs with increasing national income (Figure 3.6) [15].

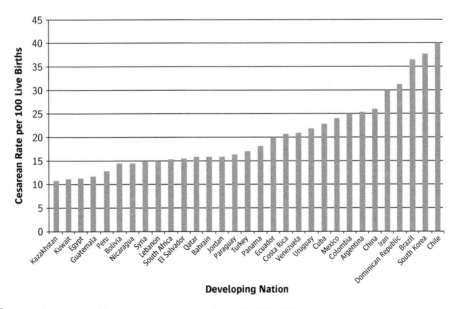

Figure 3.3 Developing nations with caesarean rates greater than 10%, 1996–2003.

Adapted from Reprinted from Clinics in perinatology, 35(3), Wylie BJ, Mirza FG., Caesarean delivery in the developing world, 571–82, Copyright (2008) with permission from Elsevier

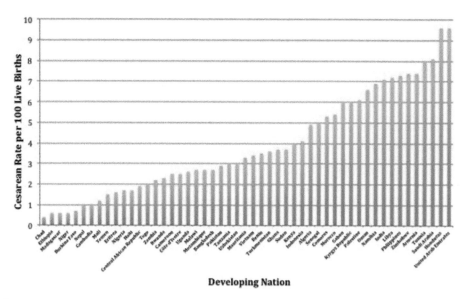

Figure 3.4 Developing nations with caesarean rates less than 10%, 1996–2003.

Adapted from Reprinted from Clinics in perinatology, 35(3), Wylie BJ, Mirza FG. Caesarean delivery in the developing world, 571–82, Copyright (2008) with permission from Elsevier

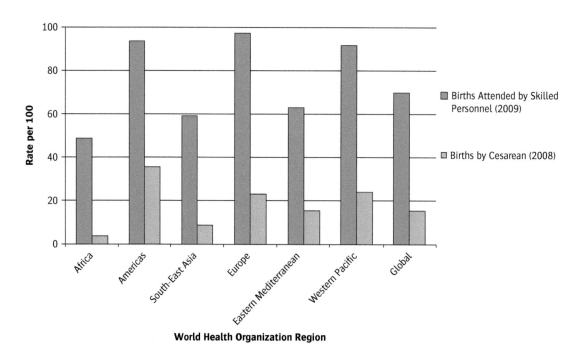

Figure 3.5 World Health Organization rates of births attended by skilled personnel, and births by caesarean by region.

Source: World Health Organization, Global Health Observatory Data Repository

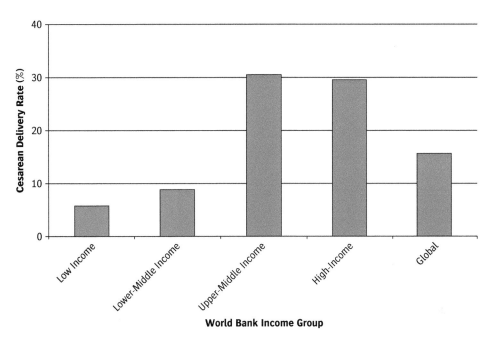

Figure 3.6 International caesarean delivery rate by World Bank income group, in 2008.
Source: World Health Organization, Global Health Observatory Data Repository

Indications for caesarean section

As a result of advances in the field of obstetrics and gynaecology, the number of indications for caesarean delivery has significantly increased over time. In the 1800s, the procedure was considered so dangerous that its use was limited to absolute cephalopelvic disproportion. Half a century later, acceptable indications had evolved to include dystocia, malpresentation, maternal illnesses, and obstetric diagnoses ranging from placenta praevia to toxaemia or pre-eclampsia [16]. Currently, there is a myriad of recognized indications for caesarean delivery.

In 2012, the Eunice Kennedy Shriver National Institute of Child Health and Human Development, the Society for Maternal–Fetal Medicine, and the American College of Obstetricians and Gynecologists detailed specific indications for caesarean section. These indications are generally applicable in both developed and developing country settings and can be classified into absolute and relative categories [17]. While absolute indications mandate caesarean delivery and therefore will always contribute to the baseline caesarean rate, they are uncommon. Examples of absolute indications include conditions such as prior classical caesarean section, complete placenta praevia, cord prolapse, vasa praevia, and prior or current uterine rupture. Relative indications represent potentially modifiable conditions that may or may not always lead to a caesarean section. Such relative indications can be subdivided into maternal, obstetric, and fetal categories (Table 3.1). The listed indications are not mutually exclusive and ultimately require interpretation by a practitioner when determining whether or not to pursue caesarean delivery.

A large majority of caesarean deliveries worldwide are due to relative indications. The aforementioned Consortium on Safe Labor report on 228,668 deliveries across 19 US hospitals provided insight into the extent that various indications contribute to the overall caesarean rate in the

Table 3.1 **Relative indications for caesarean section**

Maternal	Obstetric	Fetal
Maternal request	Arrest of labour	Malpresentation (non-vertex)
Infections (HIV, herpes simplex virus)	Multiple gestation	Fetal malformations (e.g. large omphalocele)
Medical co-morbidities (aortic stenosis, obesity)	Cephalopelvic disproportion	Fetal size (e.g. >5000 g)
Prior myomectomy	Placenta praevia	Non-reassuring antepartum testing
Prior third/fourth degree laceration	Prior caesarean section	Non-reassuring intrapartum fetal testing

Adapted from: Spong CY, Berghella V, Wenstrom KD, Mercer BM, Saade GR. Preventing the first cesarean delivery: summary of a joint Eunice Kennedy Shriver National Institute of Child Health and Human Development, Society for Maternal-Fetal Medicine, and American College of Obstetricians and Gynecologists Workshop. Obstetrics and gynecology. 2012;120(5):1181–93.

United States (Table 3.2). The most frequently cited indications for caesarean delivery were previous uterine scar, failure to progress, and non-reassuring fetal heart tones [5]. More than half (53%) of all caesarean section were performed prior to labour, and a large proportion—more than a quarter—of prelabour caesarean section in this US population were performed for 'elective' indications. Furthermore, hypertensive disorders, which alone should not be an indication for caesarean delivery, accounted for a tangible proportion of caesarean section. Such circumstances are unlikely to be found in developing countries where access to caesarean delivery facilities and supplies is limited.

Data from the World Health Organization suggest that similar trends regarding indications for caesarean delivery are occurring in developing nations. The global survey on maternal and perinatal health in Latin America revealed that the most commonly cited indications for caesarean delivery were cephalopelvic disproportion, dystocia, failure to progress, malpresentation, fetal distress, and history of prior caesarean section. Additionally, hypertensive disorders were noted to contribute significantly [9].

Table 3.2 **Common indications for prelabour and intrapartum caesarean in the United States (Consortium on Safe Labor)**

Indication	Prelabour caesarean (%)	Intrapartum caesarean (%)
Previous uterine scar	45.1	8.2
Failure to progress/cephalopelvic disproportion	2.0	47.1
Elective	26.4	11.7
Non-reassuring fetal testing/fetal distress	6.5	27.3
Fetal malpresentation	17.1	7.5
Hypertensive disorders	3.1	1.6
Fetal macrosomia	3.3	1.2
Multiple gestation	2.8	0.8

Reprinted from American journal of obstetrics and gynecology., Vol/edition, Zhang J, Troendle J, Reddy UM, Laughon SK, Branch DW, Burkman R, et al., Contemporary cesarean delivery practice in the United States, 326 e1–e10, Copyright (2010) with permission from Elsevier

Risk factors for caesarean section

The rising global rates of caesarean section have focused attention on how the increase may affect maternal and neonatal morbidity and mortality [18]. In an attempt to further understand why the rate of caesarean delivery has increased so rapidly, it is useful to examine key factors that are associated with caesarean delivery.

Prior caesarean section

Perhaps the most concerning contribution to the current utilization of caesarean delivery is a history of a prior caesarean section (see Chapter 11). The presence of a uterine scar was the reason for 45.1% of prelabour caesareans documented in the United States [5]. In the late twentieth century, multiple studies demonstrated the relative safety associated with trial of labour after previous caesarean (TOLAC) and discredited the dictum that 'once a caesarean always a caesarean' [19–21]. In the United States, a 50% increase in the vaginal birth after caesarean (VBAC) rate occurred between 1989 and 1996 [22], but the continuation of this paradigm shift was limited because of increasing concerns regarding the safety of TOLAC [23]. The rate of VBAC in the United States subsequently dropped 66% between 1996 and 2003 and has remained low despite large multicentre studies confirming the relatively low frequency of morbidity (Figure 3.7) [22, 24, 25].

The declining rate of VBAC has concomitantly led to a significant increase in the rate of caesarean delivery among women with a prior caesarean delivery (Figure 3.8). The rate of repeat caesarean delivery in the United States has remained stable at nearly 90% [26]. It is important to note that although the rate of VBAC is low, TOLAC remains a viable and at times preferred option for appropriate patients [27]. This preference is particularly important in settings with limited facilities and resources (see Chapter 13). However, it is prudent for TOLAC to occur in facilities where urgent caesarean delivery can be undertaken.

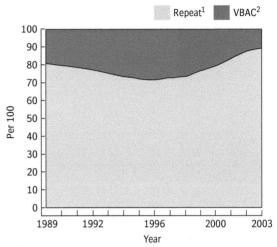

[1]Number of repeat cesarean births per 100 live births to women with a previous cesarean delivery.

[2]Number of vaginal births after previous cesarean delivery per 100 live births to women with a previous cesarean delivery.

Figure 3.7 US rates of repeat caesarean delivery and vaginal birth after caesarean delivery, 1989–2003.

Martin JA, Hamilton BE, Sutton PD, Ventura SJ, Menacker F, Munson ML., Births: final data for 2003. National vital statistics reports: from the Centers for Disease Control and Prevention, 54(2). Hyattsville, MD: National Center for Health Statistics. 2005.

Maternal demographics

Maternal demographic characteristics, including parity and age, have been independently associated with an increased caesarean delivery rate. Specifically, an increased rate of caesarean has been documented among nulliparous American women compared to their multiparous counterparts [28, 29]. Increased caesarean delivery has likewise been documented as maternal age increases. In developed nations, the increased risk of caesarean section related to these maternal characteristics is particularly notable given that an increasing number of mothers are delaying their first pregnancy and that higher rates of caesarean delivery have been documented in nulliparous patients with advanced maternal age than in those without (odds ratio 1.97; confidence interval 1.95, 2) [30, 31].

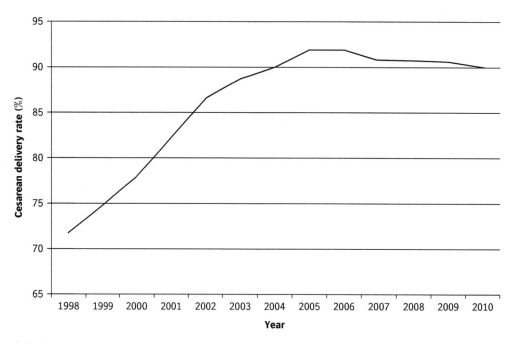

Figure 3.8 US caesarean delivery rate among women with a prior caesarean delivery, 1998–2010.

Data sourced from: National Vital Statistics System-Natality: Centers for Disease Control and Prevention, National Center for Health Statistics

Maternal medical co-morbidities

Beyond maternal demographic factors, medical conditions including obesity, diabetes mellitus, and hypertensive disorders each have implications for the rate of caesarean section. Compared to women with a normal BMI, obese and morbidly obese women, even without other co-morbidities, have an approximately twofold increased risk of caesarean delivery, including emergency caesarean section [32, 33]. The implications of a patient's BMI on the risk for caesarean delivery is compounded by an increased incidence of hypertensive disorders of pregnancy and gestational diabetes among obese and morbidly obese patients, as hypertensive diseases of pregnancy and diabetes are also associated with an increased risk of caesarean delivery [34–38].

Fetal characteristics

Characteristics of the fetus, including gestational age, malpresentation, and macrosomia, also raise the caesarean delivery rate. Specifically, early gestational ages are associated with increased rates of caesarean delivery, with as many as 60% of pregnancies being delivered by caesarean section at a gestational age of 28 weeks [5].

In modern obstetrics, fetal malpresentation is increasingly associated with caesarean delivery. Following publication of the Term Breech Trial at the turn of the twenty-first century, fetuses with breech presentation at term increasingly underwent scheduled caesarean section [39]. Between the years 1997–2003, an estimated 3.8% of term gestations (greater than 37 weeks) were breech, and over 85% of such pregnancies were delivered by caesarean section in the United States [40]. In resource-constrained countries lacking in caesarean facilities, a breech delivery remains a viable option for breech presentations.

Fetal macrosomia represents a risk factor for caesarean delivery as well. Specifically, birth weights greater than 4500 g are associated with at least a twofold increase in risk of caesarean [41].

This trend also applies in the developing world, across all World Health Organization regions [42]. The reason for this trend is not only because labour arrest is more common in the presence of large fetuses, but also because estimated fetal weights greater than 4500–5000 g, depending on diabetic co-morbidity, are considered potential indications for caesarean delivery even without labour [43].

Non-reassuring fetal heart rate

Since its advent in the 1960s, the prevalence of continuous electronic fetal monitoring during labour has become increasingly widespread [44]. While the ability of electronic fetal monitoring to reduce adverse outcomes has not been clearly demonstrated, it has been clearly associated with an increased risk of caesarean section. A recent Cochrane review that utilized international data cites a relative risk of 1.63 for caesarean section when continuous electronic fetal monitoring, as compared to intermittent auscultation, is performed [45].

Whereas induction of labour has been classically associated with increased risk of caesarean delivery, such an association has more recently been disputed [46]. Therefore we do not identify labour induction as a risk factor for caesarean delivery. Suffice it to say that the typical use of an incorrect comparison group (those who undergo spontaneous labour) rather than the true alternative to induction (expectant management) is a major reason why reported associations of caesarean section with induction may be spurious. This area is an important subject of ongoing study.

Prevention of caesarean section

Given the implications of a primary caesarean section on mode of delivery in subsequent pregnancies, it is proposed that future efforts to limit the rate of caesarean delivery will depend primarily upon reducing the rate of primary caesarean sections. Relative indications for caesarean delivery currently play an integral role in determining the rate of caesarean delivery [5]. Consequently, several authorities have published guidelines to minimize the effect of relative indications on the rate of caesarean delivery. Beyond recognizing the vital role of primary caesarean rate reduction, these proposals recommend standardized definitions of arrest disorders and quality control for subjective areas such as fetal heart tracing interpretation [17]. The significance of these efforts extends to developing nations as well, where the World Health Organization has demonstrated an association between caesarean section without a medical indication and increased maternal morbidity and mortality [9, 10].

Public perception of caesarean section represents another challenging aspect of caesarean prevention. The perceived benefits and/or prestige (in some settings) associated with the procedure are exemplified by a trend towards caesarean delivery on maternal request. In the United States, up to 26% of all cases of prelabour caesarean section have been reportedly performed in response to maternal request [47, 48]. Studies indicate that caesarean delivery on maternal request is occurring internationally as well [49–51]. One proposed method for addressing both patients' and practitioners' perception of caesarean deliveries that are performed without clear medical indications is to require documentation of consent for a 'non-indicated caesarean' delivery [17].

A consensus may never be reached regarding the optimal level of caesarean section or when caesarean delivery is clearly indicated for a relative indication. However, a combination of concerted efforts to reduce unnecessary caesareans (particularly in developed settings) and to make caesarean facilities and supplies available for necessary caesareans (particularly in developing settings) seems important for optimal short- and long-term maternal and infant outcomes. Towards these goals, WHO proposes the 10-group 'Robson' classification as a global standard for assessing, monitoring and comparing caesarean section rates within and between facilities.

Key learning points

1. Caesarean section is one of the most commonly performed major surgical procedures worldwide, with an estimated 18.5 million cases performed annually.
2. Multiple factors, including resource availability, contribute to significant variation in the rates of caesarean section between developed and developing nations.
3. Risk factors for caesarean section include a history of prior caesarean section, nulliparity, increasing maternal age, maternal medical co-morbidities, prematurity, malpresentation, suspected macrosomia, and non-reassuring fetal heart monitoring.
4. Recent health initiatives have established guidelines regarding the absolute and relative indications for caesarean section; these guidelines are applicable globally.
5. Efforts to reduce rates of caesarean delivery emphasize decreasing the number of primary caesarean section performed for relative indications, and altering public perception of the procedure.
6. The WHO recommends the 10-group (Robson) classification as the global standard for comparing varying cesarean section rates across facilities.

References

1. Hall MJ, DeFrances CJ, Williams SN, Golosinskiy A, Schwartzman A. National Hospital Discharge Survey: 2007 summary. Natl Health Stat Reports 2010; 29(29): 1–20.
2. Gibbons L, Belizan JM, Lauer JA, Betran AP, Merialdi M, Althabe F. Inequities in the use of cesarean section deliveries in the world. Am J Obstet Gynecol 2012; 206(4): 331.e1–19.
3. Lancet. Appropriate technology for birth. Lancet 1985; 2(8452): 436–7.
4. WHO Statement on Caesarean Section Rates. Geneva: World Health Organization; 2015 (WHO/RHR/15.02).
5. Zhang J, Troendle J, Reddy UM, Laughon SK, Branch DW, Burkman R, et al. Contemporary cesarean delivery practice in the United States. Am J Obstet Gynecol 2010; 203(4): 326.e1–10.
6. Osterman MJ, Martin JA. Changes in cesarean delivery rates by gestational age: United States, 1996–2011. NCHS Data Brief 2013; 124(124): 1–8.
7. Healthy People.gov. Maternal, Infant, and Child Health. 2014. http://www.healthypeople.gov/2020/topics-objectives/topic/maternal-infant-and-child-health.

8. Organisation for Economic Co-operation and Development. Health at a Glance 2013. 2015. http://www.oecd.org/health/health-systems/health-at-a-glance.htm.
9. Villar J, Valladares E, Wojdyla D, Zavaleta N, Carroli G, Velazco A, et al. Caesarean delivery rates and pregnancy outcomes: The 2005 WHO global survey on maternal and perinatal health in Latin America. Lancet 2006; 367(9525): 1819–29.
10. Lumbiganon P, Laopaiboon M, Gülmezoglu AM, Souza JP, Taneepanichskul S, Ruyan P, et al. Method of delivery and pregnancy outcomes in Asia: The WHO global survey on maternal and perinatal health 2007–8. Lancet 2010; 375(9713): 490–9.
11. Shah A, Fawole B, M'Imunya JM, Amokrane F, Nafiou I, Wolomby JJ, et al. Cesarean delivery outcomes from the WHO global survey on maternal and perinatal health in Africa. Int J Gynaecol Obstet 2009; 107(3): 191–7.
12. Betran AP, Merialdi M, Lauer JA, Bing-Shun W, Thomas J, Van Look P, et al. Rates of caesarean section: Analysis of global, regional and national estimates. Paediatr Perinat Epidemiol 2007; 21(2): 98–113.
13. Stanton CK, Holtz SA. Levels and trends in cesarean birth in the developing world. Stud Fam Plann 2006; 37(1): 41–8.
14. Wylie BJ, Mirza FG. Cesarean delivery in the developing world. Clin Perinatol 2008; 35(3): 571–82.
15. World Health Organization. World Health Statistics 2013. 2013. http://www.who.int/gho/publications/world_health_statistics/EN_WHS2013_Full.pdf?ua=1.
16. Cosgrove SAN, Norton JF. Cesarean section: Indications for and relative merits of the classic, low, and extraperitoneal operations. JAMA 1942; 118(3): 201–4.
17. Spong CY, Berghella V, Wenstrom KD, Mercer BM, Saade GR. Preventing the first cesarean delivery: Summary of a joint Eunice Kennedy Shriver National Institute of Child Health and Human Development, Society for Maternal–Fetal Medicine, and American College of Obstetricians and Gynecologists Workshop. Obstet Gynecol 2012; 120(5): 1181–93.
18. Gregory KD, Jackson S, Korst L, Fridman M. Cesarean versus vaginal delivery: Whose risks? Whose benefits? Am J Perinatol 2012; 29(1): 7–18.
19. Lavin JP, Stephens RJ, Miodovnik M, Barden TP. Vaginal delivery in patients with a prior cesarean section. Obstet Gynecol 1982; 59(2): 135–48.

20. Flamm BL, Newman LA, Thomas SJ, Fallon D, Yoshida MM. Vaginal birth after cesarean delivery: Results of a 5-year multicenter collaborative study. Obstet Gynecol 1990; 76 (5 Pt 1): 750–4.

21. Miller DA, Diaz FG, Paul RH. Vaginal birth after cesarean: A 10-year experience. Obstet Gynecol 1994; 84(2): 255–8.

22. Martin JA, Hamilton BE, Sutton PD, Ventura SJ, Menacker F, Munson ML. Births: Final data for 2003. Natl Vital Stat Rep 2005; 54(2): 1–116.

23. McMahon MJ, Luther ER, Bowes WA Jr, Olshan AF. Comparison of a trial of labor with an elective second cesarean section. N Engl J Med 1996; 335(10): 689–95.

24. Landon MB, Hauth JC, Leveno KJ, Spong CY, Leindecker S, Varner MW, et al. Maternal and perinatal outcomes associated with a trial of labor after prior cesarean delivery. N Engl J Med 2004; 351(25): 2581–9.

25. Macones GA, Peipert J, Nelson DB, Odibo A, Stevens EJ, Stamilio DM, et al. Maternal complications with vaginal birth after cesarean delivery: A multicenter study. Am J Obstet Gynecol 2005; 193(5): 1656–62.

26. Curtin SC, Gregory KD, Korst LM, Uddin SFG. Maternal morbidity for vaginal and cesarean deliveries, according to previous cesarean history: New data from the birth certificate, 2013. Natl Vital Stat Rep 2015; 64(4): 1–13.

27. American College of Obstetricians and Gynecologists. ACOG Practice Bulletin No. 115: Vaginal birth after previous cesarean delivery. Obstet Gynecol 2010; 116(2 Pt 1): 450–63.

28. Menacker F, Declercq E, Macdorman MF. Cesarean delivery: Background, trends, and epidemiology. Semin Perinatol 2006; 30(5): 235–41.

29. Heffner LJ, Elkin E, Fretts RC. Impact of labor induction, gestational age, and maternal age on cesarean delivery rates. Obstet Gynecol 2003; 102(2): 287–93.

30. Hamilton BE, Martin JA, Ventura SJ. Births: Preliminary data for 2012. Natl Vital Stat Rep 2013; 62(3): 1–20.

31. Mularz A, Gutkin R. Maternal age and successful induction of labor in the United States, 2006–10. Obstet Gynecol 2014; 123(Suppl 1): 73S.

32. Lynch CM, Sexton DJ, Hession M, Morrison JJ. Obesity and mode of delivery in primigravid and multigravid women. Am J Perinatol 2008; 25(3): 163–7.

33. Poobalan AS, Aucott LS, Gurung T, Smith WC, Bhattacharya S. Obesity as an independent risk factor for elective and emergency caesarean delivery in nulliparous women: Systematic review and meta-analysis of cohort studies. Obes Rev 2009; 10(1): 28–35.

34. Casey BM, Lucas MJ, McIntire DD, Leveno KJ. Pregnancy outcomes in women with gestational diabetes compared with the general obstetric population. Obstet Gynecol 1997; 90(6): 869–73.

35. Naylor CD, Sermer M, Chen E, Sykora K. Cesarean delivery in relation to birth weight and gestational glucose tolerance: pathophysiology or practice style? JAMA 1996; 275(15): 1165–70.

36. Gorgal R, Goncalves E, Barros M, Namora G, Magalhaes A, Rodrigues T, et al. Gestational diabetes mellitus: A risk factor for non-elective cesarean section. J Obstet Gynaecol Res 2012; 38(1): 154–9.

37. Weiss JL, Malone FD, Emig D, Ball RH, Nyberg DA, Comstock CH, et al. Obesity, obstetric complications and cesarean delivery rate: A population-based screening study. Am J Obstet Gynecol 2004; 190(4): 1091–7.

38. The HAPO Study Cooperative Research Group. Hyperglycemia and adverse pregnancy outcomes. N Engl J Med 2008; 358(19): 1991–2002.

39. Hannah ME, Hannah WJ, Hewson SA, Hodnett ED, Saigal S, Willan AR. Planned caesarean section versus planned vaginal birth for breech presentation at term: a randomised multicentre trial. Lancet 2000; 356(9239): 1375–83.

40. Lee HC, El-Sayed YY, Gould JB. Population trends in cesarean delivery for breech presentation in the United States, 1997–2003. Am J Obstet Gynecol 2008; 199(1): 59.e1–8.

41. Spellacy WN, Miller S, Winegar A, Peterson PQ. Macrosomia: Maternal characteristics and infant complications. Obstet Gynecol 1985; 66(2): 158–61.

42. Koyanagi A, Zhang J, Dagvadorj A, Hirayama F, Shibuya K, Souza JP, et al. Macrosomia in 23 developing countries: An analysis of a multicountry, facility-based, cross-sectional survey. Lancet 2013; 381(9865): 476–83.

43. American College of Obstetricians and Gynecologists. Practice Bulletin No. 22: Fetal Macrosomia. Washington, DC: American College of Obstetricians and Gynecologists, 2000.

44. Martin JA, Hamilton BE, Sutton PD, Ventura SJ, Menacker F, Munson ML. Births: Final data for 2002. Natl Vital Stat Rep 2003; 52(10): 1–113.

45. Alfirevic Z, Devane D, Gyte GM. Continuous cardiotocography (CTG) as a form of electronic fetal monitoring (EFM) for fetal assessment during labour. Cochrane Database Syst Rev 2013; 5: CD006066.

46. Mishanina E, Rogozinska E, Thatthi T, Uddin-Khan R, Khan KS, Meads C. Use of labour induction and risk of cesarean delivery: A systematic review and meta-analysis. CMAJ 2014; 186(9): 665–73.

47. National Institutes of Health. National Institutes of Health State-of-the-Science Conference statement: Cesarean delivery on maternal request March 27–29, 2006. Obstet Gynecol 2006; 107(6): 1386–97.

48. American College of Obstetricians and Gynecologists. ACOG committee opinion no. 559: Cesarean delivery on maternal request. Obstet Gynecol 2013; 121(4): 904–7.

49. Akintayo AA, Ade-Ojo IP, Olagbuji BN, Akin-Akintayo OO, Ogundare OR, Olofinbiyi BA. Cesarean section on maternal request: The viewpoint of expectant women. Arch Gynecol Obstet 2014; 289(4): 781–5.

50. Shaaban MM, Sayed Ahmed WA, Khadr Z, El-Sayed HF. Obstetricians' perspective towards cesarean section delivery based on professional level: Experience from Egypt. Arch Gynecol Obstet 2012; 286(2): 317–23.

51. Zhang J, Liu Y, Meikle S, Zheng J, Sun W, Li Z. Cesarean delivery on maternal request in southeast China. Obstet Gynecol 2008; 111(5): 1077–82.

CHAPTER 4
The modern caesarean section

Eric Jauniaux and Vincenzo Berghella

Introduction

The choice of which technique to use for a caesarean section is determined by many factors, including clinical indication, risks of intraoperative complications, whether the operation is an emergency or a repeat procedure, and the preferences of the operator. The last factor is highly variable and very often not evidence-based. Nevertheless, some technical aspects of the modern caesarean section have been rigorously assessed in randomized controlled trials (RCTs) and, when available, these aspects should form the basis on which clinical decisions are made. Moreover, additional well-designed, adequately powered trials on the specific technical aspects of caesarean section are warranted such that evidence-based practices can be extended to all aspects of the operation [1].

Caesarean section techniques have changed considerably over the last two centuries (see Chapter 1). In the last four decades, the main caesarean section procedure has been the so-called Pfannenstiel caesarean section (also known as the Pfannenstiel–Kehrer–Kerr caesarean section or the Monro Kerr caesarean section). This procedure is based on a technique described by Hermann Johannes Pfannenstiel (1862–1909) in 1900 to open the abdomen horizontally, and also described by Ferdinand Adolf Kehrer (1837–1914) in 1881 to open the lower segment of the uterus transversely (see Chapter 1). It became widespread following strong support by John Martin Munro Kerr (1868–1960), who was the first to combine the suprapubic transverse incision described by Pfannenstiel and the low transverse uterine opening described by Kehrer. This

technique has progressively replaced the midline vertical incision of the abdomen, as well as the uterine vertical incision (now called a 'classical caesarean section') used by surgeons of the nineteenth and early twentieth centuries. Interestingly, vertically opening the abdomen was still the main technique used in the 1970s, although it was known from the beginning of the twentieth century to be associated with high rates of long-term post-operative complications such as wound dehiscence and abdominal incision hernia [2], as well as being cosmetically less pleasing. The midline vertical skin incision is still considered faster for entry into the abdomen, compared to other techniques, and therefore is often used in developing countries where visibility may not be as optimized and operating time may be more of a pressing concern (see Figure 4.1). A recent prospective cohort study comparing transverse skin incision and vertical skin incision for emergency caesarean delivery in the United States found that delivery occurs more quickly by 1 minute after vertical skin incision than after transverse skin incision, although the total median operative time was longer by 3–4 minutes after vertical skin incision than after transverse skin incision [3]. As noted above, however, because of the long-term surgical complications it causes for the mother, midline vertical skin incision should only be used in special circumstances. Similarly, the classical vertical uterine incision should only be used in rare cases of very early preterm birth (23–25 weeks), placenta praevia accreta (Chapter 9) or for the delivery of conjoined twins.

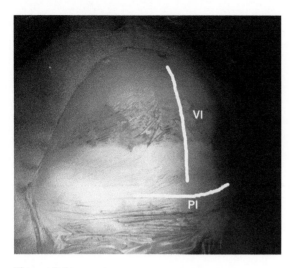

Figure 4.1 General view of a maternal abdomen showing a Pfannenstiel incision (PI) and a vertical incision (VI).

In the 1990s, simplified caesarean section procedures, including the Pelosi minimalist caesarean section [4] in the Americas, and the Vejnović modified caesarean section [5] and Misgav Ladach caesarean section [6] in Europe and Israel, respectively, were described and started to be more widely used than before. The latter procedure is now the main alternative to the Pfannenstiel–Kehrer caesarean section and is used worldwide (see Chapter 5). Historically, the extraperitoneal approach also has been used, particularly in cases with infection in an attempt to limit the spread of sepsis prior to the advent of effective antibiotics [7]. A recent single-blinded prospective trial suggested that the extraperitoneal approach reduces postoperative pain, usage of analgesics and intraoperative nausea without an increase in significant complications [8]. However, the data available supporting the routine use of extraperitoneal caesarean section are limited and insufficient to provide reliable evidence for its routine use; thus, this procedure is seldom used today.

For most of the twentieth century, caesarean section operations were mainly performed as an emergency procedure. Over the last two decades, with an increasing number of women with a previous caesarean section being offered another caesarean delivery in their subsequent pregnancies and others requesting a caesarean section for non-medical reasons, the number of planned (elective) caesarean sections is higher than the number of emergency caesarean sections in many parts of the world.

A survey of obstetricians in the United Kingdom found a wide variation in caesarean section techniques and that this variation was dependent upon the circumstance of the caesarean section [9]. For planned caesarean section, more than 80% of obstetricians used the Pfannenstiel abdominal entry and the double-layer uterine closure. For emergency caesarean section, more used the Misgav Ladach technique with a single-layer closure and administration of prophylactic antibiotics and heparin than those that did not. A survey of obstetric residents in the United States found that 77% used a horizontal skin incision for urgent or emergency caesarean section, 55% used single-layer closure of the uterine incision, 37% used double-layer uterine closure, and 11% used single-layer closure only in women undergoing simultaneous sterilization [10]. A recent survey on uterine closure and other techniques for caesarean section among Quebec's obstetrician–gynaecologists found that double-layer closure was the most common type of uterine closure used by them and that the first layer is locked by two-thirds of Quebec's obstetricians and unlocked by the remainder [11].

The immediate surgical complications of caesarean section that may occur include haemorrhage, infection, thromboembolism, and intraoperative damage to pelvic or abdominal organs such as the bladder or the bowel (see Chapter 8). Long-term complications include a risk of abnormal placentation (placenta praevia and placenta accreta) in future pregnancies, abnormal uterine bleeding due to scar defects, and secondary infertility and other adverse effects due to post-operative adhesions (see Chapter 9). The present chapter reviews the different steps of the Pfannenstiel–Kehrer caesarean section and the best available data to support practice of each technical step of the procedure, as well as the impact of the steps on intra- and post-operative complications. A comparison with the Misgav Ladach technique is presented in Chapter 5. The technical description of the procedure is also based on national and international guidelines (see http://www.guidance.nice.org.uk/; http://www.evidence.nhs.uk/evidence-update-35; http://www.rcog.org.uk/; http://www.acog.org; http://www.resources/sogc.org/publications/).

Preparation for caesarean section

Preparedness may vary depending on the urgent or emergency need to perform the caesarean section. Overall, emergency caesarean section should be performed as soon as feasible in case of immediate threat to the life of the woman or fetus, in a safe environment, by a skilled team including a practitioner skilled in the resuscitation of the newborn. When possible, pregnant women should be offered evidence-based information including indication for caesarean section, associated risks and benefits, and implications for future pregnancies.

Clinical assessment prior to caesarean section

Obstetricians must first review the indication and ensure that vaginal delivery is unlikely. If not previously done, confirm fetal viability by listening to the fetal heart rate and assess fetal presentation. Review the operative care principles including evidence-based informed consent and anaesthetic assessment. For high-risk cases, oral intake restriction should be applied when caesarean section is anticipated (see Chapter 7). Pregnant women in the United Kingdom and several other countries are entitled to decline the offer of caesarean section, even when recommended as a means to prevent fetal or maternal morbidity or morbidity. This situation varies around the world according to local legal regulations.

The 2008 World Health Organization Surgical Safety Checklist (http://www.who.int/patient safety/safesurgery/checklist/en/) was introduced to improve the safety of surgical procedures and has been widely accepted (see Editorial). Modified versions of the checklist for obstetrics have been recently proposed (see http://www.nrls.npsa.nhs.uk/resources/type/guidance and http://sogc.org/wp-content/uploads/2013/04/JOGC-Jan2013-CPG286-ENG-Online.pdf). The most important modification of the checklist seems to be adoption of classification of the level of urgency of caesarean section (caesarean section grades).

Blood tests prior to caesarean section

A full blood count should be performed before the caesarean section to exclude severe anaemia and thrombocytopenia. A rhesus group and antibody screen, testing for syphilis and HIV, a clotting screen, blood compatibility testing, and cross-matching of blood should in general be performed only in high-risk cases or when clinically indicated (severe maternal anaemia).

Preoperative preparation for caesarean section

In the operating theatre, the fetal lie and presentation are checked and the presence of fetal heartbeat confirmed. The indication for caesarean section is reviewed, as the obstetric situation may have changed since the original decision was made.

Regional analgesia (spinal and epidural) has largely replaced general anaesthesia in many maternity services. Issues regarding anaesthesia and caesarean section are presented in Chapter 7. In brief, for women having a caesarean section under regional anaesthesia, preloading intravenous (IV) fluids (crystalloid or colloid) and, when needed, ephedrine or phenylephrine should be offered to reduce the risks of maternal hypotension. To reduce the acidity of stomach contents and thus the risk of lung aspiration, women should also receive antiacid drugs when possible.

Pubic hair in the region of the proposed skin incision may be clipped (depilatory preparation). The reason for hair removal is mainly to prevent interference with wound approximation, as there is no evidence that is reduces the risks of wound infection.

The operating table should have a lateral tilt of 15° or a pillow or folded linen should be placed under the woman's right lower back to avoid vena caval compression and supine hypotension syndrome.

It is now well established that parenteral antibiotic prophylaxis (ampicillin or first-generation cephalosporins) 30–60 minutes before the skin incision reduces the risk of post-partum endometritis and total maternal infectious morbidity by half, with no significant effect on neonatal sepsis or admission to intensive care unit [1, 12, 13]. There is no evidence that a double or triple combination of antibiotics improves outcome compared to standard cephalosporin prophylaxis [1].

Fixing an indwelling urethral catheter (Foley catheter) is routinely performed for elective and emergency caesarean section in most countries around the world. Different types of catheters can be used, for example, the standard Foley catheter, a Nelaton catheter, and antibiotic-impregnated or silver alloy-impregnated catheters. The drainage tube is inserted into the urinary bladder through the urethra when analgesia is established and is then left in situ for 12–24 hours until the patient is able to be mobile. This tube is connected to a closed collection system and aims to evacuate urine and decompress the urinary bladder. This procedure may improve visualization of the lower uterine segment, minimize bladder injury, and facilitate the development of a bladder flap if required. In haemodynamically unstable women, the catheter and collection system are pivotal to monitor urine output and help evaluate the fluid balance.

If the fetal head is deep in the pelvis, assisted caesarean delivery may be necessary. This procedure is done by asking an assistant wearing sterile gloves to reach into the vagina and push the baby's head up through the vagina as soon as the uterus is opened. Within this context, vaginal preparation with povidone–iodine solution immediately before caesarean delivery reduces the risk of post-operative endometritis [1, 14]. This benefit is

higher for women undergoing caesarean section after prolonged rupture of the membranes. No data are available demonstrating whether vaginal preparation reduces morbidity in women who have received a single dose of antibiotics before the caesarean section.

A recent meta-analysis of RCTs that evaluated skin preparation in preventing caesarean-associated infection has found little evidence to support the use of specific preparations, concentrations, or methods of application [15]. Another recent meta-analysis evaluating whether preoperative skin antisepsis immediately prior to surgical incision for clean surgery prevents surgical site infection identified only one RCT that showed that preoperative skin preparation with 0.5% chlorhexidine in methylated spirits was associated with lower rates of site infection than preparation with alcohol-based povidone–iodine paint was [16]. The perceived efficacy of chlorhexidine is in fact based on evidence for the efficacy of the chlorhexidine–alcohol combination. The role of alcohol has frequently been overlooked in evidence assessments [17]. Therefore, it is not yet clear what sort of skin preparation may be most efficient for preventing surgical site infection in the context of caesarean section.

Drapes should not be adhesive, because adhesive drapes have been associated with a higher rate of wound infections, compared with nonadhesive drapes [1].

(Module 1; Module 1 MAF video. To access this video please visit http://medicalaidfilms.org/our-films/obstetric-care/. In order to obtain access to all videos in this set, please contact info@medicalaidfilms.org).

Abdominal/pelvic entry for caesarean section

The skin incision described by Pfannenstiel is slightly curved (the 'smile' incision) and performed two-fingers width (1 inch or 2.5 cm) above the pubic symphysis, if possible in a natural skin fold (Figure 4.1). The knife blade is angled at 90° to the skin, and an incision approximately 15 cm long is made to allow adequate exposure of the underlying tissues. The subcutaneous tissues are rapidly incised bluntly, sharply, or

with cautery. No RCTs comparing these techniques in caesarean section have been performed to suggest one technique is preferable. Bleeding vessels are cauterized or suture ligated, as necessary. Particular attention should be paid to branches of the epigastric vessels, which are usually located around both ends of the suprapubic incision. The corresponding anatomy is described in Chapter 2.

Once the rectus sheath or fascia is exposed, it is incised in the midline and then cut out laterally with heavy curved Mayo scissors or separated by finger dissection and gentle lateral tension (Figure 4.2). The upper and lower edges of the cut fascia are then grasped with toothed clamps, such as Kocher clamps, and elevated. Under tension, the sheath is then separated from the muscle by blunt and sharp dissection using scissors or pushing upwards between the rectus sheath and the corresponding muscle. This process should free the sheath vertically and transversely. The use of scissors dissection is often required in repeat caesarean section because of the presence of fibrous tissue between the layers. Perforating vessels are suture ligated and cut or cauterized, as necessary. The need for, benefits, and risks of sheath separation have not been assessed in an RCT, and its use is therefore not based on Level 1++ data (high level of certainty).

The peritoneum can be opened bluntly with finger dissection or sharply. In the latter case, the peritoneum is grasped with fine clamps, elevated to ensure that no bowel is incised on opening, and then entered using scissors. All the layers of the abdominal wall are then stretched manually (Figure 4.3) to the extent of the skin incision (eight-finger pull opening).

The creation of a bladder flap was routinely performed in the past during low transverse caesarean section as Pfannenstiel described it for his urological procedure. The flap is developed by lifting the visceral peritoneum (the vesico-uterine fold of the peritoneum), retracting the uterus cephalad (towards the diaphragm) to expose the bladder reflection, and entering the vesicocervical space. The bladder flap is then created by extending the peritoneal incision outwards with fine scissors or fingers and manually pushing the

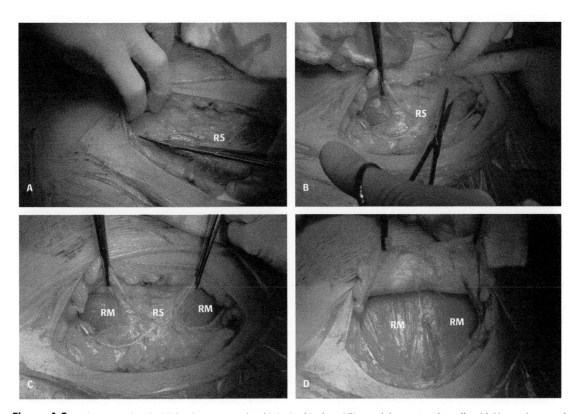

Figure 4.2 A. The rectus sheath (RS) has been exposed and is incised in the midline and then cut out laterally with Mayo scissors and gentle lateral tension. B, The upper and lower edges of cut fascia are grasped with clamps and elevated. C. Under tension, the sheath is then separated from the muscle by blunt and sharp dissection using scissors or pushing a swap upward between the rectus sheath and the corresponding muscle. D. The sheath is freed vertically and transversely, exposing the rectus muscle (RM).

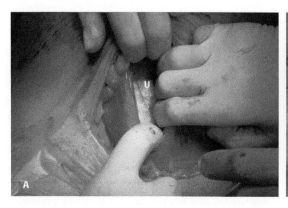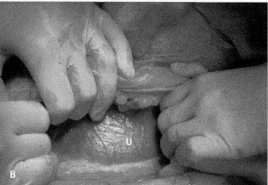

Figure 4.3 A. The layers of the abdominal wall are stretched manually to the extent of the skin incision. B. An 8-finger pull opening of the abdomen.

bladder downward. Recent RCTs have questioned the value of creating a bladder flap. A recent meta-analysis of RCTs examining the benefits of bladder flap formation during term elective caesarean section found that omission of the bladder flap step at caesarean section reduces the skin incision–delivery interval without leading to differences in bladder injury, total operating time, blood loss, or duration of hospitalization [18]. The creation of a bladder flap may be required in repeat caesarean section if the bladder is covering the lower uterine segment.

(○ Videos 1 & 2 at www.oxfordmedicine.com/textbookofcaesareansection, and Module 2 MAF video. To access this module please visit http://medicalaidfilms.org/our-films/obstetric-care/. Please note that in order to request permission to view this video you will be required to contact info@medicalaidfilms.org).

Opening the uterus in caesarean section, and delivery

Following the surgical technique described by Kehrer, the uterus is opened with a transverse lower segment hysterotomy. A small (about 3–5 cm) transverse lower segment incision using a scalpel is made through the lower segment myometrium. It should be about 1 cm below the level where the vesico-uterine serosa was incised to bring the bladder down (Figure 4.4). The uterine incision is enlarged by placing a finger at each edge and gently pulling upwards and downwards at the same time. Blunt expansion using fingers remains preferred to sharp dissection, as it results in less maternal blood loss [1]. In rare cases in which the lower uterine segment is thick and narrow, the incision may be extended in a crescent shape, using scissors instead of fingers to avoid extension into the uterine vessels. The uterine incision should be large enough (>10–12 cm) to deliver the head and body of the baby without tearing the incision and damaging the lateral uterine circulation.

The baby is delivered by placing one hand inside the uterine cavity between the uterus and the baby's head (Figure 4.5). The head is grasped, flexed, and gently lifted through the incision, taking care to try and avoid extending the incision. External fundal pressure is essential to help deliver the head and sometime the shoulders and body. This procedure can be performed by the operator using his/her other hand or by asking an assistant to press on the abdomen over the top of the uterus. Clamp and cut the umbilical cord, and hand the baby to an assistant for initial care.

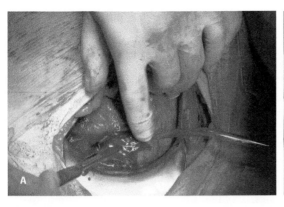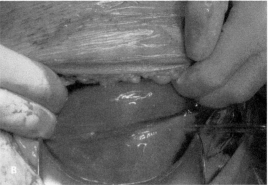

Figure 4.4 A. A small 3–5 cm transverse lower segment incision through the lower segment myometrium is made with a scalpel. B. The uterine incision is enlarged by placing a finger at each edge and pulling upwards and downwards at the same time.

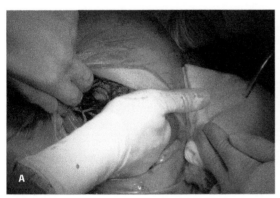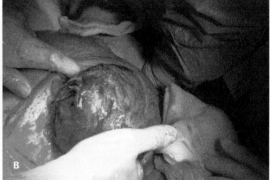

Figure 4.5 A. The baby is delivered by placing one hand inside the uterine cavity between the uterus and the baby's head. B. The head is grasped, flexed, and lifted through the incision.

Prevention of post-partum haemorrhage (PPH) has been pivotal in decreasing maternal morbidity and mortality for both vaginal and caesarean deliveries. Traditionally, at caesarean section, an oxytocin bolus is administered IV by the anaesthetist, the placenta is removed after spontaneous separation and/or gentle traction on the cord, and the uterus is massaged. Numerous trials have evaluated the role of different uterotonics in preventing uterine atony at delivery but unfortunately an optimal regiment has not been established [1]. The main drugs that have been used are oxytocin, carbetocin, tranexamic acid, and misoprostol. Oxytocin infusion (10–40 IU in 500–1000 ml crystalloid over 2–8 hours) remains the first line in uterine atony prevention at caesarean section [1]. Carbetocin has been shown to be a superior prophylactic in some RCTs but still remains not widely used [1]. Initial trials of tranexamic acid have also shown additional prevention of PPH when given at the start of caesarean section, but this intervention is still not widely supported by current guidelines. Misoprostol is inferior to oxytocin as first-line prevention for PPH [1].

It has been suggested that the method of delivering the placenta may contribute to an increase or decrease in the morbidity of caesarean section. A meta-analysis of 15 RCTs comparing manual and spontaneous delivery of the placenta at caesarean section has found that spontaneous delivery is associated with less endometritis, less blood loss, a smaller decrease in haematocrit levels post-operatively, and shorter duration of hospital stay than manual delivery is [19]. There are only two RCTs comparing uterine massage with no massage following delivery of the placenta, but both of these were in the context of vaginal birth with active management of the third stage of labour, including the use of oxytocin [20]. Data do not exist to guide best practice regarding uterine massage specifically at the time of caesarean. Technically, the massage of the uterus during a caesarean section is easy and with limited discomfort for the mother.

It can be performed more efficiently with externalization of the uterus.

It is pivotal that the operator ensures that all retained placental tissue and membranes are removed with a clean swab before starting the closure of the uterus.

(⊙ Videos 1 & 2 at www.oxfordmedicine.com/textbookofcaesareansection, and Modules 2 & 3 MAF video. To access this module please visit http://medicalaidfilms.org/our-films/obstetric-care/. Please note that in order to request permission to view this video you will be required to contact).

Closure techniques for caesarean section

Surgical wounds generally heal by primary intention during which the wound edges are brought together so that they are adjacent to each other. Wound closure is usually assisted by the use of sutures or staples. For decades, obstetricians have been closing all the layers that they opened during caesarean delivery. Thus, the uterine incision was closed with two layers of sutures, both peritoneal layers were closed with continuous sutures, and the rectus sheath was closed with continuous or interrupted sutures. More recently, many operators have advocated closing the myometrial incision with a single-layer continuous suture and avoiding closing the visceral and parietal peritoneum.

If the uterus is not externalized, closure of the uterine incision should start with the insertion of a medium-to-large retractor in order to provide a clear view of the lower segment and the bladder (Figure 4.6). Both corners of the myometrial incision should be visualized and grasped with clamps. Any extensions of the uterine opening should be identified and repaired. If required to establish adequate visualization, the bottom edge of the incision should be grasped with clamps as well. Most surgeons now use either polyglycolic sutures or synthetic absorbable braided sutures coated with polyglycolic acid, polycaprolactone, or calcium stearate, while chromic catgut is avoided.

The closure of the uterine incision is performed starting from the far angle, using a continuous unlocked suture until the near angle suture is reached. If the uterus is not exteriorized and the visibility is limited, the angle of the uterine incision closest to the surgeon can be sutured first, with a long length of suture left before cutting. The far angle is then sutured by applying a clip to the long cut end, and the uterine edges are closed with a continuous interlocking suture until the near angle suture is reached. The end of the continuous stitch is tied to the first angle suture. The first layer closure should take the full thickness of the uterine muscle in each suture, avoiding the peritoneal lining. Before closing the facia, the surgeon should make sure that there is no bleeding from the hysterotomy site and that the uterus is firm. Also, the bladder, the ovaries, and the fallopian tubes should be examined. If there is any further bleeding from the incision site, the site is best closed with figure-of-eight sutures.

Swabs on sticks are often used to clean out both paracolic gutters (the space along the outer side walls of the abdomen) before closing the abdomen. A sub-rectus sheath drain can be considered in women at risk of secondary abnormal clotting (pre-eclampsia).

As with the closure of the myometrial incision, it is suggested to clearly identify the angles of the rectus sheath (Figure 4.7) and to clip or insert a single stitch in the proximal end (the end nearest to the surgeon). The far angle is then sutured,

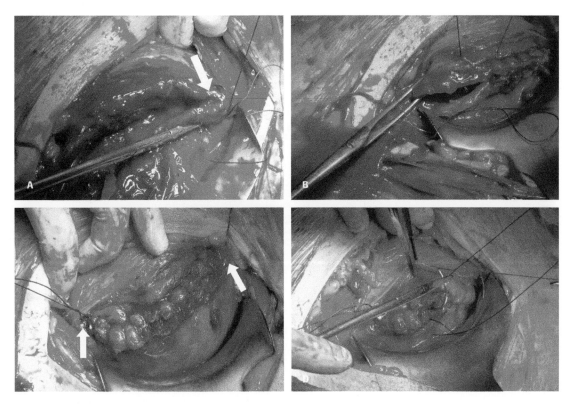

Figure 4.6 Uterine incision closure in two layers. A. The far angle (arrow) of the first layer is sutured. B. The uterine edges are closed with a continuous interlocking suture until the near angle suture is reached. C. The near angle suture. D. Closure of the second layer.

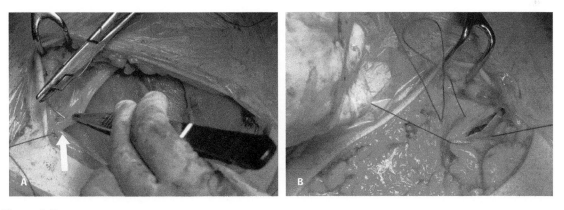

Figure 4.7 A. Closure of the rectus sheath starting from the near angle (arrow). B. Continuous interlocking suture until the far angle is reached.

and the sheet is sutured with a continuous absorbable suture (Table 4.1) until the near angle suture is reached.

The loose connective tissue just beneath the skin is called the subcutaneous tissue or the hypoderm and consists primarily of adipose cells (fat), with fibrous bands that anchor the skin to the deep fascia. It also contains blood vessels, lymphatic vessels, and cutaneous nerves, as well as collagen and elastin fibres that attach the tissue to the dermis. Many surgeons have

Table 4.1 Characteristics of suture material commonly used during caesarean section

Suture type	Tissue reaction	Tensile strength
Absorbable		
Vicryl (braided polyglactin)	Low	Good
Vicryl Rapide (monofilament polyglactic acid)	Low	Good
Monocryl (monofilament polyglecaprone)	Low	Good
PDS (monofilament polydioxanone)	Low	Highest
Dexon (braided or monofilament polyglycolic acid)	Low	Good
Catgut (twisted)	Moderate	Lowest
Non-absorbable		
Prolene (monofilament polypropylene)	Lowest	Good
Mersilene (braided polyester)	Low	High
Nylon (monofilament)	Low	High
Silk (braided or twisted)	Highest	Low

advocated the closure of subcutaneous tissue. Its closure in patients with subcutaneous space ≥2 cm and/or when haemostasis is difficult to control leads to a decrease in wound complications [21], as large subcutaneous spaces can easily fill with blood and thus create a large hematoma and a secondary abscess.

If there are no signs of infection, the skin should be closed with continuous subcutaneous synthetic absorbable suture [22].

At the end of the procedure, a sterile dressing is applied to the closed skin incision, and gentle pushes are applied to the fundus of the uterus to remove clots.

A detailed description of closure is presented in ◉ Videos 1 and 2 at www.oxfordmedicine.com/textbookofcaesareansection, and the Medical Aid Films video 'Caesarean Section: Module 4–Closure of Uterus and Abdomen' To access this module, please visit http://medicalaidfilms.org/our-films/obstetric-care/?v=94496087. Please note that in order to request permission to view this video you will be required to contact info@medicalaidfilms.org).

Further discussion of techniques used in caesarean section

Caesarean section is one the most established major operations but has evolved with little evaluation of the numerous technical changes developed over the last century. These changes only have only been evaluated recently in RCTs and thus their impact on long-term complications of caesarean section, such as pelvic adhesion, scar defects, or placenta accreta in subsequent pregnancies cannot be assessed yet. Therefore, more research is needed in this area. The know levels of certainty from RCTs for the main technical steps used in a caesarean delivery are displayed in Box 1.

Uterine exteriorization during caesarean section

Uterine exteriorization, or temporary removal of the uterus from the abdominal cavity after the baby has been born, has been advocated by many surgeons over the last three decades as a valuable

> ### Box 4.1 **Moderate and high levels of certainty for caesarean section technical steps**
>
> #### Preparation
>
> - Prophylactic antibiotics: single dose of ampicillin or first-generation cephalosporins, 15 to 60 min prior to skin incision (High level of certainty).
> - Not placing or early removal of indwelling bladder catheter (Moderate level of certainty).
> - Vaginal preparation with povidone-iodine scrub after prolonged ruptured of the membranes (Moderate level of certainty).
>
> #### Opening & Delivery
>
> - Omission of bladder flap development (Moderate level of certainty).
> - Blunt expansion of the uterine incision (High level of certainty).
> - Prevention of uterine atonia with oxytocin infusion at 10–40 IU in 500 to 1 L crystalloid over 2–8 hours (High level of certainty); with misoprostol at 200–800 μg rectal or sub-lingual (Moderate level of certainty); with tranexamic acid at 10 mg/kg IV prior to incision (Moderate level of certainty); carbetocin at 100 μg IV after delivery (Moderate level of certainty).
>
> #### Closure
>
> - Uterine exteriorization for hysterotomy repair (High level of certainty).
> - Non-closure of parietal and/or visceral peritoneal on the risk of secondary adhesions (Moderate level of certainty).
> - Closure of a subcutaneous tissue of ≥2 cm (High level of certainty).
>
> Reprinted from Am J Obstet Gynecol., 209, Dahlke JD, Mendez-Figueroa H, Rouse DJ, Berghella V, Baxter JK, Chauhan SP., Evidence-based surgery for cesarean delivery: an updated systematic review., 294–306, Copyright (2013) with permission from Elsevier

technique to facilitate repair of the uterine incision. Uterine exteriorization is particularly useful when exposure/visualization of the incision is difficult, as in obese women or when there is poor haemostasis. Several RCTs have been performed to evaluate whether exteriorization is helpful, but these have had varied results with respect to whether there are reductions in the rate of post-operative infection and perioperative haemorrhage. A meta-analysis of RCTs published between 1966 and 2003 found no evidence to make definitive conclusions about which method of uterine closure offers greater advantages [23]. RCTs and prospective studies published after 2003[24–26] have shown shorter mean operative time, shorter time to the first bowel movement, and shorter length of hospital stay as well as lower rates of surgical site infection when the uterus is exteriorized than when it is not. By contrast, moderate and severe pain at 6–48 hours is less frequent with in situ uterine repair [24, 25]. In conclusion, uterine exteriorization is safe, but there is not good evidence to suggest it is clearly preferable, and it should be performed as per the operator preference.

Closure of the uterus and the peritoneum during caesarean section

There is mounting data in the international literature on immediate and long-term outcomes associated with the different techniques and suture materials used to close the uterus and abdomen during caesarean section. The potential effects of these different surgical techniques on long-term outcomes, including the functional integrity of the uterine scar during subsequent pregnancies and the side effects of intra-abdominal adhesions, are now becoming increasingly important for guiding clinical practice and are reviewed in Chapter 9.

Several prospective studies and RCTs have evaluated the advantages and disadvantages of single- versus double-layer closure of the uterine incision, and closure versus non-closure of the peritoneum [1, 27–30]. A meta-analysis of RCTs published before 2008 found that single-layer closure of the uterine incision, compared with double-layer closure, is associated with a statistically significant reduction in mean blood loss, in the duration of the operative procedure, and in the presence of post-operative pain [27]. However, two recent RCTs found no difference between the two methods in terms of post-operative maternal infectious morbidity, pain, and blood transfusion [28, 29].

In addition to the immediate post-operative risks of single-layer versus double-layer closure of the uterus, several authors have also investigated its impact on the risk of uterine rupture in trial of labour (TOLAC) after caesarean section. The results of these investigations have been varied. A large, multicentre, case-control study has shown that a prior single-layer closure carries more than twice the risk of uterine rupture than double-layer closure does [31]. A systematic review of the best available evidence regarding the association between single-layer closure and uterine rupture found that locked but not unlocked single-layer closures are associated with a higher uterine rupture risk than double-layer closures are in women attempting TOLAC [32]. A recent small retrospective study found that the use of monofilament suture for hysterotomy closure in prior caesarean section significantly reduced the chance of having placenta praevia in the index pregnancy [33]. Thus, there is a need for high-quality, properly designed RCTs with large sample sizes to evaluate the impact of different suture materials on uterine scar defects, including rupture risk in TOLAC and the development of placenta praevia/accreta in subsequent pregnancies.

A meta-analysis on the evidence on the effects of non-closure versus closure of the peritoneum at caesarean section has shown that there is improved short-term post-operative outcome when the peritoneum is not closed [34]. However, there is no evidence for any short-term or long-term advantage in peritoneal closure for non-obstetric operations [30] and thus it cannot be recommended to close the peritoneum at caesarean section.

Finally, no difference in immediate post-operative outcome has been found based on whether chromic catgut or polyglactin [28] is used to close the uterine incision or whether a sub-rectus sheath drain [29] is used; this result suggests that any of these surgical techniques is acceptable.

Preventing adhesions following caesarean section

Long-term studies on the risks of abdomino-pelvic adhesions following caesarean section are limited. Repeat caesarean delivery increases the risks of adhesions [35] and other long-term uterine and pelvic complications (Chapter 9). There is at present no evidence to justify the time and cost of peritoneal closure (parietal or visceral) in terms of preventing adhesions [36], although a prospective cohort study has found that a single-layer uterine closure is associated with a sevenfold increase in the odds of developing bladder adhesions [37].

Adhesion prevention products are becoming commonly used in general and gynaecologic surgery. Two membrane/adhesion barriers have been approved in the United States [38], although not specifically for caesarean delivery. A barrier consisting of oxidized regenerated cellulose (Interceed absorbable adhesion barrier) has been shown to reduce adhesions during microsurgery. The same benefits may not be seen following caesarean section because complete haemostasis is crucial to its efficacy. The Seprafilm adhesion barrier, composed of hyaluronic acid and carboxymethylcellulose, is approved for use in abdominal or pelvic laparotomy. However, the use of these synthetic barriers for caesarean section has only been studied in two small, non-blinded, nonrandomized trials, both of which were underpowered and subject to bias [39]. Neither demonstrated improvement in meaningful clinical outcomes. Two recent cohort studies have shown that placing a carboxymethylcellulose barrier is not associated with total operative time blood loss, or adhesion scores at first repeat caesarean delivery between women who had a hyaluronate–carboxycellulose barrier film placed at the time of their primary caesarean delivery and those who did not [40, 41]. A systematic review of the literature on the use of adhesion barriers in the context of caesarean section yielded only a few studies, most of which are lacking in methodology [42]. Overall, the available evidence does not support the routine use of adhesion barriers during caesarean delivery.

Subcutaneous and skin closure following caesarean section

There is uncertainty about closure of the subcutaneous tissue after surgery. For most surgeons, the systematic closure of subcutaneous tissue is an unnecessary step that increases operating time and uses additional suture material without offering any benefit. A recent meta-analysis of RCTs comparing subcutaneous closure with no subcutaneous closure in non-caesarean section surgical procedures has shown that the current evidence is of very low quality and therefore insufficient to support or refute the benefits of subcutaneous closure after non-caesarean operations [43]. As previously noted, however, there is evidence that closure of the subcutaneous layer at caesarean section is beneficial in all women with subcutaneous tissue of a depth of 2 cm or greater to reduce the risks of subcutaneous haematomas and scar dehiscence [1, 21].

The primary function of suturing the skin is to maintain tissue approximation during healing, and preferably skin edges must just touch each other. There are many ways to close the skin surgical incision, including continuous or interrupted sutures, staples, tissue adhesives, or tapes. A recent meta-analysis of RCTs on the benefits and harms of continuous compared with interrupted skin closure techniques in non-obstetric surgery found that, irrespective of the differences in the nature of the suture materials used in the two groups, wound dehiscence was reduced by using continuous absorbable subcuticular sutures [44]. Staples are associated with similar outcomes in terms of wound infection, pain, and cosmetic effects, compared with sutures [45, 46], but staples removed on the third day after the operation are associated with an increased incidence of skin separation and the need for re-closure, as compared with absorbable sutures [45]. A recent RCT showed that staples are preferred to subcuticular suture for skin closure by women after caesarean section and are therefore the main suturing technique used by most operators [43]. However, another recent RCT has shown that suture closure of the skin is associated with a 57% decrease in wound complications compared to staple closure [47].

No use or immediate versus delayed removal of urinary catheter for caesarean section

Emerging evidence indicates that omitting the use of urinary catheters during and after caesarean section could reduce the associated increased risk of urinary tract infections and risk of catheter-associated pain/discomfort to the woman and could lead to earlier ambulation and a shorter stay in hospital than when catheters are used. A review of five RCTs of moderate quality indicates that there is currently insufficient evidence to assess the routine use of indwelling bladder catheters in women undergoing caesarean section [48]. The use of indwelling urinary catheters for caesarean delivery remains essential in haemodynamically unstable patients.

A systematic review of previous RCTs has suggested that early removal of the indwelling bladder catheter may be considered for caesarean section, as no benefits, and some harm, mainly from increased post-operative urinary infection rates, have been associated with long durations of catheter placement [1]. A recent RCT has also shown that immediate removal of urinary catheter after elective caesarean section is associated with lower risk of urinary infection and earlier post-operative ambulation than delayed catheter removal is, with no differences in the incidence of urinary retention necessitating re-catheterization [49].

A detailed description of post-operative care is presented in the Medical Aid Films video 'Caesarean Section: Module 6–Post Operative Care'. To access this module please visit http://medicalaidfilms.org/our-films/obstetric-care/?v=94497033. Please note that in order to request permission to view this video you will be required to contact info@medicalaidfilms.org.

Delayed cord clamping following caesarean section

Immediate umbilical cord clamping within the first seconds after vaginal or caesarean birth, regardless of whether the cord pulsation has ceased, is routine in the United States and in Europe [50]. Delayed cord clamping (DCC) for 30 to 120 seconds and/or umbilical cord milking has been shown to increase placental transfusion and thus lead to an increase of approximately 30% in neonatal blood volume at birth. In preterm neonates, there is strong evidence that DCC decreases the need for blood transfusions, the incidence of necrotizing enterocolitis, and the risks of intraventricular haemorrhage and late-onset sepsis [51, 52].

In the term newborn, there is growing evidence that DCC increases early haemoglobin concentrations and iron stores, but it may also adversely increase the risk of jaundice and the need for phototherapy [53]. Thus, in healthy term babies, DCC is likely to be beneficial as long as access to treatment for jaundice requiring phototherapy is available. DCC may also theoretically increase the length of the third stage and therefore the likelihood of maternal bleeding. However, there is no significant difference between immediate cord clamping and DCC for severe PPH, mean maternal blood loss, and haemoglobin values [53]. The optimal umbilical cord clamping practice among neonates requiring immediate resuscitation remains uncertain and there are very limited data on DCC at the time of caesarean section [54, 55]. The potential for harm caused to the mother by DCC at the time of term caesarean section needs to be weighed by clinicians in the context of its technical difficulty and the risk of PPH associated with the surgical procedure and within the settings in which they work.

High-risk caesarean deliveries

The main operative complication associated with high-risk caesarean section is maternal haemorrhage during or immediately after delivery. Anterior placenta praevia, multiple pregnancies, and severe pre-eclampsia are all associated with a high risk of major PPH requiring immediate blood transfusion. When massive bleeding is anticipated, appropriate equipment for major gynaecologic surgery, including a self-retaining retractor and instrumentation to perform a major laparotomy, should be available in the operating room. Hysterectomy remains the most commonly performed procedure for the control of PPH.

The incidence of relaparotomy/reopening after caesarean section is around 0.2%, and the risk factors include previous caesarean section, severe pre-eclampsia, placenta praevia, uterine rupture, placental abruption, cervical tear, and PPH [56, 57]. Hysterectomy may be required to control life-threatening bleeding in about a third of the patients [57]. In many tertiary care centres, these surgeries are performed in the main operating room, as opposed to in labour and delivery units, to ensure the availability of equipment, blood bank support, and nursing staff trained in advanced abdominal surgery.

In cases of placenta praevia accreta (see Chapter 9), maternal bleeding can rapidly become life-threatening. Referral of all women diagnosed antenatally with this condition to a tertiary care centre with experience in the management of complex caesarean section (caesarean hysterectomy) is essential. In all cases of placenta accreta, the use of a multidisciplinary care team is therefore recommended by professional organizations, including the American College of Obstetricians and Gynecologists (ACOG), the American Society of Anaesthesiologists (ASA), the Royal College of Anaesthetists (RCA) and the Royal College of Obstetricians and Gynaecologists (RCOG).

Caesarean section at full dilatation

Caesarean section at full dilatation is performed when delivery is required in the second stage or pushing phase of labour. A recent cohort study has indicated that nulliparous women in the second stage of labour at our institution are twice as likely to undergo caesarean delivery [58]. Women with a full-term second-stage caesarean delivery have a significantly higher than expected rate of subsequent. Spontaneous preterm birth in a subsequent pregnancy compared to women with a first-stage caesarean delivery [59].

In second-stage caesarean delivery, the fetal head can be impacted into the pelvis, making the surgical procedure technically difficult by leading to excessive manipulation of the stretched lower segment and thus resulting in angle extension and obstetrics haemorrhage. Caesarean section at full dilatation is associated with longer operative times, epidural analgesia, chorioamnionitis, and higher birth weight, compared to caesarean section during the first stage of labour [60]. Delays in delivering the impacted fetal head can contribute to an increased requirement for neonatal resuscitation and admission to the neonatal intensive care unit. The maternal composite risk index is also increased in women undergoing caesarean delivery in the second stage of labour, primarily because of uterine atony, uterine incision extension, and incidental cystotomy [60–62]. Overall, the neonatal composite morbidity in the second stage of labour is not increased compared with the first stage but second-stage caesarean section deliveries after a failed forceps or vacuum attempt have the highest rate (6.9%) of fetal injuries of all caesarean section deliveries [63].

If the fetal head is deep in the pelvis, as in obstructed labour at full dilatation, there may be a need for assisted caesarean delivery. Techniques vary internationally and there are no national guidelines or formal training for this common situation. The most commonly used method is the 'push' method. This procedure is performed by asking an assistant wearing sterile gloves to reach into the vagina and 'push' the fetus's head (disimpacting it) up through the vagina as soon as the uterus is opened. Pressure at a single point should be avoided as it is likely to cause fetal trauma and, if possible, the head should be flexed to narrow the diameter and ease delivery. Other methods have been described, such as the 'pull' method (reverse breech extraction), which involves grasping one or both fetal feet at the fundus of the uterus and applying steady traction downwards, delivering the feet first [64, 65]. Although some authors have reported lower risks of fever, urinary tract infection, and extension of the uterine incision after the pull method as compared to after the push method, there is currently insufficient evidence to support the use of any one method. The method chosen should depend on the skill and experience of the surgeon. Various devices such as the Fetal Disimpacting System (Eurosurgical Ltd, Guildford, UK) and/or the C-Snorkel have been described to aid delivery by elevating the head or alleviating the vacuum between the fetal head and the vagina. These devices have theoretical benefits but neither their efficacy nor their safety has been evaluated against the simpler and faster manual push/pull methods.

Multiple repeat caesarean deliveries

An estimated 40% of the 1.3 million caesarean deliveries performed each year in the United States are repeat procedures. Repeat caesarean sections are associated with higher maternal morbidity, and the risk of serious maternal morbidity increases with an increasing number of caesarean deliveries [66–68], mainly because of an increased risk of placenta praevia and/or accreta. The data of a prospective observational cohort of 30,132 women in the United States are summarized in Table 4.2 [64]. The incidence of placenta praevia increased from 10 in 1000 deliveries with 1 previous caesarean delivery to 28 in 1000 deliveries with ≥3 caesarean deliveries [67]. A recent meta-analysis has shown a calculated summary odds ratio of 1.47 for placenta praevia, and 1.96 for placenta accreta after 1 caesarean section [68].

The presence of adhesions during a repeat caesarean section (see Chapter 9) can make fetal extraction lengthy and the procedure challenging and may increase the risk of injury to adjacent organs. Repeated caesarean section increases the risk of uterine rupture and intraoperative complications,

Table 4.2 Relationship between maternal complication risks (%) and caesarean section number

Complications	Risk for 1st caesarean section	% risk for 2nd caesarean section	3rd	4th	5th	≥6th
Placenta accreta	0.24	0.31	0.57	2.13	2.33	6.74
Hysterectomy	0.65	0.42	0.90	2.41	3.49	8.99
Praevia + accreta	3.00	11.00	40	61	67	

including long operating times with excessive blood loss and blood transfusion [69, 70]. The incidence of a single major complication is higher in women with ≥4 caesarean sections [70].

Difficult delivery of the neonate is also more common in women who underwent ≥2 elective caesarean sections [67], but with no increase in the rate of neonatal admission to intensive care. In women with a prior caesarean delivery, when the ToS with an unsuccessful trial of forceps or vacuum results in an emergency caesarean section, the rate of fetal injury is much higher than in the elective repeat caesarean group [61]. However, data on repeat caesarean section are limited, and thus no absolute upper limit for the number of repeat caesarean deliveries can be given.

Caesarean section for placenta praevia (non-accreta)

Rapid accumulation of blood from the placental separation site during caesarean delivery for placenta praevia may obscure the surgical field and quickly leads to major maternal blood loss. Compared to epidural anaesthesia, general anaesthesia increases the estimated blood loss, is associated with a lower post-operative haemoglobin concentration, and increases the need for blood transfusion, [71]. Elective caesarean section deliveries do not differ from emergency caesarean sections in terms of estimated blood loss, the post-operative haemoglobin concentration, or the incidence of intraoperative and anaesthesia complications [71]. In the absence of abnormally invasive placental tissue, blood loss requiring transfusion remains an important cause of maternal morbidity in both anterior and posterior placenta praevia [72].

Specific surgical and additional procedures have been described for caesarean section for placenta praevia. Avoiding incision of the anterior placenta praevia by circumventing the placenta and passing a hand around its margin reduces the frequency of maternal blood transfusions during or after caesarean delivery [73]. Insertion of interrupted circular sutures at the placental separation site via the lower segment uterine incision has been shown to lead to a marked decrease in intraoperative bleeding [74].

The vessels are ligated using interrupted 2–3 cm sutures at 1 cm intervals in a circle around the bleeding area on the external (serosa) surface of the uterus. The sutures are placed as deeply as possible in order to reach the endometrium [74]. Similarly, antero-posterior compressive suture of the lower uterine segment has been shown to successfully control the bleeding in caesarean section for placenta praevia [75, 76]. The local injection of vasopressin into the placental implantation site can significantly reduce blood loss without increasing morbidity [77]. Finally, the prophylactic use of a Bakri balloon could be of benefit as an additional medical/surgical measure to control blood loss [78].

Caesarean section and obesity/ high BMI

The World Health Organization classification separates BMI (weight in kilograms/(height in metres)^2) into five categories: underweight, <18.5; normal, 18.5–24.9; overweight, 25.0–29.9; obese, 30.0–39.9; and morbidly obese, ≥40 (see http://www.who.int/mediacentre/factsheets/fs311). Worldwide obesity has nearly doubled since 1980. In 2008, more than 1.4 billion adults ≥20 years old were overweight. Of these, nearly 300 million were women. Not surprisingly, maternal obesity has become a global issue associated with perinatal risks. Overweight is now exceeding underweight in women of childbearing age, in both urban and rural areas of many low-income countries [79]. Obese and morbidly obese women have a higher rate of caesarean section than other women do and pose many surgical, anaesthetic, and logistical challenges [21, 79, 80].

Caesarean section in obese patients is associated with an increased risk for blood transfusion, and low one-minute Apgar scores [81]. Composite neonatal morbidity rises with increasing BMI from 23.0% for <30.0 kg/m^2 to 29.8% and 32.1% for 40.0–49.9 kg/m^2 and ≥50.0 kg/m^2, respectively [82]. This observation can be explained by the fact that increasing maternal BMI is related to increased incision-to-delivery interval and total operative time at caesarean delivery [82, 83]. Morbidly obese BMI exposes women to the highest risk of prolonged incision-to-delivery interval [82, 83]. Obese patients are more likely to have a caesarean delivery after labour and to have a vertical skin incision [84], and morbidly obese women have a twofold to fourfold increase in post-operative complications, including primary infectious outcome (18.8%; adjusted odds ratio, 2.7) and wound infection (18.8%; adjusted odds ratio, 3.4). Vertical skin incision is associated with a higher rate of wound complications than a transverse incision is in obese women [85] but not in morbidly obese women [86]. Overall, low transverse skin incisions and transverse uterine incisions should be the first option in obese women but there are currently insufficient data to support the utilization of transverse versus vertical skin incision depending on the level of obesity. Closure of the subcutaneous layer is recommended [1, 21] but the placement of subcutaneous drains remains controversial. Thromboprophylaxis adjusted to body weight, as well as prophylactic antibiotics, help in reducing post partum morbidity [21].

Obese women are also at higher risk of secondary deep or superficial wound infection [84]. The use of negative pressure wound therapy (NPWT), a closed, sealed system that applies negative pressure (suction) to the wound surface has been advocated in these cases. However, there are currently no suitably powered, high-quality trials to evaluate the effects of the newer NPWT products to justify their use for patient with a low risk of postcaesarean delivery surgical site infections [87].

Some of the situations described in this section and frequent intraoperative complications are presented in Module 5 of the caesarean section series produced by Medical Aid Films. To access this module please visit http://medicalaidfilms.org/our-films/obstetric-care/. Please note that in order to request permission to view this video you will be required to contact info@medicalaidfilms.org.

Key learning points

1. Parenteral antibiotic given 30–60 minutes before the skin incision reduces the risk of maternal infection by half, with no significant effect on neonatal sepsis or admission to intensive care unit.
2. Skin preparation with 0.5% chlorhexidine in methylated spirits is associated with lower rates of site infection than alcohol-based povidone–iodine paint is.
3. Omission of the bladder flap step at caesarean section reduces the skin incision–delivery interval and is not associated with differences in the risks of bladder injury, total operating time, blood loss, or duration of hospitalization.
4. Oxytocin infusion (10–40 IU in 500–1000 ml crystalloid over 2–8 hours) is the most effective pharmacologic prophylaxis in uterine atony prevention at caesarean delivery.
5. Spontaneous delivery of the placenta at caesarean section is associated with less endometritis, less blood loss, and a shorter duration of hospital stay than manual removal is.
6. Uterine exteriorization is safe and is particularly useful when visualization of the incision is difficult.
7. Single-layer closure of the uterine incision is associated with shorter operative procedure time than double-layer closure in women attempting vaginal birth after caesarean section, and locked (but not unlocked single-layer) closure is associated with a higher risk of uterine rupture.
8. Short-term post-operative outcome is improved when the peritoneum is not closed at caesarean section.
9. Closure of the subcutaneous layer at caesarean section is recommended in all women with a subcutaneous tissue of ≥2 cm.
10. Staples and sutures are associated with similar outcomes in terms of wound infection, pain, and cosmetic effects; however, compared to sutures, staples are associated with an increased incidence of skin separation and the need for re-closure if removed on Day 3, particularly in obese women.

References

1. Dahlke JD, Mendez-Figueroa H, Rouse DJ, Berghella V, Baxter JK, Chauhan SP. Evidence-based surgery for cesarean delivery: An updated systematic review. Am J Obstet Gynecol 2013; 209(4): 294–306.
2. Baskett TF, Calder AA, Arulkumaran S. Munro Kerr's Operative Obstetrics: Centenary Edition. Philadelphia: Elsevier, 2007.
3. Wylie BJ, Gilbert S, Landon MB, Spong CY, Rouse DJ, Leveno KJ, et al. Comparison of transverse and vertical skin incision for emergency cesarean delivery. Obstet Gynecol 2010; 115(6): 1134–40.
4. Pelosi MA, Ortega I. Cesarean section: Pelosi's simplified technique. Rev Chil Obstet Ginecol 1994; 59(5): 372–7.
5. Furau C, Furau G, Dascau V, Ciobanu G, Onel C, Stanescu C. Improvements in cesarean section techniques: Arad's obstetrics department experience on adapting the Vejnovic cesarean section technique. Maedica (Buchar) 2013; 8(3): 256–60.

6. Stark M, Finkel AR Comparison between the Joel-Cohen and Pfannenstiel incisions in cesarean section. Eur J Obstet Gynecol Reprod Biol 1994; 53(2): 121–2.

7. Haesslein HC, Goodlin RC. Extraperitoneal cesarean section revisited. Obstet Gynecol 1980; 55(2): 181–3.

8. Tappauf C, Schest E, Reif P, Lang U, Tamussino K, Schoell W. Extraperitoneal versus transperitoneal cesarean section: A prospective randomized comparison of surgical morbidity. Am J Obstet Gynecol 2013; 209(4): 338.e1–8.

9. Tully L, Gates S, Brocklehurst P, McKenzie-McHarg K, Ayers S. Surgical techniques used during caesarean section operations: Results of a national survey of practice in the UK. Eur J Obstet Gynecol Reprod Biol 2002; 102(2): 120–6.

10. Dandolu V, Raj J, Harmanli O, Lorico A, Chatwani AJ. Resident education regarding technical aspects of cesarean section. J Reprod Med 2006; 51(1): 49–54.

11. Demers S, Roberge S, Afiuni YA, Chaillet N, Girard I, Bujold E. Survey on uterine closure and other techniques for Caesarean section among Quebec's obstetrician-gynaecologists. J Obstet Gynaecol Can 2013; 35(4): 329–33.

12. Tita AT, Rouse DJ, Blackwell S, Saade GR, Spong CY, Andrews WW. Emerging concepts in antibiotic prophylaxis for cesarean delivery: A systematic review. Obstet Gynecol 2009; 113(3): 675–82.

13. Bhattacharjee N, Saha SP, Patra KK, Mitra U, Ghoshroy SC. Optimal timing of prophylactic antibiotic for cesarean delivery: A randomized comparative study. J Obstet Gynaecol Res 2013; 39(12): 1560–8.

14. Haas DM, Morgan S, Contreras K. Vaginal preparation with antiseptic solution before cesarean section for preventing postoperative infections. Cochrane Database Syst Rev 2014; 12: CD007892.

15. Hadiati DR, Hakimi M, Nurdiati DS. Skin preparation for preventing infection following caesarean section. Cochrane Database Syst Rev 2012; 9: CD007462.

16. Dumville JC, McFarlane E, Edwards P, Lipp A, Holmes A, Liu Z. Preoperative skin antiseptics for preventing surgical wound infections after clean surgery. Cochrane Database Syst Rev 2015; 4: CD003949.

17. Maiwald M, Chan ES. The forgotten role of alcohol: A systematic review and meta-analysis of the clinical efficacy and perceived role of chlorhexidine in skin antisepsis. PLoS One 2012; 7(9): e44277.

18. O'Neill HA, Egan G, Walsh CA, Cotter AM, Walsh SR. Omission of the bladder flap at caesarean section reduces delivery time without increased morbidity: A meta-analysis of randomised controlled trials. Eur J Obstet Gynecol Reprod Biol 2014; 174: 20–6.

19. Anorlu RI, Maholwana B, Hofmeyr GJ. Methods of delivering the placenta at caesarean section. Cochrane Database Syst Rev 2008; 6: CD004737.

20. Hofmeyr GJ, Abdel-Aleem H, Abdel-Aleem MA. Uterine massage for preventing postpartum haemorrhage. Cochrane Database Syst Rev 2013; 7: CD006431.

21. Machado LS. Cesarean section in morbidly obese parturients: Practical implications and complications. N Am J Med Sci 2012; 4(1): 13–18.

22. Mackeen AD, Berghella V, Larsen ML. Techniques and materials for skin closure in caesarean section. Cochrane Database Syst Rev 2012; 11: CD003577.

23. Jacobs-Jokhan D, Hofmeyr G. Extra-abdominal versus intra-abdominal repair of the uterine incision at caesarean section. Cochrane Database Syst Rev 2004; 18: CD000085.

24. Nafisi S. Influence of uterine exteriorization versus in situ repair on post-Cesarean maternal pain: a randomized trial. Int J Obstet Anesth 2007; 16(2): 135–8.

25. Coutinho IC, Ramos de Amorim MM, Katz L, Bandeira de Ferraz AA. Uterine exteriorization compared with in situ repair at cesarean delivery: A randomized controlled trial. Obstet Gynecol 2008; 111(3): 639–47.

26. Gode F, Okyay RE, Saatli B, Ertugrul C, Guclu S, Altunyurt S. Comparison of uterine exteriorization and in situ repair during cesarean sections. Arch Gynecol Obstet 2012; 285(6): 1541–5.

27. Dodd JM, Anderson ER, Gates S. Surgical techniques for uterine incision and uterine closure at the time of caesarean section. Cochrane Database Syst Rev 2008; 16: CD004732.

28. The CORONIS Collaborative Group. Caesarean section surgical techniques (CORONIS): A fractional, factorial, unmasked, randomised controlled trial. Lancet 2013; 382(9888): 234–48.

29. The CAESAR Study Collaborative Group. Caesarean section surgical techniques: A randomised factorial trial (CAESAR). BJOG 2010; 117(11): 1366–76.

30. Bamigboye AA, Hofmeyr GJ. Closure versus non-closure of the peritoneum at caesarean section. Cochrane Database Syst Rev 2003; 4: CD000163.

31. Bujold E, Goyet M, Marcoux S, Brassard N, Cormier B, Hamilton E, et al. The role of uterine closure in the risk of uterine rupture. Obstet Gynecol 2010; 116(1): 43–50.

32. Roberge S, Chaillet N, Boutin A, Moore L, Jastrow N, Brassard N, et al. Single- versus double-layer closure of the hysterotomy incision during cesarean delivery and risk of uterine rupture. Int J Gynaecol Obstet 2011; 115(1): 5–10.

33. Chiu TL, Sadler L, Wise MR. Placenta praevia after prior caesarean section: An exploratory case-control study. Aust N Z J Obstet Gynaecol 2013; 53(5): 455–8.

34. Gurusamy KS, Cassar Delia E, Davidson BR. Peritoneal closure versus no peritoneal closure for patients undergoing non-obstetric abdominal operations. Cochrane Database Syst Rev 2013; 7: CD010424.

35. Lyell DJ. Adhesions and perioperative complications of repeat cesarean delivery. Am J Obstet Gynecol 2011; 205(6 Suppl): S11–18.

36. Kapustian V, Anteby EY, Gdalevich M, Shenhav S, Lavie O, Gemer O. Effect of closure versus nonclosure of peritoneum at cesarean section on adhesions: A prospective randomized study. Am J Obstet Gynecol 2012; 206(1): 56.e1–4.

37. Blumenfeld YJ, Caughey AB, El-Sayed YY, Daniels K, Lyell DJ. Single- versus double-layer hysterotomy closure at primary caesarean delivery and bladder adhesions. BJOG 2010; 117(6): 690–4.

38. Bates GW, Shomento S. Adhesion prevention in patients with multiple cesarean deliveries. Am J Obstet Gynecol 2011; 205(6): S19–24.

39. Albright CM, Rouse DJ. Adhesion barriers at cesarean delivery: Advertising compared with the evidence. Obstet Gynecol 2011; 118(1): 157–60.

40. Edwards RK, Ingersoll M, Gerkin RD, Bodea-Braescu AV, Lin MG. Carboxymethylcellulose adhesion barrier placement of primary cesarean delivery and outcomes at repeat cesarean delivery. Obstet Gynecol 2014; 123(5): 923–8.

41. Gaspar-Oishi M, Aeby T. Cesarean delivery times and adhesion severity associated with prior placement of a sodium hyaluronate-carboxycellulose barrier. Obstet Gynecol 2014; 124(4): 679–83.

42. Walfisch A, Beloosesky R, Shrim A, Hallak M. Adhesion prevention after cesarean delivery: Evidence, and lack of it. Am J Obstet Gynecol 2014; 211(5): 446–52.

43. Gurusamy KS, Toon CD, Davidson BR. Subcutaneous closure versus no subcutaneous closure after non-caesarean surgical procedures. Cochrane Database Syst Rev 2014; 2: CD010425.

44. Gurusamy KS, Toon CD, Allen VB, Davidson BR. Continuous versus interrupted skin sutures for non-obstetric surgery. Cochrane Database Syst Rev 2014; 2: CD010365.

45. Huppelschoten AG, van Ginderen JC, van den Broek KC, Bouwma AE, Oosterbaan HP. Different ways of subcutaneous tissue and skin closure at cesarean section: A randomized clinical trial on the long-term cosmetic outcome. Acta Obstet Gynecol Scand 2013; 92(8): 916–24.

46. Aabakke AJ, Krebs L, Pipper CB, Secher NJ. Subcuticular suture compared with staples for skin closure after cesarean delivery: A randomized controlled trial. Obstet Gynecol 2013; 122(4): 878–84.

47. Mackeen AD, Khalifeh A, Fleisher J, Vogell A, Han C, Sendecki, J, et al. Suture compared with staple skin closure after cesarean delivery. Obstet Gynecol 2014; 123(6): 1169–75.

48. Abdel-Aleem H, Aboelnasr MF, Jayousi TM, Habib FA. Indwelling bladder catheterisation as part of intraoperative and postoperative care for caesarean section. Cochrane Database Syst Rev 2014; 4: CD010322.

49. El-Mazny A, El-Sharkawy M, Hassan A. A prospective randomized clinical trial comparing immediate versus delayed removal of urinary catheter following elective cesarean section. Eur J Obstet Gynecol Reprod Biol 2014; 181: 111–14.

50. McAdams RM. Time to implement delayed cord clamping. Obstet Gynecol 2014; 123(3): 549–52.

51. Rabe H, Diaz-Rossello JL, Duley L, Dowswell T. Effect of timing of umbilical cord clamping and other strategies to influence placental transfusion at preterm birth on maternal and infant outcomes. Cochrane Database Syst Rev 2012; 8: CD003248.

52. Backes CH, Rivera BK, Haque U, Bridge JA, Smith CV, Hutchon DJ, et al. Placental transfusion strategies in very preterm neonates: A systematic review and meta-analysis. Obstet Gynecol 2014; 124(1): 47–56.

53. McDonald SJ, Middleton P, Dowswell T, Morris PS. Effect of timing of umbilical cord clamping of term infants on maternal and neonatal outcomes. Cochrane Database Syst Rev 2013; 7: CD004074.

54. Pivetti V, Cavigioli F, Lista G, Napolitano M, Rustico M, Paganelli A, et al. Cesarean section plus delayed cord clamping approach in the perinatal management of congenital high airway obstruction syndrome (CHAOS): A case report. J Neonatal Perinatal Med 2014; 7(3): 237–9.

55. McDonnell M, Henderson-Smart DJ. Delayed umbilical cord clamping in preterm infants: A feasibility study. J Paediatr Child Health 1997; 33(4): 308–10.

56. Levin I, Rapaport AS, Salzer L, Maslovitz S, Lessing JB, Almog B. Risk factors for relaparotomy after cesarean delivery. Int J Gynaecol Obstet 2012; 119(2): 163–5.

57. Kessous R, Danor D, Weintraub YA, Wiznitzer A, Sergienko R, Ohel I, et al. Risk factors for relaparotomy after cesarean section. J Matern Fetal Neonatal Med 2012; 25(11): 2167–70.

58. Fitzwater JL, Owen J, Ankumah NA, Campbell SB, Biggio JR, Szychowski JM, Edwards RK. Nulliparous Women in the Second Stage of Labor: Changes in Delivery Outcomes Between Two Cohorts From 2000 and 2011. Obstet Gynecol. 2015; 126(1): 81–6.

59. Levine LD, Sammel MD, Hirshberg A, Elovitz MA, Srinivas SK. Does stage of labor at time of cesarean delivery affect risk of subsequent preterm birth? Am J Obstet Gynecol. 2015; 212: 360.e1–7.

60. Alexander JM, Leveno KJ, Rouse DJ, Landon MB, Gilbert S, Spong CY, et al. Comparison of maternal and infant outcomes from primary cesarean delivery during the second compared with first stage of labor. Obstet Gynecol 2007; 109(4): 917–21.

61. Lurie S, Raz N, Boaz M, Sadan O, Golan A. Comparison of maternal outcomes from primary cesarean section

during the second compared with first stage of labor by indication for the operation. Eur J Obstet Gynecol Reprod Biol 2014; 182: 43–7.

62. Giugale LE, Sakamoto S, Dunn S, Krans EE. Risk factors for inadvertent extension of the hysterotomy during cesarean delivery. Obstet Gynecol 2014; 123 (Suppl 1): 146S–7S.

63. Alexander JM, Leveno KJ, Hauth J, Landon MB, Thom E, Spong CY, et al. Fetal injury associated with cesarean delivery. Obstet Gynecol 2006; 108(4): 885–90.

64. Chopra S, Bagga R, Keepanasseril A, Jain V, Kalra J, Suri V. Disengagement of the deeply engaged fetal head during cesarean section in advanced labor: Conventional method versus reverse breech extraction. Acta Obstet Gynecol Scand 2009; 88(10): 1163–6.

65. Bastani P, Pourabolghasem S, Abbasalizadeh F, Motvalli L. Comparison of neonatal and maternal outcomes associated with head-pushing and head-pulling methods for impacted fetal head extraction during cesarean delivery. Int J Gynaecol Obstet 2012; 118(1): 1–3.

66. Silver RM, Landon MB, Rouse DJ, Leveno KJ, Spong CY, Thom EA, et al. Maternal morbidity associated with multiple repeat cesarean deliveries. Obstet Gynecol 2006; 107(6): 1226–32.

67. Marshall NE, Fu R, Guise JM. Impact of multiple cesarean deliveries on maternal morbidity: a systematic review. Am J Obstet Gynecol 2011; 205(3): 262.e1–8.

68. Klar M, Michels KB. Cesarean section and placental disorders in subsequent pregnancies: A meta-analysis. J Perinat Med 2014; 42(5): 571–83.

69. Nisenblat V, Barak S, Griness OB, Degani S, Ohel G, Gonen R. Maternal complications associated with multiple cesarean deliveries. Obstet Gynecol 2006; 108(1): 21–6.

70. Gasim T, Al Jama FE, Rahman MS, Rahman J. Multiple repeat cesarean sections: Operative difficulties, maternal complications and outcome. J Reprod Med 2013; 58(7–8): 312–8.

71. Frederiksen MC, Glassenberg R, Stika CS. Placenta previa: A 22-year analysis. Am J Obstet Gynecol 1999; 180(6 Pt 1): 1432–7.

72. Young BC, Nadel A, Kaimal A. Does previa location matter? Surgical morbidity associated with location of a placenta previa. J Perinatol 2014; 34(4): 264–7.

73. Verspyck E, Douysset X, Roman H, Marret S, Marpeau L. Transecting versus avoiding incision of the anterior placenta previa during cesarean delivery. Int J Gynaecol Obstet 2015; 128(1): 44–7.

74. Cho JY, Kim SJ, Cha KY, Kay CW, Kim MI, Cha KS. Interrupted circular suture: Bleeding control during cesarean delivery in placenta previa accreta. Obstet Gynecol 1991; 78(5 Pt 1):876–9.

75. Penotti M, Vercellini P, Bolis G, Fedele L. Compressive suture of the lower uterine segment for the treatment of postpartum hemorrhage due to complete placenta previa: A preliminary study. Gynecol Obstet Invest 2012; 73(4): 314–20.

76. Matsubara S, Kuwata T, Baba Y, Usui R, Suzuki H, Takahashi H, et al. A novel 'uterine sandwich' for haemorrhage at caesarean section for placenta praevia. Aust N Z J Obstet Gynaecol 2014; 54(3): 283–6.

77. Kato S, Tanabe A, Kanki K, Suzuki Y, Sano T, Tanaka K, et al. Local injection of vasopressin reduces the blood loss during cesarean section in placenta previa. J Obstet Gynaecol Res 2014; 40(5): 1249–56.

78. Beckmann MM, Chaplin J. Bakri balloon during cesarean delivery for placenta previa. Int J Gynaecol Obstet 2014; 124(2): 118–22.

79. Okafor UV, Efetie ER, Nwoke O, Okezie O, Umeh U. Anaesthetic and obstetric challenges of morbid obesity in caesarean deliveries: A study in South-eastern Nigeria. Afr Health Sci 2012; 12(1): 54–7.

80. Tonidandel A, Booth J, D'Angelo R, Harris L, Tonidandel S. Anesthetic and obstetric outcomes in morbidly obese parturients: A 20-year follow-up retrospective cohort study. Int J Obstet Anesth 2014; 23(4): 357–64

81. Mourad M, Silverstein M, Bender S, Melka S, Klauser CK, Gupta S, et al. The effect of maternal obesity on outcomes in patients undergoing tertiary or higher cesarean delivery. J Matern Fetal Neonatal Med 2015; 28(9): 989–93.

82. Conner SN, Tuuli MG, Longman RE, Odibo AO, Macones GA, Cahill AG. Impact of obesity on incision-to-delivery interval and neonatal outcomes at cesarean delivery. Am J Obstet Gynecol 2013; 209(4): 386. e1–6.

83. Girsen AI, Osmundson SS, Naqvi M, Garabedian MJ, Lyell DJ. Body mass index and operative times at cesarean delivery. Obstet Gynecol 2014; 124(4): 684–9.

84. Stamilio DM, Scifres CM. Extreme obesity and postcesarean maternal complications. Obstet Gynecol 2014; 124(2 Pt 1): 227–32.

85. Wall PD, Deucy EE, Glantz JC, Pressman EK. Vertical skin incisions and wound complications in the obese parturient. Obstet Gynecol 2003; 102(5 Pt 1): 952–6.

86. Marrs CC, Moussa HN, Sibai BM, Blackwell SC. The relationship between primary cesarean delivery skin incision type and wound complications in women with morbid obesity. Am J Obstet Gynecol 2014; 210(4): 319.e1–4.

87. Echebiri NC, McDoom MM, Aalto MM, Fauntleroy J, Nagappan N, Barnabei VM. Prophylactic use of negative pressure wound therapy after cesarean delivery. Obstet Gynecol. 2015; 125(2): 299–307.

CHAPTER 5
The Misgav Ladach caesarean section

Michael Stark and Eric Jauniaux

Introduction

Over the last 100 years since the modern caesarean section was promoted by John Martin Munro Kerr (1868–1960; see Chapter 1), many variations in the procedure have been introduced. There are scores of different technical variations of the caesarean section, if one includes the many different ways of opening the skin and the rectus sheath, and the ways of opening and closing the uterus, the peritoneum, and the subcutaneous tissue. In addition, for the closure of the different layers, it is possible to use different suture materials, either in a continuous locked or unlocked manner or as interrupted sutures, or staples. The main difference between the modern standard caesarean section and the traditional caesarean section is the more frequent use since the 1970s of the Pfannenstiel lower abdominal incision instead of the vertical incision. The main disadvantages of the vertical midline incision mainly include the greater risk of post-operative wound dehiscence and of incision hernia (see Chapter 4). The vertical scar also is aesthetically less pleasing than that resulting from the Pfannenstiel incision; however, it is interesting to note that vertical midline incision was the preferred technique until the 1970s and is still performed in some countries more than 100 years after Pfannenstiel described his lower abdominal transverse incision.

Major technical changes to the standard caesarean section procedure were proposed in the 1980s and 1990s. One of these major changes, proposed by Sidney Joel-Cohen, was the use of a transverse incision that was higher than the one that had been used for opening the abdomen in abdominal hysterectomy [1, 2]. Like Pfannenstiel, who was a uro-gynaecologist, Joel-Cohen was mainly a gynaecological surgeon and never described a new method to perform a caesarean section. The modified Joel-Cohen incision (JCI) technique to open the abdomen was first evaluated and implemented for routine caesarean section at Misgav Ladach General Hospital in Jerusalem, Israel, at the end of the 1980s [3–5]. In addition to the JCI on the skin, the 'Misgav Ladach caesarean section' also includes variations in which manual manipulation is used instead of sharp instruments and in which less suture material is used, compared to other methods. This chapter reviews the different surgical steps of the Misgav Ladach caesarean section. Short training technical video clips comparing the different steps of the Misgav Ladach caesarean section with those of the standard caesarean section utilizing a Pfannenstiel incision (detailed in Chapter 4) are available as supplements to this book (see ◉ Videos 2 and 3 at www.oxfordmedicine.com/textbookofcaesareansection.).

Abdominal/pelvic entry in the Misgav Ladach caesarean section

The straight horizontal skin incision described by Joel-Cohen is performed three finger-widths (4–5 cm) above the pubic symphysis, 3 cm below the line that joins the anterior superior iliac spines. This skin incision thus is more cephalad than the Pfannenstiel incision (Figure 5.1). The cut is then deepened in the midline to expose the rectus sheath (fascia). The anterior rectus sheath is opened transversely 2–3 cm only in the midline (Figure 5.2A). The rectus sheath incision is extended laterally with the slightly opened tip of round-tip straight scissors (Figure 5.2B). The rectus muscles and subcutaneous tissue are then separated by finger bilateral traction (Figure 5.3). By contrast with the Pfannenstiel incision, in the JCI the facial plate is not freed upwards

and the peritoneum is opened transversally (rather than longitudinally) by repeated bi-digital stretching (Figures 5.4 and 5.5).

The JCI does not require separating the rectus sheath from the muscles and there is no deep incision with the scalpel of the subcutaneous tissue. As the JCI is positioned higher than the Pfannenstiel incision is and includes blunt separation of tissues along natural tissue planes with a minimum of sharp dissection, it is less likely to compromise the main branches of the epigastric arteries than the Pfannenstiel incision is (see Chapter 2). No retractors are used and only a scalpel and straight scissors are used to open the abdomen.

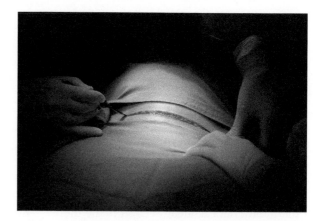

Figure 5.1 General view of the Joel-Cohen incision, showing the straight horizontal skin incision 4–5 cm above the pubic symphysis or 2.5 cm below the line that joins the anterior superior iliac spines.

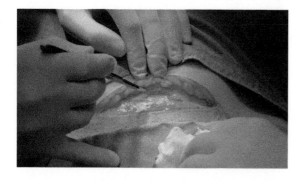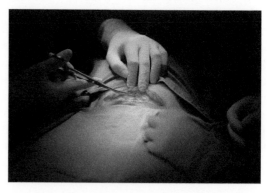

Figure 5.2 A. The cut is then deepened in the midline to expose the rectus sheath, which is then opened transversely only a few centimetres in the midline. B. The rectus sheath incision is extended laterally with the slightly opened tip of round-tip scissors.

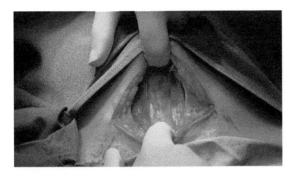

Figure 5.3 Separation of the rectus muscles and subcutaneous tissue by finger bilateral traction.

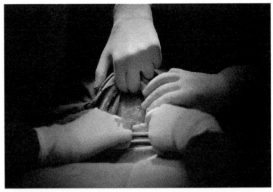

Figure 5.4 Opening the peritoneum transversally (rather than longitudinally) by repeated bi-digital stretching.

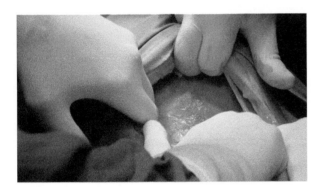

Figure 5.5 Separation of the rectus muscles and subcutaneous tissue by finger bilateral traction.

Opening the uterus during a Misgav Ladach caesarean section, delivery, and closure

The opening of the uterus in the Misgav Ladach caesarean section is similar to that described by Kehrer and Kerr, and the rest of the procedure consists of a number of surgical techniques adopted from various sources [3]. In brief, the uterine incision is performed in the lower segment of the uterus after pushing down the vesico-uterine plica (the peritoneal fold extending from the uterus to the posterior portion of the bladder) to enter directly the uterine cavity in an anatomical level where the uterine wall contains mainly fibrous tissue rather than muscle tissue. Subsequently, the fetus is extracted and the placenta is delivered.

In the Misgav Ladach caesarean section, the uterus is exteriorized in order to facilitate the stitching, enabling manual contraction of the uterus and examination of the ovaries (Figure 5.6). The uterine wall incision is closed with a single-layer continuous locking suture including the decidua and the visceral peritoneum; the parietal peritoneums are not sutured. The fascia is sutured with a continuous suture. The skin is closed with as few as possible mattress silk sutures (Figure 5.7). Between these sutures, the skin edges are approximated with Allis forceps if necessary (Figure 5.8), which are left in place for about 5 minutes.

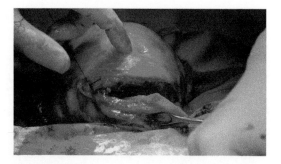

Figure 5.6 The uterus is exteriorized, and the myometrial incision is closed with a single-layer continuous locking suture including the decidua.

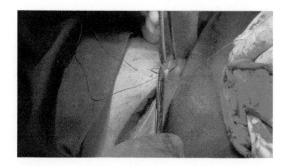

Figure 5.7 The skin is closed with two or three mattress silk sutures.

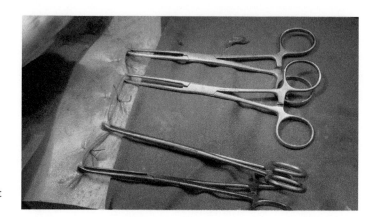

Figure 5.8 The skin edges are approximated with Allis forceps, which are left in place for about 5 minutes while the drapes are being removed.

Further discussion of techniques used in the Misgav Ladach caesarean section

As reported by the first Misgav Ladach General Hospital study in which the JCI and Pfannenstiel skin incision were compared, the main advantages of the JCI method for opening the abdomen are that it is slightly faster than the Pfannenstiel skin incision and that it reduces the risks of post-operative febrile morbidity and pain [3]. The Misgav Ladach caesarean section procedure is faster than the standard caesarean section procedure because of the fact that there are fewer steps to perform than in the standard procedure, and sharp dissection is minimized so that there is less trauma and therefore lower febrile morbidity than with the standard procedure. Estimated intraoperative blood loss was also reported to be less with the Misgav Ladach caesarean section compared with the Pfannenstiel incision but these measurements are notoriously subjective [6]. It is unclear if these advantages are due solely to the JCI on the skin or to the entire Misgav Ladach caesarean section technique. A recent meta-analysis has confirmed these initial findings (Box 5.1) but could only find two randomized controlled trials (RCTs) of intention to perform caesarean section using the different abdominal incisions to include in the review [6].

Another early study from the Misgav Ladach General Hospital [4] showed that adhesions were found in 6.3% of repeat operations after the Misgav

Ladach caesarean section compared with 28.8% after the standard caesarean section. More recent studies have confirmed that caesarean section procedures such as the Misgav Ladach caesarean section but with the modification of not creating a bladder flap and without closure of the visceral and parietal peritoneum reduce inflammatory processes and subsequent intraperitoneal adhesions [7, 8].

Two meta-analyses and two recent RCTs have compared different caesarean section techniques [9–12]. Overall, the meta-analyses found that the Misgav Ladach caesarean section was associated with less blood loss, reduced operating time, reduced time to mobilization, and reduced length of post-operative stay for the mother in the hospital, compared to the traditional caesarean section (Box 5.2). By contrast, the RCTs showed no statistically significant differences between any of the different techniques (e.g. blunt vs sharp entry; exteriorization vs intra-abdominal uterine repair; single-layer vs double-layer uterine closure; closure vs non-closure of the peritoneum) for the incidence of serious adverse events, including haemorrhage and infections [11, 12]. However, as highlighted by

---

Box 5.1 Comparison of the Joel-Cohen incision with the Pfannenstiel incision

The Joel-Cohen incision is associated with:

- Reduced delivery time (mean difference (MD), −1.90; 95% confidence interval (CI), −2.53 to −1.27 minutes);
- Reduced operating time (MD, −11.40; 95% CI, −16.55 to −6.25 minutes);
- Less estimated blood loss (MD, −58.00; 95% CI −108.51 to −7.49 ml);
- Increased time to the first dose of analgesia (MD, 0.80; 95% CI, 0.12 to 1.48 hours);
- Reduced post-operative analgesic requirements (risk ratio (RR), 0.55; 95% CI, 0.40 to 0.76);
- Reduced total dose of analgesia in the first 24 hours (MD, −0.89; 95% CI, −1.19 to −0.59);
- A 65% reduction in post-operative febrile morbidity (RR, 0.35; 95% CI, 0.14 to 0.87);
- Less post-operative hospital stay for the mother (MD, −1.50; 95% CI, −2.16 to −0.84 days).

Modified from Mathai M, Hofmeyr GJ, Mathai NE., Abdominal surgical incisions for caesarean section, 2013, Wiley

---

Box 5.2 Comparison between the Joel-Cohen based caesarean section and the Pfannenstiel caesarean section, and between the Misgav Ladach caesarean section and the traditional lower midline abdominal caesarean section

Compared to the Pfannenstiel caesarean section, the Joel-Cohen based caesarean section is associated with:

- Shorter time from skin incision to birth of the baby (n = 575; weighted mean difference (WMD), −3.84 minutes; 95% confidence interval (CI), −5.41 to −2.27 minutes);
- Shorter operating time (n = 581; WMD, −18.65; 95% CI, −24.84 to −12.45 minutes);
- Less blood loss (n = 481; WMD, −64.45 ml; 95% CI, −91.34 to −37.56 ml);
- Reduced time to oral intake post-operatively (n = 481 women; WMD, −3.92; 95% CI, −7.13 to −0.71 hours);
- Less fever (n = 1412 women; relative risk (RR) 0.47; 95% CI 0.28 to 0.81);
- Shorter duration of post-operative pain (n = 172; WMD, −14.18 hours; 95% CI, −18.31 to −10.04 hours);

- Fewer analgesic injections (n = 151; WMD, −0.92; 95% CI, −1.20 to −0.63).

Compared to the traditional lower midline abdominal caesarean section, the Misgav Ladach caesarean section is associated with:

- Less blood loss (n = 339; WMD, −93.00; 95% CI, −132.72 to −53.28 ml);
- Reduced operating time (n = 339; WMD, −7.30; 95% CI, −8.32 to −6.28 minutes);
- Time to mobilization (n = 339 women; WMD, −16.06; 95% CI, −18.22 to −13.90 hours);
- Length of post-operative stay for the mother (n = 339 women; WMD, −0.82; 95% CI, −1.08 to −0.56 days).

Modified From: Hofmeyr GJ, Mathai M, Shah A, Novikova N, Techniques for caesarean section, 2008, Wiley

the investigators of the CORONIS RCT, surgeons do not always comply with the allocated intervention [12]. Compliance is an important issue when comparing the actual events in a surgical procedure as opposed to a well-defined operation with invariant steps. Furthermore, these trials do not provide information on long-term morbidity and mortality and in particular on the risks of morbidly adherent placenta (see Chapter 9) and scar rupture in trial of labour (see Chapter 11).

Smaller recent RCTs from Nigeria [13] and Turkey [14], comparing the Misgav Ladach caesarean section with the traditional Pfannenstiel method have confirmed that the Misgav Ladach caesarean section is associated with a shorter operating time, less need for suture material, and faster maternal recovery (shorter periods of hospitalization) than the standard caesarean section is. These findings highlight the cost-saving advantage of the Misgav Ladach caesarean section procedure, a feature which is particularly important for poor-resource settings. Similarly, the clinical significance of the reported difference (less than 100 ml) in estimated blood loss may be of greater significance in women suffering from anaemia [9] such as in countries where malaria is endemic. Less fever, pain, and analgesic requirements, less blood loss, and reduced duration of surgery and hospital stay are clinical advantages for all mothers, not only those living in low-income countries. Furthermore, the economic benefits associated with the Misgav Ladach procedure can be extrapolated to savings for the health system in more affluent countries.

Although the time from skin incision to delivery of the baby is shorter with the JCI, it is unclear if the difference in time to delivery is of clinical significance. The CORONIS trial found no evidence of a difference between the JCI and the Pfannenstiel methods with respect to the risk of a low Apgar score or perinatal mortality in planned caesarean section [12]. A recent prospective cohort study has evaluated the feasibility of the Misgav Ladach technique in patients with previous caesarean sections [15]. This study found that the Misgav Ladach technique is possible in over three-fourths of patients with previous caesarean sections, with a slight increase in the incision-to-birth interval as compared with patients without previous caesarean section. In that study, anterior rectus aponeurosis fibrosis and severe peritoneal adherences were the two main indications for which the full Misgav Ladach technique could not be performed.

'Modified' Misgav Ladach procedures also have been in use, including opening the skin at the level of the Pfannenstiel incision for cosmetic reasons [16], closing the uterus with a single-layer non-locking continuous suture [17, 18], not opening the visceral peritoneum and then closing the uterus with two non-locked suture layers [19], closing the skin with subcutaneous suture [20], and various other closure methods [21]. In one RCT [19] involving a small group of women (n = 116) the Misgav Ladach caesarean section was associated with a longer time from skin incision to birth of the baby than a 'modified' Misgav Ladach caesarean section. The trial found no significant differences in operating time, blood loss, time to oral intake, time to return of bowel function, post-operative pain score, or length of post-operative stay of the mother.

Most of the studies concerning the Misgav Ladach caesarean section show the benefits of the procedure as compared to other methods, some in terms of operation time, and others in terms of febrile morbidity or need for painkillers. The reason for the different results is the non-standardization of the operation, as every detail in the operation might result in different outcome. For example, for a right-handed operator, standing on the right side of the patient the extraction of the fetus can be done with the right hand and avoid accidental extension of the uterine scar but this may be more difficult to avoid for a left-hand operator. The use of big needles when closing the uterus might enable using less suture material than small needles would. As the uterus contracts, the suture material cannot contract with it, which could result in a foreign body reaction, perhaps with the outcome of a weaker scar than would be obtained with smaller needles. In addition, the use (or not) of abdominal packs might result in different types of adhesions being formed. Obviously, only standardized methods will enable future comparisons between different surgeons and institutions [22].

Key learning points

1. The Misgav Ladach caesarean section uses the JCI, which is horizontal and performed 2–3 cm higher than the Pfannenstiel incision.

2. In the JCI, the anterior rectus sheath is opened a few centimetres in the midline, the rectus sheath is opened by the round tips of the scissors, and the rectus muscles and subcutaneous tissue are separated by bilateral finger traction.

3. The JCI does not require separating the rectus sheath from the muscles and there is no incision of the subcutaneous tissue.

4. In the Misgav Ladach caesarean section, the uterus is exteriorized, the myometrial incision is closed with a single-layer continuous locking suture, the peritoneum is not sutured, and the skin is closed with a few mattress silk sutures.

5. The Misgav Ladach caesarean section procedure is shorter and results in less post-procedure fever than the traditional Pfannenstiel-based caesarean section does.

6. The Misgav Ladach caesarean section is associated with less blood loss, reduced operating time, time to mobilization and length of post-operative hospitalization than the traditional caesarean section.

7. The economic benefits associated with the Misgav Ladach procedure can result in savings for health systems in both developed and developing countries.

References

1. Joel-Cohen S. Abdominal and Vaginal Hysterectomy: New Techniques Based on Time and Motion Studies. London: William Heinemann Medical Books, 1972.

2. Joel-Cohen S. Abdominal and Vaginal Hysterectomy. 2nd Ed. Philadelphia: JB Lippincott, 1977.

3. Stark M, Finkel AR. Comparison between the Joel-Cohen and Pfannenstiel incisions in cesarean section. Eur J Obstet Gynecol Reprod Biol 1994; 53(2): 121–2.

4. Stark M, Chavkin Y, Kupfersztain C, Guedj P, Finkel AR. Evaluation of combinations of procedures in cesarean section. Int J Gynaecol Obstet 1995; 48(3): 273–6.

5. Holmgren G, Sjoholm L, Stark M. The Misgav Ladach method for cesarean section, method description. Acta Obstet Gynecol Scand 1999; 78(7): 615–21.

6. Mathai M, Hofmeyr GJ, Mathai NE. Abdominal surgical incisions for caesarean section. Cochrane Database Syst Rev 2013 31; 5: CD004453.

7. Malvasi A, Tinelli A, Farine D, Rahimi S, Cavallotti C, Vergara D, et al. Effects of visceral peritoneal closure on scar formation at cesarean delivery. Int J Gynaecol Obstet 2009; 105(2): 131–5.

8. Malvasi A, Tinelli A, Guido M, Cavallotti C, Dell'Edera D, Zizza A, et al. Effect of avoiding bladder flap formation in caesarean section on repeat caesarean delivery. Eur J Obstet Gynecol Reprod Biol 2011; 159(2): 300–4.

9. Hofmeyr GJ, Mathai M, Shah A, Novikova N. Techniques for caesarean section. Cochrane Database Syst Rev 2008; 23: CD004662.

10. Dodd JM, Anderson ER, Gates S. Surgical techniques for uterine incision and uterine closure at the time of caesarean section. Cochrane Database Syst Rev 2008; 23: CD004732.

11. CAESAR Study Collaborative Group. Caesarean section surgical techniques: A randomised factorial trial (CAESAR). BJOG 2010; 117(11): 1366–76.

12. CORONIS Collaborative Group. Caesarean section surgical techniques (CORONIS): A fractional, factorial, unmasked, randomised controlled trial. Lancet 2013; 382(9888): 234–48.

13. Ezechi O, Ezeobi P, Gab-Okafor C, Edet A, Nwokoro C, Akinlade A. Maternal and fetal effect of Misgav Ladach cesarean section in Nigerian women: A randomized control study. Ann Med Health Sci Res 2013; 3(4): 577–82.

14. Abuelghar WM, El-Bishry G, Emam LH. Caesarean deliveries by Pfannenstiel versus Joel-Cohen incision: A randomised controlled trial. J Turk Ger Gynecol Assoc 2013; 14(4): 194–200.

15. Bolze PA, Massoud M, Gaucherand P, Doret M. What about the Misgav-Ladach surgical technique in patients with previous cesarean sections? Am J Perinatol 2013; 30(3): 197–200.

16. Heimann J, Hitschold T, Muller K, Berle P. Modifizierte Misgav-Ladach-Technik der Sectio caesarea im Vergleich mit einer konventionellen Pfannenstiel-Technik: Eine prospektiv-randomisierte Studie an 240 Patientinnen eines Perinatalzentrums [Randomized trial of the modified Misgav-Ladach and the conventional Pfannenstiel techniques for cesarean section]. Geburtshilfe Frauenheilkd 2000; 60(5): 242–50.

17. Franchi M, Ghezzi F, Balestreri D, Beretta P, Maymon E, Miglierina M, et al. A randomized clinical trial of two surgical techniques for cesarean section. Am J Perinatol 1998; 15(10): 589–94.

18. Franchi M, Ghezzi F, Raio L, Di Naro E, Miglierina M, Agosti M, et al. Joel-Cohen or Pfannenstiel incision at cesarean delivery: Does it make a difference? Acta Obstet Gynecol Scand 2002; 81(11): 1040–6.

19. Li M, Zou L, Zhu J. Study on modification of the Misgav Ladach method for cesarean section. J Tongji Med Uni 2001; 21(1): 75–7.

20. Koettnitz F, Feldkamp E, Werner C. 'Die sanfte Sektio': Eine Variante der Cohen-Methode im Vergleich zum klassischen Pfannenstielschnitt ['The gentle

caesarean': A variant of the Cohen method compared to the classical Pfannenstiel]. Zentralbl Gynakol 1999; 121(6): 287–9.

21. Xavier P, Ayres-De-Campos D, Reynolds A, Guimaraes M, Costa-Santos C, Patricio B. The modified Misgav-Ladach versus the Pfannenstiel–Kerr technique for cesarean section: A randomized trial. Acta Obstet Gynecol Scand 2005; 84(9): 878–82.

22. Stark M. Optimised meta-analysis should be based on standardised methods. BJOG 2011; 118(6): 765–6.

CHAPTER 6
Complex caesarean deliveries

Susan P. Raine and Michael A. Belfort

Introduction

Caesarean section, in principle, is not a complex surgical procedure when compared to many others performed in our specialty. It does, however, involve a complex set of physiologic and anatomical circumstances that need to interact perfectly to achieve an optimal outcome. Surgical technique is one factor but is often not the primary determinant of successful outcome. In a setting where concomitant cofactors such as obstructed labour, abruptio placentae, morbid placental invasion, prior pelvic infection, chorioamnionitis/endometritis, severe chronic anaemia, inadequate or unprepared blood transfusion capability, oxytocics, anaesthetics, lack of (or failure to properly administer) antibiotics, and lack of trained or motivated personnel, less than optimal outcome is always a possibility, even when perfect surgical technique is achieved.

As the number of caesarean deliveries around the world continues to grow, it is likely that more and more challenging caesarean deliveries will become the norm rather than the exception. This fact makes it imperative that obstetric care providers receive initial and ongoing training in the recognition of scenarios leading to increased risk and that those entrusted with the surgery in such cases have special training and experience in the management of the complications frequently associated with caesarean delivery. This imperative may well entail a revision of our policies and procedures and lead to the establishment of centres of excellence and the development of appropriate guidelines for the referral of cases at risk for complications to such centres, where all of the necessary resources would exist.

Given that the authors of this chapter have worked in both well-resourced and low-resourced settings, the experience from which this chapter derives covers both arenas. The goal of this chapter is to highlight areas of risk, in general, and to suggest ways in which these may be mitigated in both settings.

Caesarean section in well-resourced settings

Risks of caesarean section at complete dilatation with absolute dystocia

The dangers of caesarean section at full dilatation appear to be less pronounced when there is availability of immediate (or at least urgent) access to an operating room and the necessary support services to perform the surgery. While risks are somewhat mitigated, there are still complications that should be anticipated even in the best of circumstances when prolonged labour precedes caesarean delivery.

A large retrospective cohort study performed in Nova Scotia [1] studied 55,273 deliveries, of which 549 were caesarean deliveries performed at full dilation. The authors found that, compared with women who underwent caesarean delivery during the first stage of labour, those undergoing caesarean delivery at full dilation were more likely to experience intraoperative trauma (odds ratio (OR), 2.57; 95% confidence interval (CI), 1.71–3.88) and perinatal asphyxia (OR, 1.5; 95% CI, 1.06–2.14). These data confirm that, even in well-resourced hospitals, maternal and neonatal outcomes can be adversely affected by prolonged labour leading to caesarean section at full dilatation. Another study examined 627 nulliparous women with singleton pregnancies and who underwent emergency caesarean delivery in the United Kingdom; of these, 199 (18.9%) underwent caesarean delivery at full dilation [2]. The women who underwent caesarean delivery at full dilation were more likely to have an intraoperative complication (OR, 4.6; 95% CI, 2.7–7.9) and a blood transfusion (OR, 2.9; 95% CI, 1.5–5.6) than women who underwent caesarean delivery during the first stage of labour. However, there were no differences between the two groups in terms of readmission rates, hospital stays longer than 5 days, or perinatal morbidity. Another small and retrospective study conducted in Singapore on 110 emergency caesarean deliveries performed at full dilation showed no statistically significant adverse maternal or fetal outcomes [3].

It is not infrequent that the bladder may be incised or torn during a caesarean section for severe obstruction of labour. In most cases, once recognized, the bladder can be repaired in the usual fashion with a two-layer closure. Obviously, should the ureters or the trigone be damaged, urology consultation should be requested if available. If it is unavailable, the patient should be immediately referred to a centre where it can be obtained. In the event of a bladder injury and repair, an indwelling bladder catheter is recommended for at least 7–10 days.

Uterine rupture

Uterine rupture during labour has dramatic consequences for both the mother and the fetus. Once the uterus ruptures, the fetus is often spilled into the abdominal cavity, and this situation is almost always accompanied by some degree of placental abruption. As opposed to uterine scar dehiscence, in a true rupture of the uterus, with fetal extrusion, the chances of fetal survival are low unless rapid intervention is accomplished. If the patient is receiving care in a tertiary referral hospital, early identification (frequently based on fetal heart-rate abnormality before other signs [4]), and delivery within 18 minutes of the identified rupture [5] by laparotomy can prevent fetal death and promote intact neurologic survival. The risks of hypoxic ischaemic encephalopathy and perinatal death with ruptured uterus are on the order of 6.8% (1.8%–10.6%) and 1.8% (0.0%–4.2%) respectively [6, 7]. Women who opt to undergo a trial of vaginal delivery after caesarean section must be counselled as to the risk of uterine rupture during labour (see Chapter 11). For women with a previous Pfannenstiel incision, this risk is generally agreed to be about 1% and increases to between 4% and 9% for those with a classical scar [8]. Rarely, uterine rupture does occur in women who have never had full-thickness uterine surgery; however, this condition is most often seen in a low-resource setting after prolonged obstructed labour and augmented contractions [9].

Morbid obesity

Obesity, in and of itself, is a risk factor for caesarean delivery and, given the current epidemic of obesity (Figure 6.1) it is not surprising that obstetric care providers are increasingly called upon to perform caesarean deliveries for women who fall into one of the three categories of obesity (BMI ≥30) [10, 11] (see Table 6.1). Results of a secondary analysis of data from the FASTER trial indicate caesarean delivery is more common in obese and morbidly obese individuals when compared with controls (20.7% vs 33.8% vs 47.4%, respectively) [12]. Caesarean delivery in morbidly obese individuals carries increased risk based on a number of factors, including but not limited to, increased technical difficulty with the procedure, poor wound healing, and the raised potential for venous thromboembolism [13]. Not only are there maternal factors that may increase the chance of caesarean section,

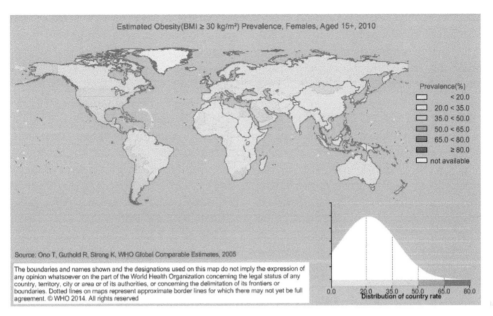

Figure 6.1 Estimated obesity (BMI ≥ 30 kg/m²) Prevalence, Females, Aged 15+, 2010.
Reprinted from Ono T, Guthold R, Strong K, WHO global estimates, Copyright (2005).

Table 6.1 International classification of adult underweight, overweight, and obesity according to BMI

Classification	BMI(kg/m²)	
	Principal cut-off points	**Additional cut-off points**
Underweight	**<18.50**	**<18.50**
Severe thinness	<16.00	<16.00
Moderate thinness	16.00–16.99	16.00–16.99
Mild thinness	17.00–18.49	17.00–18.49
Normal range	**18.50–24.99**	**18.50–22.99** **23.00–24.99**
Overweight	**≥25.00**	**≥25.00**
Pre-obese	25.00–29.99	25.00–27.49 27.50–29.99
Obese	**≥30.00**	**≥30.00**
Obese class I	30.00–34.99	30.00–32.49 32.50–34.99
Obese class II	35.00–39.99	35.00–37.49 37.50–39.99
Obese class III	≥40.00	≥40.00

Source: Reprinted from WHO, Obesity, Copyright (2004).

but fetal factors may also result in such a delivery. Given the difficulty of adequately monitoring the fetal heart rate in some obese patients coupled with the potential for labour dystocia, many practitioners are forced into performing these complicated deliveries pre-emptively.

At the time of the surgery, the surgeon must determine the type of skin incision for the patient in order to best effect delivery of the fetus and at the same time allow for optimal wound healing (Figure 6.2). Unlike a midline vertical incision, a Pfannenstiel or Joel-Cohen incision is performed under reduced tension and is not likely to become disrupted by factors that increase intra-abdominal pressure, such as a chronic cough (see Chapters 4 and 5). In a morbidly obese woman with a large abdominal panniculus adiposus that must be lifted to create a Pfannenstiel or Joel-Cohen incision, wound healing may be compromised because of a continuous presence of moisture in the area. In some cases, the panniculus may not be mobile or the anatomy of the abdomen may be altered. In these circumstances, it may be preferable to create a supra-umbilical incision located directly over the anterior and fundal portion of the uterus such that it would be possible to remove the fetus from a classical uterine incision. This approach may be best reserved for a woman also receiving a tubal ligation or, at the very least, not planning additional pregnancies due to the risk of uterine rupture in a subsequent pregnancy.

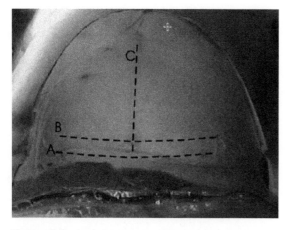

Figure 6.2 Incision types. A. Pfannensteil incision B. Joel-Cohen incision C. Vertical midline incision

Regardless of the type of incision that is ultimately chosen, current recommendations support a subcutaneous suture to prevent seroma formation and wound disruption when there is greater than 2 cm of subcutaneous fat present [14]. Furthermore, if the incision is subjected to a great deal of moisture because of the presence of skin folds, it is wise to leave a dressing in place covering the healing skin until such time that the risk for wound disruption and/or seroma formation has passed. There is no evidence that subcutaneous drain placement is effective in the prevention of post-operative morbidity (see Chapter 4).

Additional special considerations must be taken into account when performing caesarean deliveries on morbidly obese individuals. One pragmatic, and often ignored but important step, is to make sure that the operating theatre table can hold the patient's weight, especially if the patient is tilted or placed in a Trendelenberg position. Once the patient is lying in a supine position, she may experience shortness of breath, a sensation that may or may not be relieved with the insertion of a wedge to hold the patient in a left lateral tilt position relieving the pressure of the uterus on the inferior vena cava. Usually, raising the head of the bed 15°–20° is sufficient to relieve the shortness of breath sensation. Obesity affects anaesthesia choices, and it may not be possible to obtain adequate spinal or epidural analgesia because of an inadequate length of the spinal needle, an inability to ascertain the anatomic landmarks, or an uneven distribution of medication. If regional anaesthesia is ineffective or impossible, the patient must undergo general anaesthesia, which carries its own risks, including aspiration and transplacental transfer of medication to the fetus (see Chapter 7). Venous thromboembolism prophylaxis must be provided to morbidly obese women; both mechanical and pharmaceutical prophylaxis should be considered based on existing recommendations and hospital protocols. Finally, care should be taken in appropriate antibiotic dosing for morbidly obese women.

Uterine leiomyomas

Estimates of uterine leiomyomas or fibroids in pregnancy range from 0.1%–3.9% [15, 16]. Uterine leiomyomas have been implicated in a number of pregnancy complications, including recurrent abortion, preterm labour, preterm delivery, premature rupture of membranes (PROM), and malpresentation. In addition, large uterine leiomyomas are at risk for degeneration during pregnancy with the accompanying inflammation and pain that accompany the degenerative process. In a study of the hospital records of 2065 women with a diagnosis of uterine leiomyoma and who delivered between 1987 and 1993 in the US state of Washington, the prevalence of diagnosed uterine leiomyoma was 0.37% [15]. The study showed that women with uterine leiomyomas were more likely than women without uterine leiomyomas to experience pregnancy complications, including first-trimester bleeding, placental abruption, and PROM (OR, 1.87; 95% CI, 1.59–2.20). Women with uterine leiomyomas were also more likely to experience labour and delivery complications such as

dysfunctional or prolonged labour, breech presentation, and caesarean delivery (OR, 1.90; 95% CI, 1.65–2.18). Even after controlling for other indications for caesarean delivery, women with uterine leiomyomas were more likely to require caesarean delivery than women without uterine leiomyomas (OR, 7.59; 95% CI, 5.47–10.53). When medical indications for caesarean delivery were also present, women with uterine leiomyomas were still much more likely to require caesarean delivery than women without uterine leiomyomas (OR, 5.26; 95% CI, 3.98–6.95).

A systematic review looking at the impact of uterine leiomyomas across the reproductive spectrum from conception through delivery has shown that, depending on the number and location of the fibroids, caesarean delivery can be difficult [16] (see Table 6.2). Several factors must be taken into account when determining how best to enable delivery of the fetus. Women with single,

Table 6.2 Cumulative obstetric outcomes from included studies

	Fibroids	No fibroids	*P* value	Unadjusted OR (95% CI)
Cesarean	48.8% (2098/4322)	13.3% (22,989/173,052)	<0.001	3.7 (3.5–3.9)
Malpresentation	13.0% (466/3585)	4.5% (5864/130,932)	<0.001	2.9 (2.6–3.2)
Labor dystocia	7.5% (260/3471)	3.1% (4703/148,778)	<0.001	2.4 (2.1–2.7)
Postpartum hemorrhage	2.5% (87/3535)	1.4% (2130/153,631)	<0.001	1.8 (1.4–2.2)
Peripartum hysterectomy	3.3% (18/554)	0.2% (27/18,000)	<0.001	13.4 (9.3–19.3)
Retained placenta	1.4% (15/1069)	0.6% (839/134,685)	0.001	2.3 (1.3–3.7)
Chorio or endometritis	8.7% (78/893)	8.2% (2149/26,090)	0.63	1.06 (0.8–1.3)
IUGR	11.2% (112/961)	8.6% (3575/41,630)	<0.001	1.4 (1.1–1.7)
Preterm labor	16.1% (116/721)	8.7% (1577/18,187)	<0.001	1.9 (1.5–2.3)
Preterm delivery	16.0% (183/1145)	10.8% (3433/31,770)	<0.001	1.5 (1.3–1.7)
Placenta previa	1.4% (50/3608)	0.6% (924/154,334)	<0.001	2.3 (1.7–3.1)
First-trimester bleeding	4.7% (120/2550)	7.6% (1193/15,732)	<0.001	0.6 (0.5–0.7)
Abruption	3.0% (115/4159)	0.9% (517/60,474)	<0.001	3.2 (2.6–4.0)
PPROM	9.9% (123/1247)	13.0% (7319/56,418)	0.003	0.8 (0.6–0.9)
PPROM or PROM	6.2% (217/3512)	12.2% (7425/60,661)	<0.001	0.5 (0.4–0.6)

CI, confidence interval; *IUGR*, intrauterine growth rate; *OR*, odds ratio; *PPROM*, preterm premature rupture of membranes; *PROM*, premature rupture of membranes.

Reprinted from Am J Obstet Gynecol, 193/, Klatsky PC, Tran ND, Caughey AB, Fujimoto VY., Fibroids and reproductive outcomes: a systematic literature review from conception to delivery, 357–66, Copyright (2008) with permission from Elsevier.

large solitary fibroids may need to undergo primary caesarean delivery if the fetal head is unable to move past the myoma and into the pelvis. In that instance, the uterine myoma may also involve a significant portion of the lower uterine segment, thus making entry via a low transverse incision difficult or impossible. In this instance, a classical incision may be the only option to safely effect delivery of the fetus.

The safety of myomectomy at the time of caesarean delivery has long been debated because of concerns about the possibility of uncontrolled haemorrhage upon the removal of uterine leiomyomas in the presence of the increased vascularity of pregnancy [17]. A retrospective case-control study of 120 women who had uterine leiomyomas present during delivery included 40 women who underwent myomectomy at the time of caesarean delivery, and 80 controls who underwent caesarean section without myomectomy [16]. The authors defined excessive operative blood loss either as a drop in haematocrit of 10 points or more from the preoperative value, or as the need for intraoperative transfusion. Surgical technique was described as follows: 'a linear incision was made over the myoma and electro-cautery was used to remove the myomas with minimal blood loss. Myometrial closure was accomplished in one or two layers using interrupted absorbable sutures (1–0 caliber vicryl). The serosa is sutured using a continuous absorbable suture (2–0 or 3–0 caliber vicryl).' Women who underwent myomectomy at the time of caesarean delivery had statistically significantly larger uterine leiomyomas than did women who did not receive a myomectomy (8.1 ± 4.7 cm vs 5.7 ± 2.7 cm, $P \leq 0.05$). There were no statistically significant differences in the rate of haemorrhage (12.5% vs 11.3%) or post-operative fever (defined as a temperature ≥38.0°C; 7.5% vs 10%). Patients with myomectomy did have longer operations (53.3 ± 18.6 minutes vs 44.4 ± 6.7 minutes, $P < 0.05$) and longer length of hospital stay (3.3 ± 0.8 days vs 2.7 ± 0.6 days, $P < 0.05$) than those who did not undergo myomectomy.

A large teaching hospital in China adopted a policy of routine myomectomy at the time of caesarean section for women with uterine leiomyomas, and a retrospective study was conducted to evaluate the safety and efficacy of the procedure [18]. A total of 1967 pregnant women also had uterine fibromas. Of these, 1438 underwent caesarean delivery (73.1%); of the women who underwent caesarean delivery, 1242 (86.4%) underwent myomectomy at the time of caesarean section, 51 (5.3%) underwent hysterectomy at the time of caesarean section, and 145 (10.1%) underwent caesarean section only. In addition, the study examined 200 women without uterine leiomyomas who underwent caesarean delivery. Surgical technique was described extensively; no electrocautery was used. Excessive bleeding was defined as either a 10% decrease in haematocrit or the need for intraoperative transfusion. Women who underwent caesarean hysterectomy had the largest mean myoma diameter (8.1 ± 3.9 cm) compared with women who had myomectomy at the time of caesarean section (7.3 ± 4.6 cm) and women who underwent caesarean delivery without myomectomy (3.6 ± 2.1 cm). There were no significant differences between the three groups in terms of length of hospital stay, though the average length of stay in even routine caesarean delivery patients without myomas was quite long (4.9 ± 1.9 days). There were also no significant differences among the groups in the frequency of haemorrhage or incidence of post-operative fever (defined as a temperature ≥38.0°C). The length of surgery was longer in women who had myomectomy at the time of caesarean section (83.6 ± 10.8 minutes) when compared with caesarean delivery in women without uterine leiomyomas (40.2 ± 8.9 minutes) and caesarean delivery in women with uterine leiomyomas (41.9 ± 9.1 minutes).

The cumulative data suggest that, in the appropriately selected patient, myomectomy may be safely performed at the time of caesarean delivery without concerns regarding uncontrolled haemorrhage or post-operative fever. However, the optimal technique to be utilized when myomectomy is performed together with a caesarean delivery remains unclear, as different techniques are described, including the use of tourniquets and electrocautery. Patients should be counselled regarding the increased operative time and length of hospital stay if myomectomy is undertaken.

Pelvic adhesive disease

Adhesion formation is a complex process involving a disruption in the balance between fibrin deposition and fibrin breakdown during the healing process, with adhesions formed primarily during the first post-operative week (see Chapter 9).

Occasionally, the obstetrician is faced with severe pelvic adhesions on attempting to open the abdomen. These adhesions may be the result of prior caesarean delivery, pelvic inflammatory disease, or previous bowel, bladder, or gynaecologic surgery. As a general principle, unless there is immediate fetal compromise, it is best to define the anatomy prior to attempting to perform the caesarean section. In some cases, it is difficult to determine where the scar tissue ends and the abdominal cavity begins. In such situations, there is great risk of transecting underlying bowel and/or bladder. When faced with almost impenetrable scar tissue and adhesions, we advise moving higher and higher in the abdomen in a caudal direction in an attempt to expose unscarred tissue. Once the abdomen is entered and distinct structures can be recognized, a more ordered approach can be undertaken. If the original abdominal entry was through a lower transverse abdominal approach, a widened incision may be required and, in some cases, the rectus muscles may need to be cut. If necessary, an inverted-T incision or a J incision may need to be made to gain access to the upper abdomen, and in some rare cases a separate supra-umbilical incision may be the only way to access the peritoneal cavity. If the adhesions result in a virtually inaccessible anterior lower uterine segment, a fundal or even posterior uterine incision may be necessary to deliver the baby.

The presence of adhesions at caesarean delivery increases with each subsequent surgery and impacts both the time to delivery of the infant, and the overall surgical operative time (see Chapter 9). A recent study showed that, when adhesions were present, delivery times increased from the second to fourth delivery by 18.2, 20.3, and 27.5 minutes, respectively [19]. When adhesions were graded as 'severe', meaning that the words 'severe', 'extensive', or 'dense' were used in the operative report, delivery times increased by 8.4, 12.6, and 21.5

minutes, for the second to fourth caesarean deliveries as compared to the primary delivery. The authors reported decreased umbilical cord pH values in infants delivered by repeat versus primary caesarean delivery as well as decreasing Apgar scores as the number of repeat caesarean deliveries increased. They found no correlation, however, between cord pH values and the number of caesarean deliveries, the indication for caesarean delivery, or the presence of adhesions. While this study was limited by its retrospective nature and reliance on interpretation of operative reports for determination of the presence and severity of adhesions, it does seem to suggest a potential for impact on fetal well-being with increasing numbers of caesarean deliveries. These results are consistent with another retrospective chart review showing that delivery times increase by 3.0, 5.1, and 4.7 minutes, respectively, with increasing number of caesarean deliveries; all these increases were statistically significant [20].

Surgical technique focused on prevention of post-operative adhesions, including closure versus non-closure of the rectus muscles, parietal, and visceral peritoneum has been studied with varying results. Intraperitoneal adhesions and bladder adhesions have been linked to the creation of a bladder flap at the time of hysterotomy; this observation has led authors to conclude that making a bladder flap during caesarean delivery leads to an inflammatory and fibrotic reaction that results in inflammation, reactive and regenerative processes, mesothelial hyperplasia, and submesothelial fibrosis [21]. The same investigators, as well as others, have suggested that closure of the visceral peritoneum at caesarean delivery may produce an inflammatory reaction and adhesions [22, 23]. The balance of evidence thus appears to support not creating a bladder flap and not specifically closing the visceral peritoneum at the time of hysterotomy and uterine closure (see Chapters 4 and 5).

A recent study has suggested that severe striae gravidarum may indicate the presence of underlying intraperitoneal adhesions in women who have had a prior caesarean section [24]. The authors used the Davey striae gravidarum score to quantitate the severity of the striae and found that 50% of women with severe striae and a prior caesarean delivery had intraperitoneal adhesions, versus 9% of women with no striae. Similarly, the relationship between the presence of keloids and adhesion formation among women of different races has been examined [20]. While adhesion formation across races appeared to be comparable, women with keloids in the caesarean delivery scar were found to have increased adhesions between the uterus and anterior abdominal wall.

Abnormal fetal lie/unengaged fetus

Understanding fetal lie, presentation, and head position prior to entry into the abdomen or uterus can save precious minutes at the time of delivery by allowing for a strategic approach to the surgery. Benefits include planning the proper incision, hand positioning that best allows grasping and flexion of the fetal head in the case of a cephalic delivery, or feet in the case of a breech delivery, and ensuring that any additional equipment, such as forceps or a vacuum, are present in the room for quick access.

Unengaged fetal head

When an unengaged or 'floating' fetal head is encountered, it can be difficult to guide the head to a transverse uterine incision, particularly when the fetal head becomes deflexed. In this case, the use of a vacuum or forceps can be particularly useful in delivery of the fetus. It is not always possible to know when there will be a need for forceps or a vacuum in the operating room. If these instruments are not part of the routine caesarean delivery set, it is advisable to have them available in the operating room to avoid a delayed delivery as the instrument is retrieved.

To apply a vacuum at the time of caesarean delivery, the same general principles should be followed as when applying a vacuum at vaginal delivery. Almost any type of forceps can be used at the time of caesarean delivery; however, the long shanks and handles of standard forceps can create an application challenge at the time of caesarean delivery. Thus, it is advisable to obtain forceps with short shanks/handles to use during caesarean deliveries. The technique for application at caesarean delivery is also different than that used at vaginal

delivery. First, the fetal head should be palpated to determine presentation. Once presentation is confirmed, the posterior blade should be guided under the fetal head and held in place by the assistant. The anterior blade may then be placed. Depending on maternal anatomy and the type of forceps available, the blade may be placed directly on the fetal head or may need to be placed posteriorly and guided into position before locking the shanks. It is important to ensure proper placement on the fetal head before locking the shanks or placing any traction on the blades. Finally, the surgical assistant should provide fundal pressure while gentle traction is placed in an upwards direction, guiding the fetus out of the hysterotomy. Providing downwards traction towards the maternal feet may result in extensions of the hysterotomy.

Transverse back down lie

Delivery of a fetus in a transverse back down position is technically challenging and often requires a classical incision. When transverse uterine incisions are attempted for this presentation, more often than not, a J incision or a T incision on the uterus will be required to affect delivery of the infant. Extension of the uterine incision is associated with increased blood loss, broad-ligament haematoma, and uterine artery laceration [25]; thus, preoperative preparation via ultrasonographic evaluation of the fetus when presentation is uncertain is key to a safe delivery.

Perimortem caesarean delivery

The estimated incidence of cardiac arrest in pregnancy in the United States from 1998–2011 was 1 : 12,000 [26]. While this number is quite low, it is higher than the most recent estimated incidence in the United Kingdom of 1 : 20,000 [27]. This increase is potentially attributable to a number of causes, including increased numbers of pregnancies in women with heart disease, women with congenital heart disease surviving to reproductive age, and continued events such as acute haemorrhage, amniotic fluid embolism, and sepsis.

The 2010 International Consensus on Cardiopulmonary Resuscitation and Emergency Cardiovascular Care Science with Treatment Recommendations sought to determine whether any specific interventions improve the outcome of pregnant women with cardiac arrest [28]. During pregnancy at term, the occlusion of the inferior vena cava by the uterus and the fetus is significant, resulting in a stroke volume for the pregnant patient that is 30% that of a non-pregnant woman [28]. Left lateral tilt positioning in pregnant women to prevent aortocaval compression by the gravid uterus has a number of maternal and fetal benefits in non-arrest situations. For the pregnant woman, these benefits include increased blood pressure, cardiac output, and stroke volume. For the fetus, benefits include improved oxygenation and nonstress testing. Taken together, these benefits to mother and fetus suggest that left lateral tilt positioning would also be desirable in cardiac arrest to improve maternal and fetal status during the resuscitation; however, the method chosen to affect left lateral tilt position during chest compressions may be important for maternal survival.

In terms of resuscitation techniques in pregnant women, few clinical trials exist. In a systematic review [27], only two non-physiologic studies utilizing mannequins to test chest compression effectiveness were identified. These studies suggest that, while chest compressions can be delivered in a left lateral tilt position in an attempt to relieve the pressure of the uterus on the inferior vena cava, they are not as effective as those performed in the supine position. In fact, one study demonstrated that, as the angle of tilt increased, the effectiveness of the chest compressions decreased. Considering the importance of effective chest compressions in maintaining perfusion of the critical organs, and the importance of uninterrupted chest compressions, the authors recommend manual displacement of the uterus as a viable alternative to the left lateral tilt position, pointing out that manual displacement is as effective in relieving aortocaval compression during caesarean delivery in non-arrest patients [27] (see Figure 6.3).

For the mother, evacuation of the fetus and the placenta can result in a rapid improvement in haemodynamic status, including return of pulse and blood pressure. Indeed, maternal resuscitation is enhanced by delivery of the fetus, allowing for increased return of blood to the heart from the

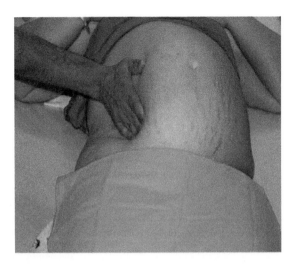

Figure 6.3 Manual leftward uterine displacement with resuscitation team.

Reprinted from Resuscitation, 82/7, Jeejeebhoy F M, Zelop C M, Windrim R, Carvalho J C, Dorian P, Morrison L J., Management of cardiac arrest in pregnancy: a systematic review, 801–9, Copyright (2011) with permission from Elsevier.

inferior vena cava once the obstructing fetus has been removed [28]. Immediate evacuation is of the uterus is even more compelling when faced with a viable fetus, as swift action can make a difference in intact survival. Based on data collected between 1900 and 1985, a viable fetus delivered within 5 minutes of the mother's cardiac arrest is likely to survive with intact neurological status [29]. Infants delivered more than 5 minutes after the onset of arrest are more likely to suffer mild to severe neurologic sequelae, though outcome is improved with increasing gestational age.

A perimortem caesarean section should proceed normally but urgently [29]. No time should be wasted in determination of fetal heart tones, as evacuation of the uterus will provide the best chance for fetal and maternal survival. The patient may or may not be moved to the operating theatre, depending on logistics and time spent in transit. As the procedure will be essentially bloodless with no cardiac output from the mother, surgery can be carried out in almost any location with relative ease. After evacuation of the uterus, as cardiac output returns, so will blood loss; thus, the patient should be closed as per standard procedure, as efficiently as possible. In general, a vertical skin incision is recommended owing to the rapidity with which fetal delivery can be affected; but, ultimately, providers should proceed with whichever type of incision they believe can be performed most rapidly.

Where defibrillation is required, the observation that there was no difference in transthoracic impedance during pregnancy suggests that standard adult energy settings are appropriate [26], although the study was later shown to be underpowered [27].

Management of morbid attachment of the placenta (MAP)

Morbid attachment of the placenta (MAP) takes many forms ranging from small focal areas of attachment that may go unrecognized at the time of delivery, to frank trophoblastic invasion of bladder and/or other structures (see Chapter 9). Complications may, and do, occur at both ends of this spectrum.

Difficult removal of a placenta at the time of caesarean section should always prompt consideration of MAP and preparation for possible ongoing haemorrhage prior to, during, and after hysterotomy closure, a need for blood transfusion, and the development of coagulopathy. Even small focal areas of placenta accreta may weaken uterine integrity and predispose to placental-bed rupture, haemorrhage into the broad ligament, and intramyometrial haematoma development. When focal MAP is recognized at the time of caesarean section, observation of the placental bed and thorough assessment of the uterine wall become very important. In most cases haemostatic sutures will suffice to control the bleeding. If these are not successful, the use of O'Leary-type uterine artery ligation [30] or uterine compression sutures (B-Lynch or some modification thereof) may improve matters (see Chapter 8). Stepwise devascularization may also be useful [31]. Ongoing haemorrhage despite these efforts should force reassessment of the strategy. When clearly life-threatening bleeding persists, the decision for hysterectomy should be taken and appropriate steps taken to initiate protocols for this type of surgery. In such cases, arterial embolization is not an option, given the set-up time required for this procedure, and the risk of delay.

We strongly recommend the development of algorithms of care for post-partum haemorrhage (including time limits and other agreed-upon trigger points) and the institution of regular simulation training to ensure staff readiness and familiarity with the process. Once the decision for emergency hysterectomy is taken, pressure over the bleeding areas can contain the haemorrhage sufficiently to allow resuscitation and preparation (line insertion, arrival of more personnel, receipt of adequate blood products, etc.) for the procedure. In those cases where safe and rapid surgical access to uterine arteries and utero-ovarian blood supply is possible, early clamping or tying (O'Leary-type sutures or progressively higher lateral uterine sutures) of these vessels may decrease blood loss. Until such time as adequate preparations are made however, proceeding with definitive surgery that could increase blood loss should be delayed if the temporizing efforts are allowing stabilization of the patient. Direct uterine compression, B-Lynch stitches [31], direct aortic compression, aortic balloon placement [32], and even aortic cross clamping have all been performed with success in order to allow haemodynamic, coagulation parameter, and electrolyte resuscitation [33].

In those situations where bleeding continues at a persistent, but not catastrophic rate, institution of haemostatic sutures (placental bed, lateral uterine, or compression) followed by inflation of a balloon catheter may control the placental-bed bleeding. This procedure is done after closure of the hysterotomy. Following inflation of the balloon with sterile saline, the hysterotomy closure can be visually inspected and its integrity checked. Attention should be paid to progressive distension of the lower uterine segment (even after contraction of the upper segment or placement of a balloon catheter), as such distension suggests ongoing bleeding and may signal the need for further procedures. In those units where in-operating-room arterial embolization is possible and the patient is haemodynamically stable, selective arterial embolization is often very effective in controlling bleeding. In those units where in-operating-room arterial embolization is not possible, we recommend proceeding with hysterectomy rather than transporting a patient with ongoing bleeding to a radiology suite where rapid hysterectomy cannot be performed in the event of need.

In some cases, focal MAP will only be recognized once most of the placenta has been removed and areas of deep invasion are encountered. When accompanied by massive bleeding, this circumstance becomes one of the most perilous situations in which we can find ourselves. Rapid haemodynamic deterioration and instability occur, and the workload of both surgical and anaesthesia teams increases exponentially, sometimes resulting in delay in communication of each other's needs. Concerted efforts at inter- and intra-team communication will ensure that both teams have minute-by-minute situational awareness and the ability to coordinate their actions. Rapid recognition of the need for hysterectomy is essential, and all efforts should be directed to performing this procedure with the least blood loss. Infrarenal aortic pressure and bimanual uterine compression can be instituted almost immediately and used to minimize ongoing bleeding while instruments and other preparations are made. If these efforts allow meaningful diminution of bleeding, they should be utilized to allow the patient to be resuscitated to the point that definitive surgery can be accomplished in a stable patient. The initiation of a massive transfusion protocol is something that all units in which caesarean delivery is being performed should practice. Baseline electrolyte levels (particularly K$^+$ and iCa^{2+}) should be measured at the same time as a full blood count and a coagulation profile are ordered. If all efforts at conservative management fail, the team have no choice but to proceed with hysterectomy with all due haste. In such cases, postoperative investigation for surgical complications (ureteric transection or ligation, bladder or bowel injury, nerve injury or haematoma development) should be carried out once the situation allows.

General principles regarding emergency surgery for placenta accreta include those outlined below. The following hints and 'pearls' are in most cases anecdotal and gleaned from a combined 50 years of operative experience and from evidence from the international literature [30–35]:

Surgical preparation for antenatal recognition of MAP

- Avoid elective surgery in a facility not set up for massive transfusion and which is without expert multidisciplinary help. It is recognized that in many situations MAP is discovered only after surgery has begun and that in many cases, even in the best of circumstances adequate resources are simply not available.

- The pregnant woman should be admitted at 33 to 34 weeks gestation, with planned preterm delivery by caesarean hysterectomy between 34 and 35 weeks.

- Preoperative consultation and prospective planning for maternal and neonatal care by a multidisciplinary team including an obstetrician, a gynaecologic surgeon, an anaesthesiologist, a urologist, an interventional radiologist, a neonatologist, a critical care specialist, and a blood bank/coagulation haematologist should be obtained. It is important to have a designated team(s) and standard operating procedures for the management of both known patients and previously unseen patients who present under emergency circumstances.

- It is crucial to establish post-partum haemorrhage and massive transfusion protocols and to have frequent simulations and/or mock drills to keep the team operationally proficient. This aspect of the preparation is a mandatory, since in those institutions where management of MAP is rare, having a protocol does not mean that the institution is always ready for such patients.

- Establishment of an arterial line, which will be used to monitor blood pressure and allow specimen collection, and insertion of central venous access catheters should precede surgery.

- We recommend that, if at all possible, bilateral ureteric stents should be placed in order to help with intraoperative identification of the ureters, which are frequently displaced or deviated by the bulging lower segment.

- Patients should be positioned in lithotomy with low Allen stirrups, to allow visualization of vaginal bleeding, if necessary, and for a third co-surgeon to have access to the surgical field.

- Abdominal entry should be via a peri-umbilical midline abdominal incision, with gentle exteriorization of the pregnant uterus to allow fundal or posterior classical hysterotomy.

- No attempts at removal of the placenta should be made when significant morbidly adherent placenta is suspected.

Intraoperative recognition of MAP

- In cases where, on opening the maternal abdomen, MAP is recognized and no preparation has been made, or no resources exist, the option of simply closing the maternal abdomen and transferring the patient to a facility with adequate resources should always be considered.
- In those situations where no higher level facility is available, the caesarean section should be performed through an incision as far as possible from the placenta. No attempt should be made to remove the placenta, and the uterus should be closed with the placenta in situ. In those cases where the placental site is not bleeding and the patient is stable, this approach is perhaps safer than proceeding with hysterectomy in an unprepared state. If the placenta remains in situ, the patient should remain in hospital for at least the first few weeks for observation since she is at risk for post-partum haemorrhage and sepsis. If at all possible, she should be transferred to a higher level facility for further management even if that requires evacuation to a different country as the patient will be transferred in a stable state.
- There are reports of resection of the placental–myometrium mass and reconstitution of the uterus in patients in whom the MAP is not a praevia and it is possible to isolate the morbidly adherent region [34]. We recognize that this procedure may be an option in some circumstances, although it is not a frequently practised or considered an option in our home institution or country. If this is done, efforts to reduce ongoing bleeding during the resection should be employed and these may include the use of a tourniquet below the region to be resected [35], use of stapler devices if available, excision with diathermy or argon beam coagulator, and use of haemostatic sutures around the border of the excision region.
- In the event that the patient begins to bleed during the caesarean delivery and a hysterectomy (or resection) has to be performed to save the patient's life, every effort to minimize bleeding should be employed, including intermittent aortic pressure, aortic cross clamping, placement of an aortic balloon catheter if available, and uterine and pelvic compression, until blood is available or help arrives.

Operative technique for MAP

- One of the most important aspects of caesarean delivery in the face of suspected or known placenta accreta is to make no attempt to remove a morbidly adherent placenta. In many cases, this decision is a considered medical judgement, but in some cases the choice is very obvious. As the risk of MAP in women with prior uterine surgery has become increasingly recognized, first and second-trimester ultrasound examination may allow early recognition of MAP and enables appropriate preparation for delivery (see Chapter 9). While MAP initially discovered at the time of delivery should become less and less common, there will still be cases where this occurs. The increasingly common practices of delayed cord clamping and allowing the placenta to spontaneously separate at the time of caesarean delivery actually may have an unintended positive safety consequence. This additional time before attempts at manual removal allows the clinician to monitor spontaneous placental separation and to carefully look at the uterus. In the event of a placenta not separating at caesarean delivery after what appears to be an appropriate amount of time, instead of attempting to find a plane and force separation, the astute clinician should consider the reason and think about MAP. This approach is a behaviour that can be taught and over time will become the norm, perhaps with measurable impact. There is an evidence base that supports this intuitively apparent course of action. Partial separation of the placenta, partial removal of the placenta in a piecemeal fashion, and forced creation of unnatural separation planes in the myometrium will all convert a stable situation with reasonable options, into an emergent and life-threatening situation with minimal options.

- Along the same lines, if areas of thinned myometrium or distended venous sinuses are seen on the surface of the uterus, even in a patient who does not have a history of multiple uterine surgeries, the prudent approach is to not apply excessive traction to the cord or attempt to manually remove a placenta that is not separating spontaneously. The recent recognition that assisted reproductive technologies significantly increase the risk of MAP may explain the increase in the incidence of MAP in women having their first delivery.

- Because of the abnormal anatomy seen in women with MAP, the technique of caesarean hysterectomy is very different than that done for an atonic uterus. Because of the very thin covering of myometrium (in some cases only a few cell layers thick) over highly vascular placental tissue, placing clamps very close to the sides of the uterus can result in tearing of the pedicle, tearing of the underlying uterine tissue, exposure of the placental mass, and resultant massive haemorrhage. For this reason, in cases of significant placenta accreta, it is essential to perform a more extensive lateral pelvic dissection of the broad ligament when a bulging lower segment (or any clearly invaded region of myometrium requiring division from surrounding tissue) is present. We ligate the round ligaments and utero-ovarian ligaments if possible after closing the uterus following the caesarean section. This step reduces to some extent the blood flow to the uterus from the fundal areas of myometrium. After this step, the majority of the blood being delivered to the uterus will be via the uterine arteries, the superior vesical arteries, the cervico-vaginal arteries, and a host of unnamed and previously unknown vessels and neovasculature that has developed via collateral circulation due to placental demand.

- Prior to performing the hysterectomy in a patient with placenta percreta and clear lateral invasion, or in cases with significant myometrial bulging (which signals almost complete myometrial replacement), we advise opening of the retroperitoneal spaces, lateral and parallel to the round ligaments. This step allows us to leave an adequate border of avascular parametrium between the thinned uterine wall and the pedicle being developed. It also allows us to identify the ureters (made easier by palpation of the stents) and other important retroperitoneal structures in a controlled fashion, devoid of any rush caused by ongoing haemorrhage. Before ligating the uterine arteries, we perform a ureterolysis and attempt to ligate the artery lateral to the ureter. We also make extensive use of a bipolar cautery device (Figure 6.4).

- We recommend early blood product replacement at the first sign of heavy bleeding; a massive transfusion protocol (transfusion of packed red blood cells and fresh frozen plasma in a 1 : 2 ratio) should be used. When the transfusion is performed, it is important that electrolyte levels are frequently measured, particularly ionized calcium and potassium. We have instituted a specific placenta percreta order set within the mass transfusion protocol that includes measurements of arterial blood gas, K^+, Ca^{2+}, complete blood count, prothrombin time and partial thromboplastin time, international normalized ratio, fibrinogen, D-dimer, glucose, and Mg^{2+} every 20–30 minutes. We usually transfuse 1 'jumbo unit' (35–50 ml) of platelets following every 8 units of packed red blood cells. We try to keep the platelet count at or above 100,000/ml.

- Placement of intra-abdominal drains to alert providers to the possibility of haemorrhage are usually not necessary but can be useful if there is any doubt.

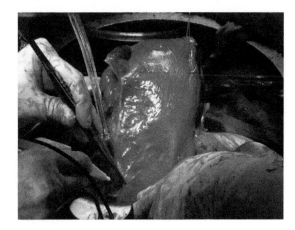

Figure 6.4 Note the coagulation line along the lateral border of the uterus.

Special considerations in placenta percreta

- It is important to understand that blood supply to the lower segment is extremely abnormal in a situation of placenta percreta. Frequently, the bladder tissue itself is actually supplying arterial blood to the placenta and draining venous blood through a network of small and tiny vessels that looked at individually seem insignificant. However, the totality of the surface area of these vessels greatly exceeds that of the uterine artery itself. The interface between the bladder tissue and the uterus involved in a placenta percreta should be treated with the same caution as a pulsating artery or distended vein. Usually, these new vessels are without significant musculature, and attempting to burn them with a diathermy device can lead to trouble. Blunt dissection of areas of invasion is contraindicated and will cause bleeding that can often cascade into an emergency situation.

- We favour the careful and painstaking dissection of the bladder tissue off the myometrium with a bipolar cautery device (LigaSure) when this is possible in order to retain as much bladder wall as we can. The device allows clamping of small pieces of vascular tissue, desiccation of the tissue mass, and ultimately bloodless separation of very vascular interfaces. Using this technique, we frequently need to buttress and oversew the bladder wall after the hysterectomy is completed because of significant thinning of the bladder wall and damage from the dissection. On occasion, we will proceed with deliberate cystotomy and excision of the piece of bladder that is attached. This approach is favoured over persistent attempts at bladder dissection in cases with deep placental invasion.

- In some rare cases, intraoperative staged arterial embolization of the placental bed (after the caesarean section but before the hysterectomy) may be deemed necessary when the placenta percreta involves the lateral pelvic side walls, and dissection without prior attempts at devascularization seems too risky.

Post-operative care

- In those facilities that have intensive care capability, we recommend that patients having had surgery for are recovered there. Not infrequently, there has been a massive transfusion and some electrolyte imbalance that requires reversal or at least close monitoring.

- Secondary haemorrhage is always a possibility as the patient awakes and in the first few hours after surgery. Close monitoring of blood pressure, heart rate, and urine output are essential.

- In those cases where there has been protracted surgery and extensive third-space fluid loss, prolonged post-operative intubation and ventilation is advised to reduce the risk of pulmonary oedema and respiratory difficulty.

- In the event of suspected oozing leading to slow intra-abdominal blood loss, we advise aggressive use of blood and blood products to resuscitate the patient and reverse any coagulopathy. Infusion of large volumes of crystalloid in such post-operative patients will expand the intravascular volume and produce a temporary increase in blood pressure and decrease in heart rate. However, the respite is usually temporary and return to the operating room inevitable, because infusing crystalloid leads to haemodilution and decreased intravascular clotting factor concentration. Decreasing the concentration of intravascular clotting factor exacerbates the continued ooze and collection of clot in the abdomen, resulting in slow distention and worsening haemoperitoneum. Once this event occurs, it is essential to remove the blood from the abdomen in order to reverse the coagulopathy. We have had to return patients to the operating room simply to drain the haemoperitoneum—there is usually no clear source of bleeding that has to be addressed and, once the blood clot and haemolysed blood has been removed, the patient can be closed without further issue.

Retroperitoneal haemorrhage during caesarean delivery

The most common cause of retroperitoneal haemorrhage at the time of caesarean delivery is extension of a hysterotomy into the broad ligament, with injury to the uterine artery. This injury can go unrecognized for some time, and often by the time it is recognized there has been significant blood loss and haematoma formation. Under most circumstances, unless there is an immediate need to open the retroperitoneum and evacuate the haemorrhage, uterine artery or other feeder artery embolization may be the safest and most effective way to control the bleeding. In our experience, attempting to locate the bleeding vessel(s) within an established retroperitoneal haematoma is difficult, if not impossible. If at all possible, and only if the patient is haemodynamically stable, selective embolization should be an option. In our institution, we prefer doing this procedure in a hybrid operating room or one equipped with a carbon fibre table and a c-arm, so that, should emergency surgery be required, it can be accomplished without delay. It is inappropriate, in our opinion, to remove a haemodynamically unstable patient to an angiography suite for embolization because, in the event of complete collapse, the challenges of anaesthesia and surgery are significantly increased. If embolization is either ineffective or impossible, and there is continued life-threatening bleeding,

it may become impossible to avoid surgery. In this case, regardless of the initial incision, a midline abdominal incision is preferred, to allow access to the upper retroperitoneum. Dealing with such situations is the purview of the vascular surgeon, and we advise the services of such an expert if at all possible. Aortic compression, aortic cross clamping, and placement of intraortic balloon devices have all been reported [32, 33, 35] and may be a consideration. It is usually best to enter the retroperitoneum high and in a region where there is no haematoma. This approach allows for proper identification of the vascular structures and a systematic search for the source of the bleeding. In an unstable patient with a coagulopathy, pressure on the pelvic structures to simply reduce blood loss and allow time for resuscitation can be life-saving. Placement of a pelvic pressure pack [36] or a balloon device to compress the pelvic side walls [37] may allow additional time for the aforesaid resuscitative efforts. A combination of pelvic pressure and embolization may sometimes be required to control the bleeding.

Caesarean section in low-resource settings

Most of the complications observed in well-resourced obstetric environments are also observed in low-resource settings, often with increased incidence. Fetal heart monitoring during labour is relatively rare in low-resource settings, and emergency caesarean delivery is uncommon for fetal compromise. Most urgent or emergent caesarean deliveries are performed for obstructed labour, antepartum haemorrhage, and uterine rupture. In many cases, there has been protracted labour and often there is attendant dehydration, anaemia, infection, and/or sepsis. The uterus is often oedematous and ischaemic, with areas of haemorrhage into the myometrium. In many such cases, fetal death has already occurred.

As a general principle, stabilization of the maternal condition prior to surgery is crucial in such precariously balanced patients. A rushed caesarean delivery in an to attempt to save a compromised

baby must be carefully weighed against the risk of losing the mother during or after the surgery because of inadequate resuscitative capability in the face of sepsis, hypovolemic shock or unexpected haemorrhage. In many cases, the mother dies from hypovolaemic shock after a technically successful caesarean delivery with average blood loss, simply because she was unable to tolerate the loss. Such a situation may exist in women with chronic severe anaemia due to malaria or other causes (i.e. malnutrition, hookworm or other helminthic infestations) in which there has been time for the mother to compensate for a haemoglobin as chronically low as 4 or 5. However, such patients are unlikely to be able to sustain an average 500 cc blood loss without catastrophic haemodynamic compromise, as their heart rate and cardiac output are already at capacity. In such cases, the blood pressure drops precipitously with minor changes in stroke volume and no compensatory response is forthcoming. Spinal or general anaesthesia administered to a woman in septic shock will also represent an often insurmountable stress.

The clinician in certain low-resource circumstances should understand that maternal outcome is primary, and that in some cases decisions not otherwise contemplated in a high-resource environment will need to be made. Thus, the algorithm for such surgery starts at a point different to that contemplated in a well-resourced environment, with the decision as to whether or not the mother can reasonably survive the anaesthesia, stress, and blood loss of a normal caesarean delivery in her current state, given the resources of the facility in which she finds herself. If she is fortunate enough to be in a hospital where an anaesthetist is available and the team has the necessary expertise, equipment, supplies, and blood products to safely undertake surgery, it may be reasonable to proceed with surgery. If she is in a poorly equipped facility with no access to emergency resuscitation, blood transfusion, and all that may be required, with no need to operate to save the mother's life, it may be that the wisest action is to delay any surgery until such time as the necessary conditions prevail or until the patient can be transported to a facility where the surgery can be safely done. This decision may have to be made with the knowledge that it will almost certainly result in the loss of the fetus.

In the event of a fetal death and an obstructed labour, destructive fetal procedure to allow vaginal delivery and avoid major abdominal surgery is an option in trained hands [38, 39]. While such procedures are uncommon and training for them is almost unknown in high-resource settings, it is our opinion that they can be life-saving and that training under appropriate circumstances should be revisited. Within this context, in women with fetal demise and abruptio placentae, abdominal surgery can be avoided and vaginal delivery safely accomplished without serious complications or loss of maternal life [40, 41]. In many low-resource settings, the rate of uterine rupture is estimated to be much higher than that seen in high-resource settings, possibly because of, in addition to prolonged labours, traditional practices encourage the use of herbs and local drugs as supplements to augment labour.

Many of the abovementioned decision points are not ones that most clinicians trained in high-resource environments have ever faced, and they should be thoroughly prepared in their home institution before being deployed to a low-resource environment. Such preparation may involve lectures, counselling by a mental health professional, simulated scenarios, and interviews with people experienced in low-resource obstetrics. Newly deployed personnel should be followed closely for signs of stress, demoralization, feelings of hopelessness, anger, and frustration with the local system, and PTSD, all of which may manifest at some time during their stay. While more detail on this topic is beyond the scope of this chapter, it is important enough that we make specific mention of it here to ensure that the reader is acutely aware of the mental strain under which clinicians in low-resource environments function.

Caesarean delivery after obstructed labour

As previously mentioned, in some cases, ceasarean delivery after obstructed labor may result in morbidity or mortality for the pregnant woman, thus if the baby is dead and a destructive procedure is possible with adequately trained personnel available, this procedure may be the most advisable course of action. In particular, if the baby is in a cephalic presentation and the skull can be breached and the cerebral material removed, the cranium will collapse and allow delivery of the baby. While aesthetically disturbing, in most cases a vaginal delivery is preferable to a caesarean delivery in these patients. These women are at particular risk for atony and post-partum haemorrhage, and delivery should only be initiated in a situation where resuscitation can be accomplished. In addition, they are frequently infected or have had an abruption (or both), and antibiotic treatment or prophylaxis is essential. Careful assessment of the vagina and cervix will be mandatory after delivery and for several days following delivery to observe for vaginal, cervical, and bladder necrosis. It has been suggested that all women who have had an extended period of obstructed labour be catheterized for 5–7 days and observed for evidence of fistula formation. However, despite some logic for such management, evidence for this suggestion remains anecdotal [42].

In those cases where there is a live fetus (or a dead fetus, under special circumstances), and an informed decision has been made to perform a caesarean delivery in a woman who has had protracted labour, there are a number of technical issues that deserve consideration. Frequently, in a low-resource setting, the baby is severely impacted into the pelvis because of prolonged labour. The lower uterine segment will be significantly thinned and may even be so retracted that the bladder fills the anatomic space where the operator expects to find the lower uterine segment. It is not rare that unsuspecting and inexperienced surgeons perform an abdominal vaginal delivery by transecting the bladder and delivering the baby abdominally through the anterior vaginal wall and bladder. The resulting damage, if not life-threatening, may result in permanent urinary tract damage. Perhaps the best way to avoid such a situation is to initially disimpact the fetal head vaginally prior to starting the caesarean section, with gentle upwards pressure on the moulded fetal head. Disimpaction may take a few minutes and will usually be announced by a loud sucking sound and movement of the fetal head upwards back into the maternal pelvis.

Overall, we recommend operating with the patient in a low lithotomy position to allow vaginal access during the surgery. A midline incision should be made with wide exposure of the lower uterine segment. The hysterotomy should be made much higher on the uterus than in a non-obstructed labour, and careful identification of the bladder is warranted prior to any incision being made. We also recommend careful entry in the midline and scoring the uterus in a narrow U shape such that the incision is directed upwards and away from the uterine arteries. The uterus should be entered in the midline bluntly if possible and then bluntly extended with caudal–caudad stretching. Prior

to delivery of the fetal head, an assistant can gently elevate the fetal head into the pelvis again. In this way, it is possible to minimize lower uterine segment and bladder trauma. Following delivery, the clinician should expect uterine atony and post-partum haemorrhage, and administration of oxytocin should be started along with uterine massage and manual compression of the myometrium between the clinician's hands. Early use of balloon tamponade, compression sutures, and concomitant other uterotonic drugs should be undertaken at the first sign of atony and persistent haemorrhage in order to aggressively minimize blood loss. In most low-resource environments, this early recognition and aggressive use of methods to reduce blood loss may mean the difference between life and death.

In many low-resource environments, caesarean delivery at full dilation may be performed hours or days after the woman enters the second stage of labour, and such delays most certainly can result in additional complications, including a long hospital stay, increased likelihood of haemorrhage, extension of the surgical incision into the vagina or uterine arteries, injury to the genitourinary and/or gastrointestinal tracts (Figure 6.5), and postoperative fever [24]. In some cases of extremely prolonged and obstructed labour, there may be necrosis of the cervix with separation of the uterus and vagina, almost always accompanied by a dead fetus, infection/sepsis, and extensive bladder destruction usually involving the trigone. Clearly, when this type of injury occurs, the potential for complications beyond the obstetric injury are increased, and acute respiratory distress syndrome and pulmonary compromise should be expected. Early transfer to a referral centre is recommended. In a low-resource setting with such significant injury and the high risk of uterine necrosis, hysterectomy may be the best option since microabscesses may already be present in the damaged myometrium. In such a case, removal of the cervix is recommended in order to minimize the necrotic tissue left in the pelvis. Special attention should be paid to the ureters to ensure patency and integrity and urologic referral is recommended. In the event that the ureters are detached and no urologic expertise

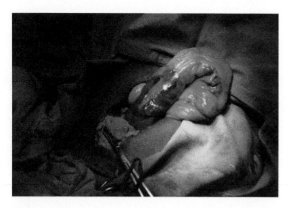

Figure 6.5 Rectal necrosis secondary to prolonged obstructed labour.

Photo courtesy of Jeffery Wilkinson, M.D.

is available, the ureters may be catheterized with ureteric stents and drained into a sterile urine bag while the patient is transported to an appropriate facility for definitive repair.

It has been recently suggested that, in case of obstructed labour in low-resourced rural areas, healthcare workers could be trained to perform symphysiotomy [43]. Symphysiotomy is an old operation in which the fibres of the pubic symphysis were partially divided to allow separation of the joint and thus enlargement of the pelvic dimensions, thereby facilitating vaginal delivery of the fetus in the presence of mild-to-moderate cephalopelvic disproportion. It can be performed with local anaesthesia and does not require an operating theatre or advanced surgical skills [43, 44]. A recent review has concluded that symphysiotomy can be a life-saving procedure in certain circumstances and that professional and global bodies should provide guidelines, which are based on the best available evidence, for the use (or non-use) of symphysiotomy [44].

Caesarean delivery in obese women

Overweight and obesity (BMI 30–45) now exceeding underweight in young women residing in both urban and rural areas of many low-resource countries [10], resulting in obstetric and anaesthetic risks that are similar to those observed in well-resourced countries. When the obstetric theatre records and case files were reviewed for caesarean deliveries

in the University of Nigeria Teaching Hospital, Enugu, Nigeria, from May 2008 to December 2010, an incidence of 12.4% of maternal morbid obesity was found [45]. The complication rates in obese women are similar in different parts of the world and include intra-partum and post-operative complications such as wound infection and endometritis, wound opening, hematoma or seroma, and emergency department visit (see Chapter 4).

Myomectomy at the time of caesarean delivery

As access to blood products is limited in low-resource countries, and myomectomy at the time of caesarean delivery is associated with increased blood loss there is little experience of combined caesarean section–myomectomy in low-resource countries. A brief communication detailing a prospective study performed in Accra, Ghana, comparing caesarean delivery with and without myomectomy [46] enrolled 24 women, including 12 with uterine leiomyomas and 12 without. The procedures of women who underwent myomectomy at the time of caesarean delivery took on average 11.25 minutes longer than those for women who did not undergo myomectomy at the time of caesarean delivery; this difference was not statistically significant, according to the author. The two groups experienced comparable blood loss, with an average estimated blood loss of 392 ml in the myomectomy patients versus 388 ml in the non-myomectomy patients; this similarity may be because of the use of a tourniquet around the uterine arteries and infundibulo-pelvic ligament during the myomectomy. Apart from tourniquet usage, no description was offered as to surgical technique. A systematic review of nine studies of women who underwent caesarean myomectomy and who underwent caesarean delivery alone saw a 0.30 g/dL greater drop in hemoglobin in the caesarean myomectomy group than in the control group, but the difference is not significant [47]. These data suggest that caesarean myomectomy may be a reasonable option for some women with anterior leiomyoma who are potentially at risk of bleeding post-operatively.

Key learning points

1. Caesarean delivery at complete dilation with dystocia is associated with increased risks, such as intraoperative trauma.
2. In a true rupture of the uterus with fetal extrusion, the chances of fetal survival are low unless rapid intervention is accomplished.
3. Current recommendations support a subcutaneous suture to prevent seroma formation and wound disruption when there is greater than 2 cm of subcutaneous fat.
4. The presence of adhesions at caesarean delivery increases with each subsequent surgery and impacts the time to delivery of the infant and overall surgical operative times.
5. A viable fetus delivered within 5 minutes of cardiac arrest is likely to survive with intact neurological status.
6. Algorithms of care for post-partum haemorrhage (including time limits and other agreed-upon trigger points) and regular simulation training should be used to ensure staff readiness.
7. If significant haemorrhage at the time of delivery is anticipated, patients should be positioned in lithotomy with low Allen stirrups, to allow visualization of vaginal bleeding.
8. When a significantly adherent placenta is suspected, no attempts at removal of the placenta should be made.
9. The most common cause of retroperitoneal haemorrhage at the time of caesarean section is extension of a hysterotomy into the broad ligament, with injury to the uterine artery.
10. Most of the caesarean complications observed in well-resourced obstetric environments are also observed in low-resource settings, often with an increased incidence.

References

1. Allen VM, O'Connell CM, Baskett TF. Maternal and perinatal morbidity of caesarean delivery at full cervical dilatation compared with caesarean delivery in the first stage of labour. BJOG 2005; 112(7): 986–90.
2. Selo-Ojeme D, Sathiyathasan S, Fayyaz, M. Caesarean delivery at full cervical dilatation versus caesarean delivery in the first stage of labour: Comparison of maternal and perinatal morbidity. Arch Gynecol Obstet 2008; 278(7): 245–9.
3. Radha P, Tagore S, Rahman MF, Tee J. Maternal and perinatal morbidity after Caesarean delivery at full cervical dilatation. Singapore Med J 2012; 53(10): 655–8.
4. Ayres AW, Johnson TR, Hayashi R. Characteristics of fetal heart rate tracings prior to uterine rupture. Int J Gynaecol Obstet 2001; 74(3): 235–40.
5. Leung AS, Leung EK, Paul RH. Uterine rupture after previous cesarean delivery: Maternal and fetal consequences. Am J Obstet Gynecol 1993; 169(4): 945–50.
6. Landon MB, Hauth JC, Leveno KJ, Spong CY, Leindecker S, Varner MW, et al. Maternal and perinatal outcomes associated with a trial of labor after prior cesarean delivery. N Engl J Med 2004; 351(25): 2581–9.
7. Smith G, Pell J, Cameron A, Dobbie R. Risk of perinatal death associated with labor after previous cesarean delivery in uncomplicated term pregnancies. JAMA 2002; 287(20): 2684–90.
8. American College of Obstetricians and Gynecologists. ACOG Practice Bulletin No. 115: Vaginal birth after previous cesarean delivery. Obstet Gynecol 2010; 116(2 Pt 1): 450–63.
9. Akaba GO, Onafowokan O, Offiong RA, Omonua K, Ekele BA. Uterine rupture: Trends and feto-maternal outcome in a Nigerian teaching hospital. Niger J Med 2013; 22(4): 304–8.
10. World Health Organization. Estimated Obesity(BMI ≥ 30 kg/m²) Prevalence, Females, Aged 15+, https://apps.who.int/infobase/Comparisons.aspx.
11. World Health Organization. BMI Classification. 2016. http://apps.who.int/bmi/index.jsp?introPage=intro_3.html.
12. Weiss JL, Malone FD, Emig D, Ball RH, Nyberg DA, Comstock CH, et al. Obesity, obstetric complications and cesarean delivery rate: A population-based screening study. Am J Obstet Gynecol 2004; 190(4): 1091–7.
13. Slavin VJ, Fenwick J, Gamble J. Pregnancy care and birth outcomes for women with moderate to super-extreme obesity. Women Birth 2013; 26(3): 179–84.
14. Chelmow D, Rodriguez EJ, Sabatini MM. Suture closure of subcutaneous fat and wound disruption after cesarean delivery: A meta-analysis. Obstet Gynecol 2004; 103(5 Pt 1): 974–80.
15. Coronado G, Marshall L, Schwartz S. Complications in pregnancy, labor, and delivery with uterine leiomyomas: A population-based study. Obstet Gynecol 2000; 95(5): 764–9.
16. Klatsky PC, Tran ND, Caughey AB, Fujimoto VY. Fibroids and reproductive outcomes: A systematic literature review from conception to delivery. Am J Obstet Gynecol 2008; 198(4): 357–66.

17. Kaymak O, Ustunyurt E, Okyay R, Kalyoncu S, Mol-lamahmutoglu L. Myomectomy during cesarean section. Int J Gynaecol Obstet 2005; 89(2): 90–3.

18. Li H, Du J, Jin L, Shi Z, Liu M. Myomectomy during cesarean section. Acta Obstet Gynecol Scand 2009; 88(2): 183–6.

19. Morales KJ, Gordon MC, Bates GW. Postcesarean delivery adhesions associated with delayed delivery of infant. Am J Obstet Gynecol 2007; 196(5): e461–466.

20. Tulandi T, Al-Sannan B, Akbar G, Ziegler C, Miner L. Prospective study of intraabdominal adhesions among women of different races with or without keloids. Am J Obstet Gynecol 2011; 204(2): e131–134.

21. Malvasi A, Tinelli A, Guido M, Cavallotti C, Dell'Edera D, Zizza A, et al. Effect of avoiding bladder flap formation in caesarean section on repeat caesarean delivery. Eur J Obstet Gynecol Reprod Biol 2011; 159(2): 300–4.

22. Malvasi A, Tinelli A, Farine D, Rahimi S, Cavallotti C, Vergar D, et al. Effects of visceral peritoneal closure on scar formation at cesarean delivery. Int J Gynaecol Obstet 2009; 105(2): 131–5.

23. Lyell DJ, Caughey AB, Hu E, Blumenfeld Y, El-Sayed YY, Daniels K. Rectus muscle and visceral peritoneum closure at cesarean delivery and intraabdominal adhesions. Am J Obstet Gynecol 2012; 206(6): e511–515.

24. Cakir Gungor AN, Oguz S, Hacivelioglu S, Isik S, Uysal A, Gencer, M, et al. Predictive value of striae gravidarum severity for intraperitoneal adhesions or uterine scar healing in patients with previous caesarean delivery. J Matern Fetal Neonatal Med 2013; 27(13): 1312–15.

25. Pandit SN, Khan RJ. Surgical techniques for performing caesarean section including CS at full dilatation. Best Pract Res Clin Obstet Gynaecol 2013; 27(2): 179–95.

26. Mhyre JM, Tsen LC, Einav S, Kuklina EV, Leffert LR, Bateman BT. Cardiac arrest during hospitalization for delivery in the United States, 1998–2011. Anesthesiology 2014; 120(4): 810–8.

27. Jeejeebhoy FM, Zelop CM, Windrim R, Carvalho JC, Dorian P, Morrison LJ. Management of cardiac arrest in pregnancy: A systematic review. Resuscitation 2011; 82(7): 801–9.

28. Morrison LJ, Deakin CD, Morley PT, Callaway CW, Kerber RE, Kronick SL, et al. Part 8: Advanced life support: 2010 International Consensus on Cardiopulmonary Resuscitation and Emergency Cardiovascular Care Science with Treatment Recommendations. Circulation 2010; 122(16 Suppl 2): S345–421.

29. Katz VL. Perimortem cesarean delivery: Its role in maternal mortality. Semin Perinatol 2012; 36(1): 68–72.

30. O'Leary JL, O'Leary JA. Uterine artery ligation in the control of intractable postpartum hemorrhage. Am J Obstet Gynecol 1966; 94(7): 920–4.

31. AbdRabbo SA. Stepwise uterine devascularization: A novel technique for management of uncontrolled postpartum hemorrhage with preservation of the uterus. Am J Obstet Gynecol 1994; 171(3): 694–700.

32. Sovik E, Stokkeland P, Storm BS, Asheim P, Bolas O. The use of aortic occlusion balloon catheter without fluoroscopy for life-threatening post-partum haemorrhage. Acta Anaesthesiol Scand 2012; 56(3): 388–93.

33. Belfort MA, Zimmerman J, Schemmer G, Oldroyd R, Smilanich R, Pearce M. Aortic compression and cross clamping in a case of placenta percreta and amniotic fluid embolism: A case report. AJP Rep 2011; 1(1): 33–6.

34. Chandraharan E, Rao S, Belli AM, Arulkumaran S. The Triple-P procedure as a conservative surgical alternative to peripartum hysterectomy for placenta percreta. Int J Gynaecol Obstet 2012; 117(2): 191–4.

35. Huijgen QC, Gijsen AF, Hink E, Van Kesteren P. Cervical tourniquet in case of uncontrollable haemorrhage during caesarean section owing to a placenta accreta. BMJ Case Rep 2013; doi: 10.1136/bcr-2013-009237.

36. Dildy GA, Scott JR, Saffer CS, Belfort MA. An effective pressure pack for severe pelvic hemorrhage. Obstet Gynecol 2006; 108(5): 1222–6.

37. Charoenkwan K. Effective use of the Bakri postpartum balloon for posthysterectomy pelvic floor hemorrhage. Am J Obstet Gynecol 2014; 210(6): e581–583.

38. Lawson J. Embryotomy for obstructed labour. Trop Doct 1974; 4(4): 188–91.

39. Smale LE. Destructive operations on the fetus: Review of literature and application in 10 cases of neglected dystocia. Am J Obstet Gynecol 1974; 119(3): 369–74.

40. Belfort M. A new instrument for the delivery of the impacted dead fetus. Trop Doct 1988; 18(4): 180–2.

41. Belfort M, Moore P. The use of a cephalic perforator for delivery of the dead fetus in cases of severe abruptio placentae. SAMJ 1990; 77: 80–2.

42. Creanga AA, Genadry RR. Obstetric fistulas: A clinical review. Int J Gynaecol Obstet 2007; 99(Suppl 1): S40–46.

43. Monjok E, Okokon IB, Opiah MM, Ingwu JA, Ekabua JE, Essien EJ. Obstructed labour in resource-poor

settings: The need for revival of symphysiotomy in Nigeria. Afr J Reprod Health 2012; 16(3): 94–101.

44. Hofmeyr GJ, Shweni PM. Symphysiotomy for feto-pelvic disproportion. Cochrane Database Syst Rev 2012; 10: CD005299.

45. Okafor UV, Efetie ER, Nwoke O, Okezie O, Umeh U. Anaesthetic and obstetric challenges of morbid obesity in caesarean deliveries: A study in South-eastern Nigeria. Afr Health Sci 2012; 12(1): 54–7.

46. Kwawukume E. Myomectomy during cesarean section. Int J Gynaecol Obstet 2002; 76(2): 183–4.

47. Song D, Zhang W, Chames MC, Guo J. Myomectomy during cesarean delivery. Int J Gynaecol Obstet. 2013;121(3):208–13.

CHAPTER 7
Anaesthesia for caesarean section

Desikan Rangarajan and Paul Howell

Introduction

Anaesthesia for caesarean section can pose significant risk to the mother and the fetus. However, maternal deaths related to anaesthesia for caesarean section are uncommon in resource rich countries. A recent report from the United Kingdom showed 261 maternal deaths for the 2006–2008 triennium, giving a maternal mortality rate of 11.7 per 100,000 [1, 2]. Of these, only 2.68% (7 deaths) were related to anaesthesia, giving a rate of 3.1 deaths due to anaesthesia per 1,000,000 maternities. Similarly, in the United States, only 1.6% of maternal deaths (which totalled 5375 deaths over the 12-year period) were related to anaesthesia over a 12-year period [3].

In resource-poor countries, however, there is undoubtedly a significantly higher risk of death from anaesthesia-related complications, compared to resource-rich countries. Though the numbers often are not recorded or reported, there are some clues in the literature. In South Africa, anaesthesia-related deaths accounted for 6% of all preventable deaths in 2008–2010 [4]. In one report from a teaching hospital in Nigeria, the death rate from anaesthesia was estimated to be 3.7 per 1000 [5]. In sub-Saharan Africa, the recorded death rate is as high as 1%–2% at caesarean section, with anaesthesia-related events contributing up to one-third of the observed mortality [6, 7].

These deaths in resource-poor countries largely have been attributed to a lack of resources, including the limited number of medically-qualified anaesthetists, and to deficiencies in training especially for the non-physician anaesthetic practitioner, leading to airway problems, inappropriate application of anaesthesia, and inability to recognise a sick or haemodynamically-compromised parturient.' Furthermore, a lack of essential monitoring equipment and drugs, combined with shortcomings in essential infrastructure, compound the issue and result in suboptimal care for a huge cohort of women.

Historically, the majority of anaesthesia-related deaths in the United Kingdom were due to airway problems (failed intubation and pulmonary aspiration) associated with general anaesthesia for emergency caesarean section, and many of these cases were staffed out-of-hours by poorly trained, poorly supported junior staff. Awareness of these issues has led to a widespread increase in the use of regional anaesthesia for caesarean section, and 2012 data show that only around 10% of caesarean section in the United Kingdom are now performed under general anaesthesia [8]. Reduction in the use of general anaesthesia, allied with improved training, monitoring, and support for anaesthetists has been instrumental in the significant decrease in anaesthesia-related mortality associated with caesarean section.

The purpose of this chapter is to highlight the important aspects of delivering safe anaesthesia for caesarean section in sometimes difficult circumstances.

Anaesthesia providers and standards

In resource-rich areas of the world, anaesthesia is most commonly provided by physician anaesthetists who have specialized after qualifying as a medical doctor. In the United States and some north European countries, nurse anaesthetists (usually under the supervision of a physician anaesthetist) provide a large proportion of the anaesthetics administered.

In contrast, in resource-poor areas of the world, and particularly outside of the major cities, medically qualified anaesthetists are a rare commodity, and it is usual for the vast majority of anaesthesia in surgical cases to be administered by non-physician anaesthetic technicians, often with very little or no supervision by physician anaesthetists.

Anaesthetic training

Adequate training in anaesthesia, whether for physician or non-physician providers, is crucial for providing an effective and efficient service where the focus is the safety of the mother and the fetus. Maternal mortality reports from the United Kingdom and South Africa have repeatedly highlighted the need for better healthcare worker training [1, 8]. Recommendations from the latest South African report suggest that anaesthetic providers who will care for pregnant women should complete a specific obstetric anaesthetic module, achieve competencies relevant to obstetric emergencies, and be able to use early warning scores [9].

An effective training programme requires:

1. A structured educational process;

2. Core competencies, knowledge and behavioural aspects required for the safe practice to have been identified and validated by a reputable organization (usually the regional college of anaesthesia); and

3. Competencies to be tested by examinations and while 'on the job'.

Good teamwork is a cornerstone of good care, and should be fostered and practised regularly in activities such as 'skills and drills' and simulation-based scenarios. Similarly, in emergency clinical situations, it is vital that the obstetrician and

---

Box 7.1 The World Federation of Societies of Anaesthesiologists' 'highly recommended' requirements to meet safe administration of anaesthesia for caesarean section

Preoperative

- Anaesthetic pre-assessment to tailor an appropriate and safe strategy;
- All anaesthetic equipment checked;
- Supplemental oxygen present and supply verified.

Intraoperative

- Continuous measurement of tissue oxygenation; pulse oximetry highly recommended;
- When pulse oximetry not available, dedicated personnel and adequate illumination to detect and manage hypoxia;
- Ventilation continually assessed by visual inspection;
- Capnography if intubated;

- Monitoring of the heart rate and rhythm is mandatory (ECG, pulse oximeter); continuous palpation of pulses and auscultation of the heart if monitoring is not available;
- Blood pressure at least every 5 minutes;
- Audible alarms turned on at all times.

Post-operative

- Presence of dedicated recovery with trained staff;
- Vital signs monitored; pulse oximetry highly recommended;
- Adequate analgesia prescribed and available;
- Every effort made to alleviate suffering.

Alan F. Merry, Jeffrey B. Cooper, Olaitan Soyannwo, Iain H. Wilson, and John H. Eichhorn, Can J Anaesth, 2010, 1027–1034, Springer

anaesthetist discuss the immediate management of the patient and agree a plan of action, underpinned by an understanding of and respect for each practitioner's priorities and concerns.

Standards for providing safe anaesthesia

The World Federation of Societies of Anaesthesiologists (WFSA) in 2010 has advised on the 'highly recommended' (meaning mandatory) requirements (Box 7.1) to meet safe administration of anaesthesia (including for caesarean section) worldwide [10].

While anaesthesia without the mandatory standards for elective procedures is deemed unacceptable, the WFSA recognizes that in resource-poor regions the mandated standards frequently cannot be met because of limitations of resources and organizational structure. In such situations, the WFSA strongly advises that anaesthesia only should be undertaken for life- or limb-threatening surgery.

Of note, is the current Lifebox® charitable project (established by the WFSA, the Association of Anaesthetists of Great Britain and Ireland, the Harvard School of Public Health, and the Brigham and Women's Hospital) which aims to provide simple pulse oximetry monitoring to every location worldwide in which anaesthetics are given (see http://www.lifebox.org) [11].

Technical considerations for anaesthesia during caesarean section

Pregnancy-related physiological changes pertinent for anaesthesia

The physiological changes associated with pregnancy are covered in other textbooks. Aspects particularly relevant to anaesthesia are listed in Table 7.1.

Reduction in the functional residual capacity of the lungs and increased oxygen consumption in the pregnant woman lead to rapid oxygen desaturation following induction of anaesthesia or apnoea. Airway changes can result in difficult or failed intubation (which is up to eight times more frequent in the term parturient than in the non-pregnant woman). Because of these issues, adequate preoxygenation before induction of general anaesthesia is very important.

The abdominal changes that occur during pregnancy increase the likelihood that gastric contents may be aspirated. To minimize acid-induced pneumonitis in such an event, it is accepted and expected practice in resource-rich countries to administer a histamine-receptor antagonist (e.g. ranitidine) and an oral antacid buffer (e.g. sodium citrate) prior to induction of general anaesthesia for caesarean

Table 7.1 **Pregnancy-related changes relevant to the anaesthetist**

	Issue	Risk
Airway	Engorged friable mucosa	Easily bleeds
	Enlarged breasts	Difficult laryngoscopy
	Oedema in pre-eclampsia	Failed intubation more likely
Lungs	Reduced functional residual lung capacity	Rapid desaturation
	Increased oxygen requirement	
Abdomen	Increased gastric volumes	Aspiration pneumonitis
	Delayed gastric emptying after pain/opioids	
	Passive regurgitation	

Alan F. Merry, Jeffrey B. Cooper, Olaitan Soyannwo, Iain H. Wilson, and John H. Eichhorn, Can J Anaesth, 2010, 1027–1034, Springer

section. These reduce the acid content of the stomach and the risk of morbidity and mortality if pulmonary aspiration should occur.

From around 20 weeks gestation, the gravid uterus is of sufficient size to compress the inferior vena cava and the adjacent aortic segment when the mother is supine. This compression prevents venous return to the heart, resulting in reduced cardiac output and blood pressure. The drop in blood pressure is exacerbated by regional and general anaesthesia and may lead to cardiovascular collapse if aortocaval compression is not alleviated. Furthermore, aortocaval compression can also reduce uterine blood flow and cause non-reassuring fetal status. When the mother is supine, the uterus must be displaced laterally to the left, either by placing a wedge under the mother's back or by lateral tilting the table enough to see the gravid abdomen move off the midline.

Haematological changes during pregnancy include dilutional anaemia and mild thrombocytopaenia. Additionally, reduced albumin level lowers the oncotic pressure of the blood, making the pregnant woman liable to be tipped into pulmonary oedema with intravenous fluid therapy, particularly in pre-eclampsia.

Appreciation of these risks and adaptation of anaesthetic practice has led to a significant fall in anaesthesia-related deaths in the United Kingdom over the years [12].

Choice of anaesthesia for caesarean section

Anaesthesia for caesarean section can be achieved in a number of ways, and the approach should be dictated by the clinical situation and the resources available. The two main methods are general anaesthesia and regional anaesthesia (consisting of spinal, epidural, or combined spinal–epidural techniques), but local anaesthesia and ketamine anaesthesia also have a place in resource-poor settings (Table 7.2).

Regardless of the technique used, large-bore venous access should be used, and oxygen, relevant drugs, appropriate monitoring, and resuscitation equipment should all be immediately available. Aortocaval compression should be minimized by providing left lateral uterine tilt.

There is always a risk of vomiting and pulmonary aspiration associated with unexpected maternal collapse or the need for emergency general anaesthesia. Therefore, adequate measures to reduce the risk of aspiration pneumonia should be undertaken. Such measures may include premedication to reduce stomach acid production (e.g. ranitidine) and to enhance stomach emptying (e.g. metoclopramide). Neutralization of stomach acid with a buffer such as oral sodium citrate immediately prior to starting the procedure is also recommended.

Table 7.2 **Contraindications to regional anaesthesia**

Issue	Reason
Patient refusal	Poor cooperation, litigation
Haemorrhage	Hypotension, coagulopathy
Coagulopathy	Spinal haematoma
Hypovolaemia	Cardiovascular collapse
Generalized sepsis	Hypotension, epidural abscess
Infection at site of insertion	Meningitis, epidural abscess
Raised intracranial pressure	Coning
Spinal cord abnormalities (e.g. spina bifida)	Spinal cord damage
Allergy to local anaesthetics	Anaphylaxis
Extremely non-reassuring fetal status	General anaesthesia should be quicker

NB: Contraindications may be *relative* or *absolute*.

Regional anaesthesia (neuraxial techniques) for caesarean section

Regional anaesthesia has become the clearly preferred technique for caesarean section in resource-rich countries and also is being widely encouraged in resource-poor areas. It has distinct advantages over general anaesthesia, primarily because it avoids the adverse risks and side effects of general anaesthesia [13].

Neuraxial blocks can be achieved by the deposition of local anaesthetic with or without opioid into the subarachnoid space (spinal) or into the epidural space. In either case, the sensory block (often tested with cold sensation) ideally should be between the level of T4 (i.e. at the nipples) and the sacral roots. There is some evidence that testing the sensory block with light touch and ensuring a block to the T6 level (costal margin) prior to incision is more reliable than using cold sensation, but this method is not in widespread practice [14]. Achieving these levels is recommended so as to avoid pain during the procedure. Not only is pain during caesarean section extremely unpleasant for the mother, it is also a leading cause of litigation in obstetric anaesthesia in resource-rich countries. During the period 1995–2007 in the United Kingdom, inadequate anaesthesia accounted for 31% of litigation claims related to obstetric regional anaesthesia [15].

There are a number of contraindications to regional anaesthesia (Table 7.3), but the results of the third National Audit Project (NAP3) conducted by the Royal College of Anaesthetists in the United Kingdom has shown that regional anaesthesia in obstetric patients overall is extremely safe [16]. The risk of healthy patients developing the most feared of complications, a vertebral canal or epidural haematoma, following a neuraxial block was shown to be extremely small, with an incidence of 0.85 : 100,000 [16].

In patients with coagulopathy, it is generally accepted that the incidence of spinal haematoma would be higher than in patients without this condition. However, because of the rarity of spinal haematoma, definitive risk quantification is not possible. Consensus opinion suggests that the risk of this complication should be viewed as a continuum and be balanced against benefit [17].

Table 7.3 Core drugs for obstetric anaesthesia

Purpose	Drugs
Antacid prophylaxis	Sodium citrate Ranitidine Omeprazole
Induction agent	Thiopentone Propofol Etomidate Ketamine
Muscle relaxant	Suxamethonium Atracurium Vecuronium Rocuronium
Inhalational agent	Isoflurane Sevoflurane Desflurane (Halothane) (Ether)
Reversal	Neostigmine Glycopyrronium Atropine Sugammadex
Antiemetic	Ondansetron Metoclopramide Cyclizine
Analgesia	Opioids NSAIDs Paracetamol
Vasopressor	Ephedrine phenylephrine Metaraminol
Uterotonic	Oxytocin Ergometrine Carboprost

Timing of heparin is particularly relevant here, as the use of unfractionated and low molecular weight heparin (LMWH) to prevent thromboembolic events is commonplace in resource-rich countries and may increase the risk of developing a spinal haematoma after regional anaesthesia.

Guidelines from the Royal College of Obstetricians and Gynaecologists as well as wide consensus opinion recommend an interval of 12 or 24 hours after prophylactic or therapeutic LMWH administration, respectively, before performing neuraxial blockade [18], and LMWH should not be administered for 4 hours after a neuraxial procedure. There is no evidence that low-dose aspirin treatment (e.g. 75 mg per day) or truly prophylactic dosing of unfractionated heparin (e.g. 5000 U twice a day) is a contraindication for regional anaesthesia.

Thrombocytopaenia is a concern for anaesthetists when considering regional anaesthesia, because of the possibility of causing a spinal haematoma. There is still no reliable, easily available, test of platelet function, and obstetric anaesthetists therefore mostly rely on platelet count as a surrogate for platelet function. Correspondingly, anaesthetists generally consider regional anaesthesia safe if the platelet count is above 75–80 × 10^9/l. However, trends are considered as important as absolute values, as platelets may fall precipitously in situations such as severe pre-eclampsia or HELLP syndrome. Although platelet counts are not usually required in healthy women prior to neuraxial blockade, in those at risk of thrombocytopaenia, a platelet count should ideally be performed within the preceding 6 hours. It is appreciated that in rural or low-resourced settings, access to quick laboratory tests may not be available. In such circumstances, the low risk of a spinal haematoma should be weighed against the clinical situation. For example a spinal technique in the context of a borderline-low platelet count may be preferable to general anaesthesia for a parturient with a difficult airway and with an inexperienced anaesthesia provider.

Localized infection at the site of the neuraxial needle insertion carries with it a risk of seeding pathogens into the central nervous system and is hence a contraindication to neuraxial anaesthesia. In the case of systemic infection, or sepsis originating elsewhere, in women that have been treated with antibiotics *and where no overt signs of systemic sepsis (e.g. tachycardia, hypotension, and ongoing pyrexia) are manifest*, it is reasonable to consider regional anaesthesia.

Spinal anaesthesia for caesarean section

Single shot spinal anaesthesia (SSS) is the most common technique used worldwide for caesarean section. In skilled hands, it is safe, quick, and reliable. In this technique, local anaesthetic with or without a synergistic additive (usually opioid) is deposited into the intrathecal space by using a fine needle. The spinal cord ends at the L1 to L2 level in most individuals and hence the needle should be inserted below L2 to prevent inadvertent cord damage. Typically the L3–L4 or L4–L5 interspaces are recommended, since it is well recognized that anaesthetists often actually insert spinal needles at interspaces higher than expected [19, 20].

The most common potentially serious complication of spinal anaesthesia is post-dural-puncture headache due to continuing cerebrospinal fluid (CSF) leakage. This complication is dependent on the needle size and configuration of the needle tip. The short bevelled tip of the traditional Quincke needle cuts through the dural fibres but results in a relatively high incidence of post-dural-puncture headache, especially in pregnant women. The use of a 22-gauge Quincke needle for SSS has a post-dural-puncture headache rate of up to 36%. This rate can be reduced to less than 5% when the 27-gauge size is used. However, Quincke needles have been superseded in modern obstetric anaesthetic practice by pencil-point spinal needles (e.g. Whitacre, Sprotte), which incorporate a non-cutting needle tip. This tip separates the dural fibres instead of cutting them and is associated with significantly lower post-dural-puncture headache rates than Quincke needles are. Standard practice has therefore become to use a 25-gauge (or smaller) pencil-point needle for spinal anaesthesia in pregnant women. The use of 25- or 27-gauge needles has lowered the incidence of post-dural-puncture headache to less than 1% [21].

The most common local anaesthetic used for spinal anaesthesia is 0.5% hyperbaric bupivacaine. However, bupivacaine 0.75%, lidocaine 2% or 5%, and ropivacaine 0.5% or 0.75% are alternatives. Hyperbaric preparations (with added glucose to make the solution 'heavy') are popular, as gravity helps direct the spread of local anaesthesia selectively and produces a more predictable block.

The addition of short-acting, lipid soluble opioids (e.g. fentanyl, sufentanil) improve the quality and success of the spinal block and reduces the total amount of local anaesthetic required. The latter effect is desirable as large local anaesthetic doses are associated with increased hypotension (see 'Hypotension'). Moreover, the addition of a long-acting opioid (e.g. morphine, diamorphine) provides excellent post-operative analgesia.

Other additives which may improve the quality or duration of the spinal block include epinephrine (adrenaline) and clonidine, although these are not used widely.

All the quantities of drugs used in spinal anaesthesia are small and hence there is insignificant amount of transfer to the fetus.

In experienced hands, spinal anaesthesia can be administered quickly, and there may be little difference between the time of decision to caesarean section and delivery when compared with general anaesthesia. The decision to delivery time in Category 1 sections has been shown to be prolonged by 7–8 minutes when SSS anaesthesia is used [22, 23]. There are insufficient data to suggest that this time difference causes adverse outcomes for the fetus, although there is evidence to show that excessive use of ephedrine to correct hypotension induced by spinal anaesthesia is associated with increased fetal acidosis [24].

The time from decision to delivery is dependent on the coordinated efforts of a number of individuals, including midwives, obstetricians, operating theatre staff, paediatricians, and anaesthetists. Attempts to shorten the anaesthetic time without addressing other contributing factors will very likely lead to an increased incidence of anaesthesia-related maternal complications. Certainly, some clinical scenarios, for example prolonged fetal bradycardia, will necessitate rapid delivery.

Despite the relatively small difference in speed between spinal and general anaesthesia, in extremely urgent situations it may be preferred to use general anaesthesia, since spinals are sometimes unexpectedly difficult to perform or slow in onset, irrespective of the experience of the anaesthetist. The decision to use general anaesthesia is best made by personnel (i.e., the anaesthetist and obstetrician) present at the time of the urgent situations (Category 1 caesarean section), as they must collectively balance the risks between general anaesthesia (i.e. mostly airway and intubation issues) and spinal anaesthesia (unexpected difficulty or slow onset of block).

Epidural anaesthesia for caesarean section

In epidural anaesthesia, local anaesthetic drugs are administered into the epidural space to inhibit sensory nerve roots, either via a one-shot technique, or more commonly via a catheter for multiple dosing. The epidural space is found by a 'loss-of-resistance' technique using air or saline in a special low-resistance syringe attached to a relatively large-bore (16- or 18-gauge) Tuohy (epidural) needle; the epidural catheter is then threaded into the epidural space through the epidural needle and can remain in situ throughout labour.

Epidural anaesthesia is rarely used de novo for elective caesarean section but, in resource-rich countries, epidurals are commonly used for analgesia in labour. If caesarean section becomes necessary, additional doses of anaesthetic solutions can be administered through the epidural catheter to achieve surgical anaesthesia for emergency caesarean section. However, a poorly functioning epidural in labour should alert the anaesthetist to the possibility of failure to produce surgical anaesthesia through the use of the epidural catheter, and alternative techniques should be considered.

Local anaesthetic agents such as bupivacaine, ropivacaine, lidocaine, and 2-chloroprocaine are used for epidural anaesthesia in caesarean section, with opioids and/or other supplemental drugs often added. The speed of onset of anaesthesia for these agents is variable, and a recent meta-analysis [25] suggested the fastest onset is achieved when 2% lidocaine with epinephrine is used; a block to T4 can be achieved within 10 minutes (mean). This time may be further reduced if fentanyl is added to the mixture, and it is not uncommon for anaesthetists to use complex mixtures including bupivacaine, lidocaine, epinephrine, opioid, and bicarbonate to create a rapid onset epidural mixture. However, if this practice is used, anaesthetists should be aware of the risks of inadvertent drugs errors being made, particularly when complex mixtures are being used in an emergency situation.

Epidural anaesthesia offers an advantage over SSS in that it can be supplemented during surgery should the mother experience pain or if surgery is prolonged. In addition, if an epidural catheter is already present for labour analgesia, it is a relatively simple procedure to add additional medication for surgery.

Disadvantages of epidural anaesthesia include the fact that the volumes and doses administered via this route are up to *ten times* the amount used in spinal blocks, and hence there is possibility of systemic toxicity.

Insertion and management of epidural anaesthesia requires considerably more skill and training than the spinal technique, is more expensive, and carries with it additional inherent risks. In the low-resource setting, the lack of appropriately skilled professionals, coupled with the additional expense, may preclude the routine use of this technique.

Combined spinal–epidural anaesthesia for caesarean section

Here, the two techniques of spinal and epidural anaesthesia are combined and can be administered sequentially (spinal followed by epidural anaesthesia, or epidural followed by spinal anaesthesia), or more commonly performed via a needle-through-needle technique: the epidural space is located with a Tuohy needle through which a fine-bore spinal needle is introduced to penetrate the dura and deposit local anaesthetic mix into the subarachnoid space. A catheter is then threaded into the epidural space.

The combined spinal–epidural anaesthesia (CSE) technique remains a source of debate among obstetric anaesthetists. Advocates argue that it couples the speed of onset of SSS, with the option of intraoperative supplementation via the epidural catheter should it be required. Furthermore, the amount of local anaesthetic administered via the spinal component can be reduced, thus reducing the incidence of hypotension. Detractors note the increased degree of training and expertise that is required, the additional costs, and the data from the NAP3, conducted by the Royal College of Anaesthetists, which suggests there to be disproportionately greater risk of long-term neurological complications from CSE than from either spinal or epidural techniques alone [16].

Again, the requirements for additional training and expertise, and the added costs of equipment reduce the attractiveness of this technique in the low-resource setting.

Complications and side effects of regional anaesthesia

Data from the NAP3 have confirmed the overall relative safety of regional anaesthesia in obstetric patients and show that there is a lower rate of serious long-term complications from regional anaesthesia when used in obstetric patients than when used in non-obstetric patients [16].

Nevertheless, the anaesthetist must be trained to recognize and deal effectively with complications when they do occur. In South Africa, maternal death related to spinal anaesthesia has been on the rise. In the last National Committee on Confidential Enquiry into Maternal Deaths triennial report (2008–2010), two-thirds of the 93 deaths attributed to anaesthesia occurred in patients having spinal blockade. Farina and Rout have suggested that this high proportion may reflect the misconception that spinal anaesthesia is inherently safe and can be administered with minimal training [26]. Additionally, in seven of the cases, the patient had spinal anaesthesia administered by the surgeon and care handed over to non-medically qualified personnel while the surgeon proceeded with the operation. Though such practice may reflect under-resourcing and may be common in resource-poor areas, it cannot be considered typically acceptable or safe.

Hypotension

Spinal anaesthesia invariably produces a degree of sudden-onset sympathetic block resulting in peripheral vasodilatation and a fall in blood pressure. This condition is often accompanied by a compensatory tachycardia and, if the drop in pressure is severe, nausea and vomiting (posing an airway risk). On occasion, the sympathetic block may be of sufficient extent to inhibit the cardiac accelerator fibres (T1–T4) and thereby precipitate cardiovascular collapse. The incidence of hypotension may be lower with epidurals and also with CSEs if smaller spinal doses are used.

Thus, strategies to promptly recognize and treat hypotension should be in place. Positioning the patient in the left lateral tilt to alleviate aortocaval compression is mandatory and, if not done, will worsen the situation by impeding venous return to the right heart. On occasion, it may be necessary to manually displace the gravid uterus to recover blood pressure. Preloading with intravenous crystalloid fluids before spinal anaesthesia has not been shown to be beneficial, although co-administration of a crystalloid *during* the development of the block is effective in the short term and is an appropriate strategy [27]. Colloids have been shown to be of increased benefit but are relatively expensive, carry a low but important risk of anaphylaxis, and may not be readily available in low-resourced environments. Other techniques such as compression stockings applied to the legs have variable success.

Vasopressors are the cornerstone of blood pressure control, and regional anaesthesia should not be performed unless they are readily available. Ephedrine, metaraminol, and phenylephrine are the most commonly used agents. Recent evidence suggests that the pure alpha-1 adrenergic agonist, phenylephrine, is the agent of choice. Phenylephrine has been shown to result in a higher fetal pH when compared to ephedrine for intraoperative blood pressure control [24]. Phenylephrine can be administered as a bolus or by infusion. Again, familiarity with the agent is required for safe practice.

Phenylephrine may cause a reflex bradycardia which is associated with a fall in cardiac output and therefore may not be the most suitable vasopressor when heart rates are low to begin with. In such cases the alpha- and beta-adrenergic effects of ephedrine may be preferable, as would be the use of a vagolytic agent such as glycopyrronium or atropine. Meticulous attention to cardiovascular parameters is required to ensure safety of mother and child.

High block/total spinal block

High sensory-motor blocks occur when the spread of local anaesthetic extends above the desired level. Such spread can occur unexpectedly during spinal or epidural anaesthesia and may be more common in obese women and those of short stature than in others. However, this event also may be a result of poor management of patient position or excessive dosing of regional anaesthetic drugs. Typically, high blocks are accompanied by hypotension and bradycardia, paraesthesia and numbness of the arms, and shortness of breath as the intercostal muscles become paralysed.

Careful monitoring of the developing sensory and motor block in the first few minutes after giving the spinal or epidural drugs is necessary. In the event of a block spreading too high and too quickly, head-up tilt may prevent further cephalad spread.

Excessively high block of the C3, C4, or C5 nerve roots may impair diaphragmatic function and airway protective reflexes and, if severely compromised, the patient is likely to require intubation and ventilation.

'Total spinal' block is the extreme version of this situation and may occur suddenly when a large dose of additional epidural drug is given through an epidural catheter which has migrated intrathecally, producing a massive dose spinal anaesthetic. Total spinal block manifests itself as a rapid loss of consciousness associated with cardiorespiratory collapse. Management is supportive.

Inadequate block/failed spinal block

Although spinal anaesthesia is widely considered the most reliable and effective regional anaesthetic technique for caesarean section, the incidence of suboptimal sensory block is not infrequent, even in resource-rich countries. In the United Kingdom, conversion to general anaesthesia because of inadequate spinal anaesthesia is required in approximately 0.5% of cases; however, in resource-poor countries, the prevalence may be as high as 6% [28]. Conversion rates for epidurals that had been used for caesarean section after being used for labour are higher than those for spinals. Hence, the anaesthesia provider relying on regional anaesthesia must also be able to deliver a safe general anaesthetic for the obstetric patient and to manage a potentially difficult airway.

Except in an emergency situation and with the patient's consent, surgery should not commence before adequate anaesthesia has been achieved. Testing of the sensory and motor block before allowing surgery to start will usually alert the anaesthetist to a suboptimal block, whereupon, if time allows, appropriate alternative strategies can be undertaken. Such strategies include repeating the spinal, adding additional medication through the epidural, or performing general anaesthesia if warranted by the clinical situation.

The difficulty for the anaesthetist arises when patients feel discomfort after the start of surgery, which occasionally happens despite an apparently adequate block at the outset. The reasons for inadequate blocks are multifactorial and include operator error, inadequate amounts of drugs, anatomical variation, and prolonged surgery. Strategies to deal with failed spinals should be in place, and failed spinal/epidural algorithms may be useful.

Effective communication between the anaesthetist and the obstetrician is important in addressing this scenario. If the patient experiences pain, surgery should stop immediately and, if the fetus has not yet been delivered, conversion to general anaesthesia is often the most appropriate response. If pain is experienced after delivery, administration of intravenous analgesics such as ketamine and/or opioids should be considered. Entonox (nitrous oxide/oxygen mixture) inhalation, if it is available, can be useful in this situation. Pain and discomfort also may be reduced if the surgeon can limit manipulation of the abdominal contents. At all times, the mother should be kept advised on the actions taken, and general anaesthesia should be offered if the pain is unresolved.

Post-dural-puncture headache

Even with smaller pencil-point needles, post-dural-puncture headache can occur after uneventful spinal anaesthesia. With epidurals, the risk of accidental dural puncture is generally considered to be in the region of 1% but, since epidural needles are of large calibre (16- to 18-gauge), there is a very high risk of consequently developing post-dural-puncture headache (70%).

The headache occurs because the continued CSF leak from the puncture site creates a state of low intracranial pressure. This low-pressure state is thought to induce traction on the intracranial meninges and veins, resulting in headache. The cardinal features are frontal and/or occipital headache worsened by standing or sitting, as gravity further enhances the traction. Additional features such as photo- or phonophobia, nausea, vomiting, or tinnitus may be present [21]. The headache presents within 48 hours in 90% of cases, although there can be a delay of up to 7 days, and usually resolves through natural healing of the dural hole in 1–2 weeks.

Management is dependent on the severity. Oral analgesics (e.g. paracetamol, NSAIDs, and/or simple opioids) may be useful in mild cases. It is important to keep the patient well hydrated. Various other therapies including caffeine have been trialled, but there is little evidence supporting their use. Caffeine may paradoxically make the clinical situation worse by keeping the mother awake.

The only potentially curative treatment for post-dural-puncture headache is epidural blood patch (EBP), and this procedure should be offered to patients with severe or prolonged post-dural-puncture headache symptoms. EBP should be performed by an anaesthetist experienced in epidural anaesthesia, to minimize the risk of further complications. The procedure involves locating the epidural space again with a Tuohy needle and giving approximately 20 ml of autologous blood into the epidural space. Resolution of the headache is often rapid, but the exact mechanism by which the blood patch has its desired effect is unknown; explanations suggesting it creates a physical plug over the offending hole may be overly simplistic.

Apart from the debilitating headache, a persistent CSF leak can cause sufficient traction on vessels to create subdural haematomas [29]. In such circumstances, the nature of the headache is likely to change and other neurological signs may present; thus, patients with unresolved post-dural-puncture headache should always be followed up.

Headaches following regional techniques should not automatically be attributed to post-dural-puncture headache. A careful history and examination should be performed to rule out other causes such as meningitis, pre-eclampsia, cortical vein thrombosis, and subarachnoid haemorrhage.

Neurological complications after neuraxial anaesthesia

The incidence of neurological deficit after delivery in the obstetric population approaches 1%. Most of these issues are transient, due mainly to the mechanics of pregnancy and delivery, and not related to neuraxial anaesthesia. Risk factors have been shown to be primiparity, prolonged second stage, and the use of forceps [30].

Neural injuries directly caused by regional anaesthesia techniques are rare in the obstetric population. The NAP3 has estimated that permanent nerve damage as a consequence of regional anaesthesia has an incidence of 0.2–1.2 : 100,000 [16]. Overall, there was evidence that the incidence of complications after neuraxial block for obstetric indications is extremely low. However, although the numbers were small, there appears to be a higher incidence of complications after combined spinal–epidural anaesthesia compared to spinal or epidural techniques alone.

The majority of obstetric-related injuries result in sensory loss, and a third involve motor fibres. The commonest lesions are areas of numbness or pain on the lateral and anterior aspects of the thigh. This is meralgia paraesthetica and is due to compression of the lateral cutaneous nerve of the thigh, sometimes with the femoral nerve, against the inguinal ligament. Risk factors include obesity, diabetes, and prolonged hip flexion. The common peroneal nerve may also be compressed while in stirrups, resulting in foot drop. Compression of the lumbosacral plexus by the descending fetal head can also result in foot drop. Other nerve palsies include obturator and femoral neuropathy.

Other common side effects of regional anaesthesia

Shivering and shaking is often seen and may interfere with monitoring and surgery, as well as cause distress to the patient. Though unpleasant, this condition usually resolves spontaneously. The cause is unknown and varies from patient to patient.

Nausea and vomiting is a common problem and can pose a risk to the airway. The cause is usually hypotension or vagal hyperactivity. Although appropriate management of hypotension will usually alleviate nausea, occasionally anti-emetics may be necessary.

Itch can also be problematic intra- or post-operatively when neuraxial opioids are used. It responds poorly to treatment with chlorpheniramine. Small doses of intramuscular naloxone (typically 2 µg/kg) may be more effective than chlorpheniramine would be.

Local anaesthetic infiltration

Local infiltration techniques may be useful when a surgeon is working alone, with no anaesthetic equipment or services, such as in low-resource areas [31]. This technique typically is not practised in resource-rich environments, and few surgeons/obstetricians are adequately trained in its use. The procedure involves the sequential infiltration of the skin, rectus sheath, peritoneum, and visceral peritoneum of the uterus with local anaesthetic (e.g. lidocaine). Epinephrine at a dilution of 1:200,000 is usually added to the lidocaine to allow a large dose to be used safely. Furthermore, epinephrine can help curtail bleeding at the incision site and facilitate an improved surgical field. Patients should be warned of discomfort, and surgery should proceed, if possible, without the use of retractors or packs.

General anaesthesia for caesarean section

Over the decades, there has been a move away from general anaesthesia for caesarean section in resource-rich countries, as regional anaesthesia is generally considered safer and better than general anaesthesia in most circumstances. However, when there is immediate threat to life of mother or baby, or regional anaesthesia is contraindicated (see Table 7.3), general anaesthesia may be needed. With adequate training and cohesive teamwork, general anaesthesia can be established promptly.

Provision for general anaesthesia is usually more complicated and more expensive than for regional anaesthesia, since considerably more equipment and drugs are required. Such provision requires financial and infrastructure investment, maintenance of equipment, and a reliable supply of drugs and anaesthetic gases (see Table 7.4).

In the knowledge that oxygen saturations fall very quickly in pregnant women after induction of anaesthesia, it is absolutely necessary to pre-oxygenate the patient properly, that is, replace as much air in the lungs with oxygen as possible, such as through application of 100% oxygen via a tight-fitting mask (i.e. one with no leaks). Where time permits, this should be for 3 minutes but, in an emergency situation, 5 vital capacity breaths are almost as effective.

Thiopentone has long been the induction agent of choice but increasingly propofol is used. In haemodynamically unstable patients, etomidate or ketamine may be chosen to provide a more stable induction (i.e. less associated hypotension).

Because of the increased risk of pulmonary aspiration, tracheal intubation following rapid sequence induction with cricoid pressure is still considered obligatory when general anaesthesia is administered for caesarean section. Suxamethonium remains the primary relaxant of choice, having the fastest onset of all relaxants. Although supraglottic airway devices (e.g. laryngeal mask, I-Gel, LMA Proseal) have become the mainstay of elective non-obstetric anaesthesia, they have no place in routine general anaesthesia for caesarean section since they do not protect the airway from aspiration.

General anaesthesia is usually maintained with an inhalational agent such as sevoflurane or isoflurane but, in resource-poor areas, halothane or ether may still be in use. Nitrous oxide is often included in the gas mix because of its vapour-sparing and

Table 7.4 **Anaesthesia for pre-eclampsia/eclampsia**

Condition	Comments
Pre-eclampsia and eclampsia	Regional anaesthesia generally preferred (coagulation permitting)
	Spinal anaesthesia commonly used
	Regional anaesthesia induced hypotension less than expected
	Higher risk of pulmonary oedema
	Pressor response of general anaesthesia needs to be controlled to reduce risks of cerebral haemorrhage/cardiac ischaemia: opioids, beta blockers, $MgSO_4$
	Risks of airway oedema/difficult intubation

analgesic properties, and a minimum of 50% oxygen is recommended before delivery of the baby to optimize fetal oxygenation in utero. Anaesthetic vapours cause relaxation of the uterus and may result in increased bleeding and, while a Cochrane review of over 1700 patients showed greater blood loss in caesarean sections under general compared to regional anaesthesia, there was no difference in transfusion requirements between the groups [32]. However, when uterine atony is present, it may be prudent to turn off the anaesthetic vapour and maintain anaesthesia with an intravenous agent instead (e.g. propofol).

An anaesthetic machine is required to provide anaesthetic vapours and ventilation; such machines range from the highly sophisticated to the simple-to-use, simple-to-maintain draw-over devices still in use in resource-poor areas (where there may be no reliable electricity or pressurized gas supplies).

There is always a balance to be drawn between giving the mother adequate anaesthesia to guarantee unconsciousness/prevent awareness and giving an excessively deep anaesthetic which then depresses the baby; for this reason, opioid analgesia is usually not given until after delivery of the baby. Ideally, a multimodal approach will be taken with respect to analgesia, incorporating opioid, non-steroidal analgesic agent, and paracetamol, as well as local anaesthesia infiltration to the wound. Recently, interest has been shown in the use of transversus abdominis plane (TAP) blocks, which can provide prolonged and effective post-operative analgesia after caesarean section (see 'Analgesia in the post-operative period following caesarean section').

At the end of the operation, residual muscle relaxant should be reversed, and the patient extubated fully awake (i.e. with good airway reflexes present) either head down on the side, or sitting upright. She should then be monitored in a monitored setting (i.e. a recovery room) until fully awake. Recent maternal mortality reports from the United Kingdom show that patients are still at risk of airway and respiratory compromise after the end of the operation and that they need close observation during this time [1]. The components of safe general anaesthesia are summarized in Box 7.2.

> **Box 7.2 Components of safe general anaesthesia**
>
> Components of safe general anaesthesia include:
> - Antacid prophylaxis (ranitidine, sodium citrate);
> - Preoxygenation (supply of oxygen);
> - Anaesthetic machine;
> - Monitoring equipment;
> - Drugs (induction agent, muscle relaxants, inhalation agent, analgesia, reversal);
> - Rapid sequence induction (training, suxamethonium);
> - Tracheal intubation (laryngoscope, tracheal tubes, difficult airway equipment);
> - Ventilation (ventilator or manual bag squeeze);
> - Inhaled vapours to maintain anaesthesia (vaporizer, agent, nitrous oxide);
> - Monitoring in immediate post-operative recovery period (training, staff).

Failed intubation

Failed intubation is one of the most stressful and acute of anaesthetic crises and, unless prompt and appropriate action is taken by the anaesthetist, the mother may die from hypoxia. An old adage is that 'women don't die from failed intubation, they die from failure to stop trying to intubate.' Thus, having failed to intubate, the main priority is to ventilate the patient to regain adequate oxygenation.

Achieving this end may mean bagging the patient with a face mask and airway. Increasingly anaesthetists are becoming familiar with supraglottic airways and may use one of these devices in order to maintain oxygenation, even though such devices do not protect against aspiration.

Assuming airway manoeuvres improve oxygenation, the anaesthetist may try to intubate again; but, if this attempt is unsuccessful, the anaesthetist will need to make a decision on whether to wake the mother up or to allow surgery to proceed with what will always be considered a suboptimal airway (and one which is unprotected from aspiration of gastric contents).

This decision will be based on the relative security of the airway, the clinical indications for caesarean section, and the experience of the anaesthetist, but there is a strong argument which says anaesthetists should always wake a mother up after failed intubation rather than proceeding with a suboptimal unprotected airway *unless the caesarean section is being performed for maternal life-saving reasons (e.g. haemorrhage, collapse).* The safety of the mother will be considered to outweigh any perceived risks to the baby, even in the case of non-reassuring fetal status.

In this situation, which is stressful not just for the anaesthetist but also for the obstetric team, good communication and collective understanding of relevant issues and needs are crucial.

If the lungs cannot be ventilated using routine rescue techniques, including the use of supraglottic airways, then cricothyroidotomy or tracheostomy is the next step. Anaesthetists can prepare for unexpected failed intubation by using simulation-based scenarios in training sessions.

Intravenous ketamine for caesarean section

Ketamine is commonly used in resource-poor countries as an induction agent and also as a sole anaesthetic agent without intubation and other aspects of traditional general anaesthesia. It causes a 'dissociative anaesthesia' by inhibiting the connections between thalamo-cortical and limbic systems, resulting in a trance-like state with profound anaesthesia. Importantly, cardiovascular stability and respiratory reflexes are maintained, and ketamine is popular in the low-resource setting, where it is sometimes used as the sole anaesthetic agent without airway control. There is still potential for aspiration of gastric contents, but the risk of this is not well quantified and probably low.

Ketamine stimulates salivary secretions, and an antisialogogue (e.g. atropine) is commonly used to control this side effect. Post-operative delirium is common and may be attenuated by a small dose of a benzodiazepine given after delivery of the baby. Ketamine does not provide optimal surgical conditions as there is no muscle relaxation, and tonic contraction of the uterus can make disengagement of the fetal head difficult in obstructed labour. Furthermore, patients under ketamine often have involuntary movements and phonate, which both surgeon and anaesthetist will need to handle.

This technique, although probably quite common in resource-poor settings, cannot be considered best practice. There is very little published data on the use of ketamine as sole anaesthetic agent for caesarean section, and the World Health Organization advises that this technique be reserved for situations when equipment and anaesthetic expertise are unavailable. However, there also is no evidence to suggest that it is any less safe than an inexperienced, poorly trained, unsupported anaesthetist trying to deliver a traditional intubation-based anaesthetic in a low-resource setting [33].

Anaesthesia for pre-eclampsia

Regional anaesthesia is the preferred technique for women presenting with pre-eclampsia or eclampsia and many may have epidural analgesia instigated in labour before presenting for caesarean section (see Table 7.5). Eclampsia is not in itself a contraindication to regional anaesthesia, providing coagulation status and level of consciousness are acceptable. Following an eclamptic convulsion, administration of $MgSO_4$ and blood pressure control should be considered a prerequisite before rushing to emergency caesarean section.

Spinal anaesthesia, which traditionally has been avoided in severe pre-eclampsia because of concerns about an increased risk of hypotension, is now considered a safe and appropriate technique to use [34].

The endothelial dysfunction in pre-eclampsia causes leaky capillaries, and patients with pre-eclampsia are at particular risk of developing pulmonary

Table 7.5 Summary of pros and cons of anaesthesia for caesarean section

	Comments	Pros	Cons
Local infiltration	'Squirt-and-cut' technique by surgeon	May be useful where no anaesthetic services are available	Few surgeons have the training to perform this now Relatively uncomfortable for patient Risk of local anaesthetic toxicity
Spinal anaesthesia	Probably commonest technique worldwide Simple, easy to learn technique Currently the commonest cause of anaesthesia-related mortality in South Africa	Quick to perform Reliable dense block Cheap Little airway risk (but NB: having an airway-competent practitioner present is essential) Generally considered very safe Mother awake, so mother–baby bonding can occur rapidly Neuraxial opioid may be given for post-op analgesia	Finite duration of block (~2 hours) Hypotension Vasopressors may be needed Fetal acidosis associated with high ephedrine use Low risk of post-dural-puncture headache
Epidural anaesthesia	Usually for women who already have an epidural for labour analgesia	Top-up is easy if epidural already in situ Duration of block may be extended ad infinitum by top-ups Mother awake. so mother–baby bonding can occur rapidly Neuraxial opioid may be given for post-op analgesia	May take longer than to work than spinal anaesthesia would Large-dose local anaesthesia More complicated than spinal anaesthesia Risk of local anaesthetic toxicity/total spinal block Risk of dural tap and post-dural-puncture headache
Combined spinal–epidural anaesthesia	Popular among a minority of enthusiasts Usually needle-thru-needle technique	Potential benefits of fast spinal with extendable titratable epidural block Mother awake, so mother–baby bonding can occur rapidly Neuraxial opioid may be given for post-op analgesia	Most complicated regional anaesthesia technique Requires additional equipment Requires a long learning curve Potential side effects/complications of both spinal and epidural anaesthesia Disproportionately high neurological complication rate compared to spinal or epidural anaesthesia alone
General anaesthesia	The default fall-back technique when regional anaesthesia not possible or contraindicated Intubation with rapid sequence induction expected Indicated for sick and unstable patients Indicated for very urgent caesarean section	Fast(est), most reliable technique Mother asleep Airway secure (once intubated) Can be used to manage unstable patients	Training required Complex equipment required Risks of failed intubation/aspiration Risk of uterine atony/increased blood loss Risk of awareness Post-op pain relief may be problematic Post-op nausea and vomiting Drug transfer to baby; neonatal depression Delayed mother–baby bonding
Ketamine (sole agent)	May be useful in resource-poor settings where no (or poorly trained/poorly equipped) anaesthetic practitioners are available Produces dissociative-type anaesthesia Frequency of use in resource-poor settings unclear, but little documentation in literature	Minimal equipment required Cheap Patients maintain their own airway Supports blood pressure	Patients may move during surgery Safety not established Small (unquantified) risk of aspiration Post-op delirium

oedema if excessive intravenous fluids are administered; correspondingly, intravenous fluid management should be prudent.

General anaesthesia is indicated in a minority of cases in which neuraxial techniques are contraindicated, most commonly when coagulopathy has developed. General anaesthesia provides particular challenges in this group of patients, compounding the usual problems of general anaesthesia with additional risks: the airway is likely to be oedematous, and visualization of the glottis may prove difficult or even impossible, leading to difficult or failed intubation [35, 36].

Importantly, the hypertensive response to laryngoscopy is exaggerated in pre-eclampsia and, unless attenuated in some way, this response may cause intracranial haemorrhage or cardiac ischaemia. Short-acting opioids (e.g. such alfentanil,

fentanyl, and remifentanil), $MgSO_4$, and beta blockers all may be used. Since no single drug or combination has been shown to be superior, the drug(s) used to control the hypertensive response should be dictated by drug availability and familiarity to the anaesthetist. If opioids are used before delivery of the baby, it is prudent to be prepared for a degree of neonatal respiratory depression, since these drugs readily cross the placenta.

Emergence from anaesthesia is also a crucial period, as the blood pressure is likely to spike during extubation. Conscientious attention to prevent undue blood pressure rises is required. In this setting, opioids may delay emergence, and short-acting beta blockers may be more appropriate. Post-operatively, these patients require increased levels of monitoring and care.

Analgesia in the post-operative period following caesarean section

Immediate post-operative monitoring in a dedicated recovery unit by staff trained in recovery skills should follow all caesarean sections, regardless of the mode of anaesthesia. This approach is to ensure that early complications of surgery and anaesthesia can be quickly detected and managed. Vital signs, including the respiratory rate, oxygen saturations, temperature, blood pressure, heart rate, and heart rhythm, are normally assessed at short intervals. Additionally, pain scores, nausea scores, and the level of consciousness are all documented [1]. Patients who have received neuraxial anaesthesia should have the residual level of block, and its disappearance, recorded before discharge.

Pain following caesarean section is both somatic (form the skin, fascia, and muscles) and visceral (peritoneum, visceral structures) in origin. Adequate pain control enables mothers to mobilize earlier, thereby reducing the risk of thromboembolic events, and enhancing bonding with her baby [37].

When regional techniques are used, opioids (e.g. morphine, diamorphine) may be administered via the intrathecal (spinal) or epidural route to confer effective analgesia, which lasts between 12 and 24

hours. This technique is very much preferred in resource-rich countries, and the dose of opioids administered is sufficiently small that there is a very low concentration systematically and transfer to the breast milk is clinically insignificant.

Parenteral opioids are the mainstay of post-operative management in those who have had a general anaesthetic for caesarean section or in those for whom opioids given through a regional technique are contraindicated. Patient-controlled analgesia systems are widely used in resource-rich areas, although cost, complexity, and security issues limit their availability in resource-poor countries.

As part of the multimodal approach, paracetamol and NSAIDs (if not contraindicated) may also be given. While opioids in general are useful in controlling visceral pain, agents such as NSAIDs will reduce inflammation in the tissue and reduce somatic pain.

The use of local anaesthetics to infiltrate around the wound and to block afferent nerves is another useful adjunct. Wound infiltration with agents such as 0.5% bupivacaine can give a few hours of post-operative analgesia, but in general the effects are relatively short-lived. Nerve blocks (e.g. ilioinguinal, hypogastric) and rectus sheath catheters may be useful in reducing opioid consumption.

Recently, there has been growing interest in the use of the TAP block, where local anaesthetics are deposited between the internal oblique and the transverse abdominis muscles, either under ultrasound guidance or blindly by using a landmark technique. TAP blocks have been shown to be effective and reduce both 24- and 48-hour opioid requirements [38, 39].

Key learning points

1. Regional anaesthesia (spinal, epidural, CSE) is the default technique for caesarean section unless contraindicated.
2. For Category 1 caesarean section (imminent threat to life of mother or baby), there should be discussion between the obstetrician and anaesthetist regarding whether there is time to attempt a regional technique or whether general anaesthesia is required.
3. Pain during caesarean section under ineffective regional anaesthesia is the commonest cause of obstetric anaesthesia-related litigation.
4. Serious long-term complications following regional anaesthesia are extremely rare.
5. The risk of aspiration of gastric contents mandates the use of rapid sequence induction and intubation when general anaesthesia is required for caesarean section.
6. In the event of failed intubation at general anaesthesia for caesarean section, consideration for the mother's life and well-being will take precedence over that of the fetus.
7. Effective team work and continual communication between anaesthetists, obstetricians, and midwives is mandatory for the safety of mother and baby.
8. Headaches after regional anaesthesia warrant full investigation and must not be solely attributed to dural puncture.
9. In women with pre-eclampsia, regional anaesthesia is preferred. General anaesthesia should only be conducted by experienced anaesthetists, and blood pressure control at induction and emergence is crucial.
10. Following a caesarean section, the mother must be observed in a dedicated recovery area by adequately trained staff prior to discharge to the ward.

References

1. Centre for Maternal and Child Enquiries. Saving Mothers' Lives: Reviewing maternal deaths to make motherhood safer: 2006–2008. The Eighth Report on Confidential Enquiries into Maternal Deaths in the United Kingdom. BJOG 2011; 118(1): 1–203.
2. Kinsella S. Anaesthetic deaths in the CMACE (Centre for Maternal and Child Enquiries) Saving Mothers' Lives report 2006-08. Anaesthesia 2011; 66(4): 243–54.
3. Hawkins JL, Chang J, Palmer SK, Gibbs CP, Callaghan WM. Anesthesia-related maternal mortality in the United States: 1979–2002. Obstet Gynecol 2011; 117(1): 69–74.
4. Farina Z, Rout C. 'But it's just a spinal': Combating increasing rates of maternal death related to spinal anaesthesia. S Afr Med J 2012; 103(2): 81–2.
5. Okafor U, Ezegwui H. Maternal deaths during caesarean delivery in a developing country: Perspective from Nigeria. Int J Third World Med 2008; 8(1): http://ispub.com/IJTWM/8/1/4858t.
6. Fenton PM, Whitty CJ, Reynolds F. Caesarean section in Malawi: Prospective study of early maternal and perinatal mortality. Br Med J 2003; 327(7415): 587.
7. Hansen D, Gausi SC, Merikebu M. Anaesthesia in Malawi: Complications and deaths. Trop Doct 2000; 30(3): 146–9.
8. Obstetric Anaesthetists' Association. National Obstetric Anaesthesia Data for 2011: A Report. 2013. http://www.oaa-anaes.ac.uk/assets/_managed/editor/File/NOAD/NOAD%202011%20final.pdf.
9. Pattinson B. Reducing maternal deaths. S Afr J Obstet Gynaecol 2012; 18(2): 30–1.
10. Merry AF, Cooper JB, Soyannwo O, Wilson IH, Eichhorn JH. International standards for a safe practice of anesthesia 2010. Can J Anesth 2010; 57(11): 1027–34.
11. Lifebox Foundation. Lifebox. 2015. http://www.lifebox.org.
12. Cooper GM, McClure JH. Maternal deaths from anaesthesia. An extract from *Why Mothers Die 2000–2002*, the Confidential Enquiries into Maternal Deaths in the United Kingdom: Chapter 9: Anaesthesia. Br J Anaesth 2005; 94(4): 417–23.
13. Bamigboye AA. Regional versus General Anaesthesia for Caesarean Section: RHL Commentary (Last Revised: 29 November 2007). The WHO Reproductive Health Library. Geneva: World Health Organization, 2007.
14. Russell IF. At caesarean section under regional anaesthesia, it is essential to test sensory block with light touch before allowing surgery to start. Int J Obstet Anesth 2006; 15(4): 294–7.
15. Szypula K, Ashpole KJ, Bogod D, Yentis SM, Mihai R, Scott S, Cook TM. Litigation related to regional

anaesthesia: An analysis of claims against the NHS in England 1995–2007. Anaesthesia 2010; 65(5): 443–52.

16. Cook TM, Counsell D, Wildsmith JAW. Major complications of central neuraxial block: Report on the Third National Audit Project of the Royal College of Anaesthetists. Br J Anaesth 2009; 102(2): 179–90.

17. Harrop-Griffiths W, Cook T, Gill H, Hill D, Ingram M, Makris M, et al. Regional anaesthesia and patients with abnormalities of coagulation. Anaesthesia 2013; 68(9): 966–72.

18. Royal College of Obstetricians and Gynaecologists. Reducing the risk of thrombosis and embolism during pregnancy and the puerperium: Green-top Guideline No. 37a. 2015. http://www.rcog.org.uk/globalassets/documents/guidelines/gtg-37a.pdf.

19. Broadbent CR, Maxwell WB, Ferrie R, Wilson DJ, Gawne-Cain M, Russell R. Ability of anaesthetists to identify a marked lumbar interspace. Anaesthesia 2000; 55(11): 1122–6.

20. Reynolds F. Damage to the conus medullaris following spinal anaesthesia. Anaesthesia 2001; 56(3): 238–47.

21. Turnbull DK, Shepard DB. Post-dural puncture headache: Pathogenesis, prevention and treatment. Br J Anaesth 2003; 91(5): 718–29.

22. Popham P, Buettner A, Mendola M. Anaesthesia for emergency caesarean section, 2000–2004, at the Royal Women's Hospital, Melbourne. Anaesth Intensive Care 2007; 35(1): 74–9.

23. Beckmann M, Calderbank S. Mode of anaesthetic for category 1 caesarean sections and neonatal outcomes. Aust N Z J Obstet Gynaecol 2012; 52(4): 316–20.

24. Veeser M, Hofmann T, Roth R, Klöhr S, Rossaint R, Heesen M. Vasopressors for the management of hypotension after spinal anaesthesia for elective caesarean section. Systematic review and cumulative meta-analysis. Acta Anaesthesiol Scand 2012; 56(7): 810–16.

25. Hillyard SG, Bate TE, Corcoran TB, Paech MJ, O'Sullivan G. Extending epidural analgesia for emergency Caesarean section: A meta-analysis. Br J Anaesth 2011; 107(5): 668–78.

26. Farina Z, Rout C. 'But it's just a spinal': Combating increasing rates of maternal death related to spinal anaesthesia. S Afr Med J 2013; 103(2): 81–2.

27. Cyna AM, Andrew M, Emmett RS, Middleton P, Simmons SW. Techniques for preventing hypotension during spinal anaesthesia for caesarean section. Cochrane Database Syst Rev 2006; 4: CD002251.

28. Adenekan AT, Olateju SO. Failed spinal anaesthesia for Caesarean section. J W Afr Coll Surg 2011; 1(4): 1–17.

29. Liang MY, Pagel PS. Bilateral interhemispheric subdural hematoma after inadvertent lumbar puncture in a parturient. Can J Anesth 2012; 59(4): 389–93.

30. Wong CA. Neurologic deficits and labour analgesia. Reg Anesth Pain Med 2004; 29(4): 341–51.

31. Nandagopal M. Local anaesthesia for cesarean section. Tech Reg Anesth Pain Manag 2001; 5(1): 30–5.

32. Afolabi BB, Lesi AFE, Merah NA. Regional versus general anaesthesia for caesarean section. Cochrane Database Syst Rev 2006; 4: CD004350.

33. Howell PR. Supporting the evolution of obstetric anaesthesia through outreach programs (Editorial). Int J Obstet Anesth 2009; 18(1): 1–3.

34. Henke VG, Bateman BT, Leffert LR. Spinal anesthesia in severe preeclampsia. Anesth Analg 2013; 117(3): 686–93.

35. Izci B, Riha RL, Martin SE, Vennelle M, Liston WA, Dundas KC, et al. The upper airway in pregnancy and pre-eclampsia. Am J Respir Crit Care Med 2003; 167(2): 137–40.

36. Munnur U, de Boisblanc B, Suresh MS. Airway problems in pregnancy. Crit Care Med 2005; 33(10): S259–268.

37. Verstraete S, Van de Velde M. Post-cesarean section analgesia. Acta Anaesthesiol Belg 2012; 63(4): 147–67.

38. Abdallah FW, Laffey JG, Halpern SH, Brull R. Duration of analgesic effectiveness after the posterior and lateral transversus abdominis plane block techniques for transverse lower abdominal incisions: A meta-analysis. Br J Anaesth 2013; 111(5): 721–35.

39. Abdallah FW, Halpern SH, Margarido CB. Transversus abdominis plane block for postoperative analgesia after Caesarean delivery performed under spinal anaesthesia? A systematic review and meta-analysis. Br J Anaesth 2012; 109(5): 679–87.

CHAPTER 8

Prevention and management of post-operative caesarean section complications

Philip J. Steer

Introduction

It is a truism that the best prevention of post-operative caesarean section complications is through the use of the most appropriate surgical technique for doing the operation in the first place. These techniques are covered in other chapters and so here I will cover additional prophylactic techniques, as well as the diagnosis and management of complications within the immediate post-operative period. In order of frequency of occurrence, the complications of caesarean section are haemorrhage, sepsis, and thromboembolism. I will therefore cover them in this order.

Haemorrhage following caesarean section

Diagnosis of post-partum haemorrhage

The commonest cause of post-partum haemorrhage following caesarean section is uterine atony, that is, a failure of the uterus to contract firmly. Uterine contraction controls haemorrhage by two mechanisms: the first is the so-called living ligatures effect, whereby the contracting myofibrils constrict the blood vessels passing through the myometrium; the second is by raising intrauterine pressure and thus arresting low-pressure venous oozing. When the contraction is deficient, excessive haemorrhage will result. Diagnosis of excessive haemorrhage is made by observing either more blood loss than expected or a deterioration in the maternal condition. The former is usually observed during the

procedure in response to surgical trauma, whereas the latter occurs after the abdomen has been closed; the uterus can accommodate so much blood that often the first signs of excessive haemorrhage are those of maternal cardiovascular decompensation, namely, tachycardia, hypotension, and ultimately loss of consciousness. It is therefore vital that all women are observed closely following caesarean section, with regular measurements of their pulse rate, blood pressure, level of consciousness, and per vaginam blood loss. Such measurements are often recorded using specially designed charts which were first developed in the mid-1990s. *The Seventh Report on Confidential Enquiries into Maternal Deaths in the United Kingdom*, which contains data from the years 2003–2005, recommends the use of a modified early warning score to assist in identifying the obstetric patient at risk of deterioration [1]. The rationale was that, in many cases, early warning signs of impending maternal collapse go unrecognized. This recommendation was reiterated in the subsequent triennial maternal mortality report [2].

The pharmacological approach to treating post-partum haemorrhage

The average blood loss at caesarean section is generally higher than estimated; for example, one detailed study of caesarean sections performed during labour showed that the average loss was 1106 ml [3]. For this reason, it is usual to give oxytocics to encourage uterine contraction/retraction. Historically, a widely used oxytocic after vaginal birth has been a combination of 5 IU of oxytocin (Syntocinon) and 0.5 mg of ergometrine (ergonovine) as Syntometrine. The addition of ergometrine reduces average blood loss, over and above the effect of oxytocin alone, by about 20% [4]. However, the use of ergometrine increases the risk of maternal complications such as a diastolic blood pressure greater than 100 mmHg, nausea and vomiting, and headache. Moreover, ergometrine has a specific effect causing spasm of the coronary arteries, and this effect can lead to acute myocardial infarction [5–8]. Other possible side effects include nausea, vomiting, abdominal pain, diarrhoea, headache, dizziness, tinnitus, chest pain, palpitation, bradycardia, dyspnoea, and rashes. For these reasons, its routine use is usually avoided, and it is particularly contraindicated in women with pre-existing heart disease.

Accordingly, the most commonly used routine regime following caesarean section is oxytocin alone (see Chapter 4). As almost all women having a caesarean section will have an intravenous infusion running, it is common to give the oxytocin intravenously as a *slow* intravenous injection. The acute administration of 5 units of oxytocin can cause an abrupt halving of maternal blood pressure from vasodilatation in the subcutaneous blood vessels [9], and in turn this drop in pressure can cause myocardial ischaemia [10]. The average reduction of the mean arterial blood pressure by the administration of a 5 IU bolus is 27 mmHg [11]. The uterotonic

efficacy of 2 IU is similar to that of 5 IU but as might be expected, it has fewer haemodynamic side effects [12], and Carvalho et al. have suggested that the optimum regime may be the injection of a bolus of 0.35 IU, plus continuing low-dose infusion at 40 mU/min [13]. The infusion can be continued for as long as necessary, although clinical experience suggests that no more than 4 hours of infusion is usually required.

In recent years, a long-acting synthetic oxytocin analogue, carbetocin, has been introduced in some countries. When given as a single dose, it has efficacy similar to that of an oxytocin infusion [14] but it is considerably more expensive and therefore is not currently widely used.

If the oxytocin infusion appears to be insufficient to maintain uterine contraction, one possible next step is to give prostaglandin E_1 (misoprostol). There are no scientific papers regarding the optimal doses for this purpose; however, FIGO guidelines [15] suggest 800 μg sublingually as a single dose. The most common and most serious complication of this approach is maternal hyper-pyrexia [16].

Another variety of prostaglandin that is sometimes used is prostaglandin $F_{2-alpha}$ (carboprost, Hemabate). The recommended dose is 0.25 mg, and it can be given by intramyometrial injection [17].

Intrauterine balloon in the treatment of post-partum haemorrhage

If myometrial contractility is impaired, one way of arresting venous (and to a lesser extent arterial) bleeding is to raise the intramyometrial pressure by tamponade within the cavity of the uterus. Traditionally, this procedure was done by packing the uterus with materials such as gauze swabs [18] but, in 2001, publications by Johanson [19] and Bakri [20] suggested the use of a hydrostatic balloon would be effective. These balloons are inserted through the cervix and then inflated with up to 500 ml of normal saline. The usual approach is to infuse the saline until the inflation pressure starts to rise or the bleeding stops, whichever is the earlier. There have been no randomized trials, but a number of case series have been published which suggest that balloons have approximately 80%–90% effectiveness in arresting post-partum haemorrhage [21, 22].

Uterine compression sutures in the treatment of post-partum haemorrhage

The concept of inserting longitudinal sutures into the uterus to raise the intramyometrial pressure was first described by Lynch and colleagues in 1997 [23]. The technique was originally developed to control bleeding following caesarean section, because it requires an anterior lower segment incision for insertion, as originally described. The concept is to raise the intramyometrial pressure without running sutures across the uterine cavity, so as to minimize the risk of the formation of subsequent adhesions (Figures 8.1, 8.2). The square suturing approach suggested by Cho et al. in 2000 [24] aims to obliterate the uterine cavity as well as raising intramyometrial pressure (Figure 8.3) but has been reported to lead to both pyometra [25] and synechiae [26, 27]. Another similar technique uses 'U' sutures rather than square sutures but also recommends multiple sutures to obliterate the uterine cavity [28] and has also been reported to result in synechiae [29]. The Hayman suture is similar in principle to the B-Lynch but does not require a lower segment incision (Figure 8.4) [30, 31]. An important point with all these sutures is that an absorbable suture should

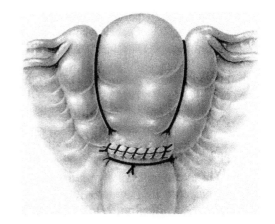

Figure 8.2 Completion of the B-Lynch uterine compression suture.

Lynch C, Coker A, Lawal AH, Abu J, Cowen MJ. The B-Lynch surgical technique for the control of massive postpartum haemorrhage: an alternative to hysterectomy? Five cases reported. BJOG 1997; 104(3):372–375.

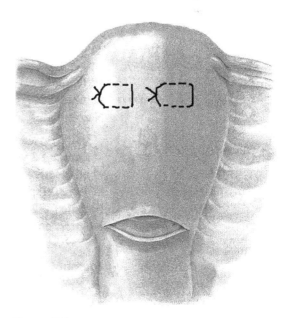

Figure 8.3 Illustration of the Cho square uterine compression suture.

Cho JH, Jun HS, Lee CN. Hemostatic suturing technique for uterine bleeding during cesarean delivery. Obstet Gynecol 2000; 96(1):129–131.

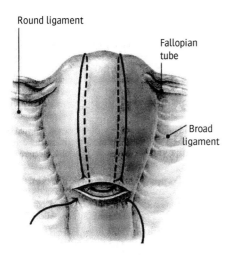

Round ligament

Fallopian tube

Broad ligament

Figure 8.1 Illustration of the suture technique for performing the original B-Lynch uterine compression suture.

Lynch C, Coker A, Lawal AH, Abu J, Cowen MJ. The B-Lynch surgical technique for the control of massive postpartum haemorrhage: an alternative to hysterectomy? Five cases reported. BJOG 1997; 104(3):372–375.

be used. Non-absorbable sutures become loose once the uterus retracts and so risk entangling the bowel or causing intra-abdominal adhesions [32]. It is also important to avoid devascularizing the uterine tissue completely, as ischaemic necrosis can result [33–38].

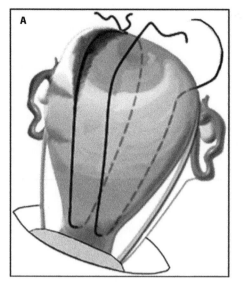 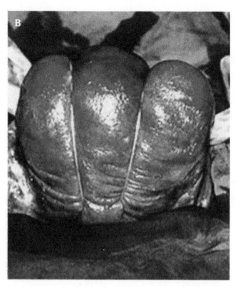

Figure 8.4 Illustration of the Hayman uterine compression suture.

Ghezzi F, Cromi A, Uccella S, Raio L, Bolis P, Surbek D. The Hayman technique: a simple method to treat postpartum haemorrhage. BJOG 2007; 114(3): 362–365.

Sometimes, the majority of uterine bleeding is from the lower segment, commonly secondary to a low implantation site of the placenta. In such cases, localized vertical compression sutures may be useful [39]; others have reported turning the cervix in upon itself and suturing it so as to include the lower segment [40].

The success rate of uterine compression sutures in controlling post-partum haemorrhage, so that a hysterectomy does not become necessary, is usually quoted as 90% or more in the case series reported. In a national UK study carried out using the UK Obstetric Surveillance System, the success rate was reported as 75% [41].There have been no randomized trials of their efficacy.

Uterine compression sutures in combination with an intrauterine balloon in the treatment of post-partum haemorrhage

The combination of uterine compression sutures and an intrauterine balloon was first suggested in 2002 and has been reported several times [42, 43] as being effective. However, there is a risk of uterine devascularization if excessive intrauterine pressure is generated against a restricting uterine compression suture. While intrauterine balloons used alone are commonly left for 24 hours before being removed, it may be wise to consider deflating the balloon after 12 hours when it is used in combination with compression sutures.

Uterine artery ligation in the treatment of post-partum haemorrhage

The uterine artery can be tied off shortly after it passes under the ureter and ascends upwards along the side of the uterus. This method has been reported to be successful in arresting bleeding, particularly if the bleeding is occurring because of an extension of the lower segment incision into the lateral part of the uterus [44]. It seems likely that uterine artery ligation is commonly performed inadvertently, when such extensions are sutured. There appear to be no serious long-term sequelae from such ligation.

Internal iliac ligation in the treatment of post-partum haemorrhage

Internal iliac ligation is a difficult technical procedure and should only be undertaken by an experienced surgeon [45]. Quoted success rates vary from 43% to 90%.

Caesarean hysterectomy in the treatment of post-partum haemorrhage

In most cases, the above manoeuvres will serve to arrest bleeding. However, if bleeding is continuing and cannot be stopped, then it may become necessary to remove the uterus (see Chapter 6). In many cases (e.g., those associated with atony) it will be sufficient to do a subtotal hysterectomy, as it is unusual for the cervix to bleed profusely. If, however, the cervix itself is bleeding (e.g. such as when a placenta praevia has been present), the cervix needs to be removed as well.

Arterial embolization in the treatment of post-partum haemorrhage

The use of micro-emboli using materials such as gel foam introduced into the internal iliac artery to block the microvasculature and arrest bleeding was first described in 1979, with a success rate in case reports of about 90% [46]. The key problem with its use is that it requires sophisticated angiography facilities and the availability of an experienced interventional radiologist 24 hours a day, 365 days a year, if it is to be relied upon as a therapy. Complications inherent in its use are radiation exposure, contrast nephrotoxicity, pelvic infections (including abscess formation), and ischaemic phenomena (tissue necrosis and buttock claudication). A 2014 audit of 117 cases in a single centre reported that 3 cases of uterine necrosis required hysterectomy (as well as 4 cases requiring hysterectomy because of a failure to control bleeding) [47].

Sepsis following caesarean section

Wound, urinary, and endometrial infections are relatively common complications of caesarean section, occurring in about 6.4% of cases [48] and higher in obese women (see Chapter 4). There are now at least 81 randomized controlled trials that have been published regarding the use of antibiotic prophylaxis at the time of caesarean section to reduce the incidence of puerperal sepsis [49]. Overall, the administration of prophylactic broad-spectrum antibiotics at the time of caesarean section results in a reduction in the incidence of episodes of fever (relative risk (RR), 0.45; 95% confidence interval (CI), 0.39–0.52), endometritis (RR, 0.39; 95% CI, 0.34–0.43), wound infection (RR, 0.41; 95% CI, 0.35–0.48), urinary tract infection (RR, 0.54; 95% CI, 0.46–0.64), and serious infection (RR, 0.42; CI, 0.28–0.65) [49]. No other prophylactic technique is known to reduce the incidence of infectious complications substantially, although preoperative skin preparation and antiseptic cleansing are usually recommended.

The most contentious issue currently is the timing of the administration of the antibiotics. Evidence summarized in the 2011 National Institute for Health and Care Excellence (NICE)/ Royal College of Obstetricians and Gynaecologists (RCOG) guideline [48] suggests that administration of the antibiotics at the start of the procedure (usually at skin incision) reduces the incidence of puerperal infection by about a third, as compared with administering the antibiotic after cord clamping. However, using this method means that a substantial amount of antibiotic will be transferred to the baby across the placenta, and the long-term implications of such transfer for the development of the baby's immune system are as yet unknown.

Wound infections and haematomas

The diagnosis of wound infection follows the classical rubric of *tumor, calor, dolor*. Translated from the Latin, this phrase means 'swelling, heat, and pain'. It is important to distinguish the swelling due to infection from that due to subcutaneous haematoma. Significant bleeding into the wound can be either behind the rectus sheath (in which case it can be substantial, cause hypotension and a significant drop in the haemoglobin concentration of the blood, and recognized by deterioration of the vital signs, i.e. tachycardia and hypotension) or between the rectus sheath and the skin. Because the latter space is limited, thus limiting the amount of blood loss, the haemodynamic effects are much less obvious but the pain is usually considerably worse because of the stretching of the tissues. If there is substantial bleeding behind the rectus sheath, the bleeding can dissect into the peritoneal cavity, causing peritonitic pain as well as acute collapse. If there is a significant deterioration in the vital signs following surgery, it is better to intervene early rather than allow the patient's condition to deteriorate and progress to a coagulopathy, which is much more difficult to correct. Re-exploration of the wound and giving the regional or general anaesthesia required in an otherwise fit patient is distressing for the patient but not usually medically dangerous; procrastination and having to operate on a patient who is already cardiovascularly collapsed is potentially lethal. In contrast, it is often better to await spontaneous resolution of subcutaneous haematomas than to reopen the wound, which often only serves to stimulate fresh bleeding. The patient should be warned that either the haematoma will resolve slowly over several weeks (often accompanied by spectacularly colourful bruising) or the clot will evacuate spontaneously through a spontaneous dehiscence of a part of the skin incision. The dehiscence will usually heal by itself by secondary intention, and resuturing is not necessary unless the dehiscence is extensive. The main complication that needs to be watched for is infection.

It should be noted in relation to wound haematomas that it was popular in the 1960s and 1970s to recommend routine drainage of the space behind the rectus sheath, sometimes with corrugated or Robertson drains, but most commonly with closed drains using suction ('Redivac'). I was personally not convinced that they were useful but instead placed emphasis on achieving thorough haemostasis before closure of the wound. In my year as a registrar, alternating with a senior registrar who routinely used drains, over the first 6 months we collected data on the incidence of haematoma in our respective patients, and when they showed no difference, he abandoned drains. This conclusion was verified by a 2013 Cochrane review which reviewed 10 trials that recruited 5248 women [50]. The review found that there was no evidence of any difference in the incidence of wound infection, other wound complications, febrile morbidity, or pain in women who had wound drains, as compared with those who did not, and some evidence that a subcutaneous drain may increase the rate of wound infection. The onset of infection is usually associated with a rise in maternal temperature. Diagnosing the cause of the maternal temperature can be difficult. Examination of the wound is useful, because the edges of the incision or bruised area will become very red, tender, and oedematous as the blood vessels become leaky and allow the transmigration of antibodies and white cells into the infected area. It can be helpful to mark the edges of the affected area with an indelible pen, and check after 12 hours to see if the area is spreading. If so, this observation suggests infection. It is important to obtain swabs for culture and then to start a broad-spectrum antibiotic in adequate dosage (it can be particularly helpful to give the first 24 or 48 hours of treatment intravenously to ensure adequate tissue levels; swelling and oedema will limit the perfusion of the area). Response should occur within 24 hours; the maternal temperature should begin to settle during the day (spikes of temperature in the evening will often persist up to 10 days, gradually becoming lower as the condition resolves), tachycardia should resolve, and the affected area should begin to shrink. If the condition remains unimproved or is worse after 48 hours, it is vital to check the results of the culture to make sure that an appropriate antibiotic is being used (check for multidrug-resistant *Staphylococcus aureus* and Group A streptococci in particular) and involve a microbiologist and a general surgeon experienced in dealing with wound infections (in many general hospitals, there is now a wound infection team which specializes in techniques such as negative pressure drainage). A particular danger is necrotizing fasciitis ('killer bug which ate my flesh') which in a previously fit patient is usually due to Group A streptococci. The incidence of this potentially lethal infection is increasing. During the twentieth century, there was a decline in its virulence, but in the last decade or so this decline appears to be reversing. The key to recognizing it is the appearance of necrotic areas of skin (these areas go grey or black); this appearance constitutes a medical/surgical emergency, as it can progress to a fatality in only a few days. Prevention, and early treatment, consists of laying open the wound with extensive debridement until healthy tissue is seen, together with intravenous high-dosage broad-spectrum antibiotics. The combination of benzylpenicillin, clindamycin, and gentamicin are commonly used (if the patient is allergic to penicillin, then meropenem can be used instead).

Endometritis following caesarean section

Following normal birth, approximately 1%–3% of women will develop an infection of the endometrium and surrounding tissues. This figure rises to approximately 5%–15% following caesarean section. If, however, there has been a caesarean following prolonged rupture of the membranes, then the incidence may be 30% or higher. Common pathogens include Group B streptococci, other streptococci, *Escherichia coli*, and *Proteus* species. Gram-negative anaerobic organisms such as *Bacteroides* species can also cause this complication. Early onset endometritis is commonly associated with a temperature in excess of 38°C, whereas late-onset endometritis is more commonly associated with small or moderate amounts of bleeding per vaginam and only a low-grade or absent fever. With early onset of a high fever, women will generally be treated with antibiotics such as penicillin/clindamycin and gentamicin, which are given intravenously.

Late-onset endometritis can be treated with oral broad-spectrum antibiotic therapy that typically uses amoxicillin and/or metronidazole.

Late-onset endometritis is often confused with bleeding due to retained products of conception. Significant retained products are very unusual following caesarean section because it is routine practice to check the uterine cavity carefully before closure to ensure that the entire placenta has been removed. A common cause of confusion is that, for up to 4–6 weeks following delivery, ultrasound scans will usually show high-level echoes because of the presence of blood clots retained within the uterine cavity. These clots may resorb completely or be passed spontaneously, particularly at the time of the first menstruation. Curettage of the uterus is not usually necessary unless there is evidence of a substantial retained placental segment (e.g. 5% or more of placental volume), or symptoms/signs fail to respond to broad-spectrum antibiotic therapy. It should be noted that fragments of endometrium removed by curettage will always show the presence of degenerating chorionic villi, as the tips of the villi remain embedded in the endometrium even after the main body of the placenta has separated. Thus, the finding of chorionic villi in evacuated material does not indicate that placenta has been 'left behind' in a negligent fashion. There is a higher risk of uterine perforation when uterine curettage is performed in the puerperium, both because of the scar left in the uterus by the procedure and because the myometrium may be softened by subsequent inflammation. Many clinicians prefer to use a blunt soft-suction catheter; monitoring the procedure with ultrasound may improve safety. Untreated or inadequately treated endometritis can result in major post-partum haemorrhage; women must be monitored until their symptoms/signs resolve.

Thromboprophylaxis following caesarean section

In pregnancy, haemostatic changes occur which reduce blood loss at the time of delivery and in the puerperium. During pregnancy, the risk of thrombosis is increased approximately 6-fold, while it is increased 11-fold in the puerperium [51]. Thrombotic risk is increased after abdominal surgery, partly because of impedance of venous return, but also because of enforced immobility. In the eighth Centre for Maternal and Child Enquiries report on maternal deaths from 2006 to 2008 in the United Kingdom [2], there were 16 deaths due to thrombosis and pulmonary embolism. This report highlighted the importance of obesity (BMI >30): nine of the affected women were obese. Six women died after caesarean section; they all died between 2 and 6 weeks after delivery (two more women died more than 42 days after caesarean section and were therefore classified as late deaths). Four of the six women were obese, and one had a BMI >40. A population-based cohort study from the United Kingdom, published in 2013, investigated the potential risk factors for venous thromboembolism; while it found that the highest risk was stillbirth, other factors, including obesity, obstetric haemorrhage, preterm delivery, and caesarean section, were also important [52]. Despite these known risks, there have been surprisingly few studies of the value of thromboprophylaxis following caesarean section. A Cochrane review published in 2014 found only one trial of thromboprophylaxis that investigated maternal mortality [53]; this trial compared 5-day versus 10-day administration of low molecular weight heparin. There were no deaths, and there were no differences seen between the two groups in terms of symptomatic thromboembolic events, symptomatic pulmonary embolism, or symptomatic deep-vein thrombosis (however, note that the number of asymptomatic cases of deep-vein thrombosis is approximately four times that of symptomatic cases). The authors estimated that about half of all post-partum acute pulmonary embolism cases follow caesarean section.

Most studies of thromboprophylaxis following caesarean section now recommend the use of low molecular weight heparin, which has a longer half-life, higher bioavailability, and a more predictable anticoagulant response than unfractionated heparin does, thus avoiding the need for dose adjustment or laboratory monitoring in most patients [53]. The main adverse effect of prophylaxis is haemorrhage. In the Cochrane review, nine studies evaluated thromboprophylaxis during and/or after caesarean section. The results suggest an approximately 60% reduction in symptomatic thromboembolic events; however, in each study, the 95% confidence intervals of the relative risks all included one and were therefore not statistically significant. The authors concluded that there was insufficient evidence on which to base recommendations for thromboprophylaxis during pregnancy and the early postnatal period. There are even fewer data on other methods of prophylaxis, such as graduated compression stockings, hydration, and early mobilization. While the 2011 NICE clinical guideline recommended the use of thromboprophylaxis following caesarean section [48], the authors of the guideline commented that 'the choice of method of prophylaxis should take into account risk of thromboembolic disease and follow existing guidelines' [54, 55]. The RCOG *Green-top Guideline 37a* recommends that all women who have had an emergency caesarean section should be considered for thromboprophylaxis with low molecular weight heparin for 7 days after delivery, as should those women who have had an elective caesarean section and who have one or more additional risk factors (such as age >35 years or BMI >30) [54]. These guidelines were graded as Level C (systematic review of case-control or cohort studies).

Bladder injury following caesarean section

The overall likelihood of bladder injury at the time of an uncomplicated caesarean is low (about 1 in 300 cases) but is more likely if there was a previous caesarean, especially with dense adhesions, when the risk rises to 1 in 25. Most injuries are to the dome of the bladder rather than the trigone, and the key is to recognize them at the time of surgery. Defects should be closed with two layers, within invagination of the initial suture line, using a 2-0 or 3-0 absorbable suture. Following such bladder injury, it is customary to put the patient on continuous bladder drainage via a urethral catheter for 7–10 days, to allow the defect to heal.

Occasionally, the injury is not recognized at the time of surgery. If urine leaks into the peritoneal cavity, there will be abdominal distension and tenderness, which is sometimes accompanied by nausea and vomiting and which will require surgical re-exploration. Sometimes the leak is via the abdominal incision, resulting in a copious watery discharge. The substance being leaked can be identified as urine by sending a specimen to the laboratory for urea measurement (a high urea content means that it is urine and not peritoneal fluid). Once a urine leak is diagnosed, surgical correction is necessary. Even more rarely, the leakage may be per vaginam; this situation is more likely following caesarean section at full dilatation, when what was intended to be a lower segment incision can in fact be through the cervix or even the vagina; subsequent infection/inflammation can erode into the base of the bladder, resulting in a fistula. In such cases, continuous bladder drainage is necessary until the infection/inflammation subsides with the aid of antibiotic therapy. Secondary repair is best deferred for some weeks until the fistula can be excised and the defect repaired, usually with overlapping layers.

Blood transfusion during caesarean section

Following delivery, the loss of the placental intervillous space, together with the contraction of the uterus, reduces the circulatory volume by approximately 500 ml. The average maternal blood loss at vaginal birth is approximately 500 ml, and therefore the average woman will not be haemodynamically compromised by the birth process. The average blood loss at caesarean section is approximately 1 l, resulting in a net reduction in circulating volume compared with the cardiovascular space of approximately 500 ml. Such a blood volume deficit is easily compensated for by a healthy adult and is, for example, the usual amount of blood taken from blood donors. Accordingly, it therefore seems logical not to consider blood replacement unless the blood loss is estimated to be more than 1 l.

Simplistically, one could therefore suggest that a blood loss of 1500 ml should prompt a transfusion of one unit of blood (500 ml), a loss of 2000 ml a transfusion of two units of blood, and so on. However, it has become apparent during the last decade that it is likely that common transfusion practices result in too much blood being given 'just in case'. For example, in obstetrics, the nostrum that 'if you need to give one unit, then better give two' is widespread in Europe and the United States. This approach is likely to be an inappropriate policy. First, if there has been an overestimate of blood loss (and estimation of blood loss is notoriously unreliable), there is a risk of overloading the circulation (a particular risk in women with cardiac disease). Moreover, each unit of blood comes from a separate donor and therefore giving two units of blood carries twice the risk of a transfusion reaction compared with giving one. In addition, each unit will carry a separate risk of introducing an infection carried by the donor; there have in the past been major outbreaks of hepatitis C and HIV from giving blood, and there continues to be concerned about the transmission of prion disease. In 2012, the US Joint Commission and the American Medical Association-convened Physician Consortium For Performance Improvement [56] listed blood transfusion as the second commonest overused intervention in medicine (for completeness, the other four were antibiotics for viral upper respiratory tract infection, tympanostomy tubes (grommets), early term delivery, and percutaneous cardiac stenting). They commented that, while blood transfusions can be life-saving, they also carry risks that range from mild complications to death. A major meta-analysis in the *BMJ* in 2015 reported on 31 trials, which included 9813 randomized subjects, of a restrictive versus liberal transfusion strategy for red blood cell transfusion [57]. In the restrictive group, only 45% of subjects were transfused compared with 86% in the liberal group, and the mean number of units transfused was 1.47 versus 2.9. There was no difference in mortality or morbidity and the authors commented that 'liberal transfusion strategies have not been shown to confer any benefit to patients and have the potential for harm'. A 2014 editorial in the *New England Journal of Medicine*

[58] recommended that the traditional transfusion threshold of 8 g/dl should be reduced to no more than 7 g/dl, and the authors commented that 'it is clearer than ever that smaller transfusions are better for many patients than larger ones'. They also commented that a restrictive transfusion policy was beneficial in patients with septic shock. It has even been suggested that blood transfusion might affect long-term mortality by changing immune function and thus potentially increasing the risk of subsequent infections and cancer recurrence, although recent evidence suggests that, if such a risk exists, it is probably small [59].

Key learning points

1. Measure blood loss carefully and, if the loss exceeds 1 l, give additional oxytocics (e.g., oxytocin infusion, misoprostol).
2. If bleeding continues after optimizing pharmacologic therapy, consider uterine compression sutures (Hayman), followed if necessary by uterine artery ligation.
3. Internal iliac artery ligation can be tried but should only be undertaken by those specifically trained in its use.
4. Arterial embolization should be considered but requires specialized facilities and expertise.
5. Maintaining a good circulating blood volume by early blood transfusion is important to prevent post-operative complications such as shock lung.
6. Antibiotic prophylaxis before skin incision is recommended to reduce maternal complications but the long-term impact on the baby's immune system development is unknown.
7. Most cases of post-operative endometritis respond to antibiotic treatment, and suction curettage of the uterus should be reserved for non-responders.
8. All women who undergo caesarean delivery should receive thromboprophylaxis.
9. Bladder injury is relatively common and so close inspection of the bladder before closure is imperative. Injuries should be repaired immediately and bladder drainage by catheter used for 10 days.
10. If blood transfusion becomes necessary (indicated by adverse changes in maternal vital signs), the minimum amount of blood necessary to restore normal vital signs should be given; extra blood should not be given 'just in case'. An appropriate level at which to consider prophylactic transfusion is 7 g/dl.

References

1. Lewis G (ed.). The Confidential Enquiry into Maternal and Child Health (CEMACH). Saving Mothers' Lives: Reviewing maternal deaths to make motherhood safer: 2003–2005. The Seventh Report on Confidential Enquiries into Maternal Deaths in the United Kingdom. London: CEMACH, 2007.
2. Centre for Maternal and Child Enquiries. Saving Mothers' Lives: Reviewing maternal deaths to make motherhood safer: 2006–2008. The Eighth Report of the Confidential Enquiries into Maternal Deaths in the United Kingdom. BJOG 2011; 118(1): 1–203.
3. Brant HA. Blood loss at caesarean section. J Obstet Gynaecol Br Commonw 1966; 73(3): 456–9.
4. Royal College of Obstetricians and Gynaecologists. Intrapartum Care of Healthy Women and their Babies during Childbirth. London: RCOG Press, 2007.
5. Yaegashi N, Miura M, Okamura K. Acute myocardial infarction associated with postpartum ergot alkaloid administration. Int J Gynaecol Obstet 1999; 64(1): 67–8.
6. Sutaria N, O'Toole L, Northridge D. Postpartum acute MI following routine ergometrine administration treated successfully by primary PTCA. Heart 2000; 83(1): 97–8.
7. Mousa HA, McKinley CA, Thong J. Acute postpartum myocardial infarction after ergometrine administration in a woman with familial hypercholesterolaemia. BJOG 2000; 107(7): 939–40.
8. Tsui BC, Stewart B, Fitzmaurice A, Williams R. Cardiac arrest and myocardial infarction induced by postpartum intravenous ergonovine administration. Anesthesiology 2001; 94(2): 363–4.
9. Jonsson M, Hanson U, Lidell C, Norden-Lindeberg S. ST depression at caesarean section and the relation to oxytocin dose. A randomised controlled trial. BJOG 2010; 117(1): 76–83.
10. Svanstrom MC, Biber B, Hanes M, Johansson G, Naslund U, Balfors EM. Signs of myocardial ischaemia after injection of oxytocin: A randomized double-blind comparison of oxytocin and methylergometrine during Caesarean section. Br J Anaesth 2008; 100(5): 683–9.
11. Thomas JS, Koh SH, Cooper GM. Haemodynamic effects of oxytocin given as i.v. bolus or infusion on women undergoing Caesarean section. Br J Anaesth 2007; 98(1): 116–9.
12. Sartain JB, Barry JJ, Howat PW, McCormack DI, Bryant M. Intravenous oxytocin bolus of 2 units is superior to 5 units during elective Caesarean section. Br J Anaesth 2008; 101(6): 822–6.
13. Carvalho JC, Balki M, Kingdom J, Windrim R. Oxytocin requirements at elective cesarean delivery: A

dose-finding study. Obstet Gynecol 2004; 104(5 Pt 1): 1005–10.

14. Larciprete G, Montagnoli C, Frigo M, Panetta V, Todde C, Zuppani B, et al. Carbetocin versus oxytocin in caesarean section with high risk of post-partum haemorrhage. J Prenat Med 2013; 7(1): 12–8.

15. FIGO. Misoprostol: Recommended Dosages 2012. 2012. http://www.figo.org/sites/default/files/uploads/project-publications/Miso/Misoprostol_Recommended%20Dosages%202012.pdf.

16. Elati A, Weeks A. Risk of fever after misoprostol for the prevention of postpartum hemorrhage: A meta-analysis. Obstet Gynecol 2012; 120(5): 1140–8.

17. Bai J, Sun Q, Zhai H. A comparison of oxytocin and carboprost tromethamine in the prevention of postpartum hemorrhage in high-risk patients undergoing cesarean delivery. Exp Ther Med 2014; 7(1): 46–50.

18. Hsu S, Rodgers B, Lele A, Yeh J. Use of packing in obstetric hemorrhage of uterine origin. J Reprod Med 2003; 48(2): 69–71.

19. Johanson R, Kumar M, Obhrai M, Young P. Management of massive postpartum haemorrhage: Use of a hydrostatic balloon catheter to avoid laparotomy. BJOG 2001; 108(4): 420–2.

20. Bakri YN, Amri A, Abdul JF. Tamponade-balloon for obstetrical bleeding. Int J Gynaecol Obstet 2001; 74(2): 139–42.

21. Dabelea V, Schultze PM, McDuffie RS Jr. Intrauterine balloon tamponade in the management of postpartum hemorrhage. Am J Perinatol 2007; 24(6): 359–64.

22. Doumouchtsis SK, Papageorghiou AT, Vernier C, Arulkumaran S. Management of postpartum hemorrhage by uterine balloon tamponade: Prospective evaluation of effectiveness. Acta Obstet Gynecol Scand 2008; 87(8): 849–55.

23. Lynch C, Coker A, Lawal AH, Abu J, Cowen MJ. The B-Lynch surgical technique for the control of massive postpartum haemorrhage: An alternative to hysterectomy? Five cases reported. BJOG 1997; 104(3): 372–5.

24. Cho JH, Jun HS, Lee CN. Hemostatic suturing technique for uterine bleeding during cesarean delivery. Obstet Gynecol 2000; 96(1): 129–31.

25. Ochoa M, Allaire AD, Stitely ML. Pyometria after hemostatic square suture technique. Obstet Gynecol 2002; 99(3): 506–9.

26. Wu HH, Yeh GP. Uterine cavity synechiae after hemostatic square suturing technique. Obstet Gynecol 2005; 105(5 Pt 2): 1176–8.

27. Rathat G, Do TP, Mercier G, Reyftmann L, Dechanet C, Boulot P, et al. Synechia after uterine compression sutures. Fertil Steril 2011; 95(1): 405–9.

28. Hackethal A, Brueggmann D, Oehmke F, Tinneberg HR, Zygmunt MT, Muenstedt K. Uterine compression U-sutures in primary postpartum hemorrhage after

Cesarean section: Fertility preservation with a simple and effective technique. Hum Reprod 2008; 23(1): 74–9.

29. Poujade O, Grossetti A, Mougel L, Ceccaldi PF, Ducarme G, Luton D. Risk of synechiae following uterine compression sutures in the management of major postpartum haemorrhage. BJOG 2011; 118(4): 433–9.

30. Hayman RG, Arulkumaran S, Steer PJ. Uterine compression sutures: Surgical management of postpartum hemorrhage. Obstet Gynecol 2002; 99(3): 502–6.

31. Ghezzi F, Cromi A, Uccella S, Raio L, Bolis P, Surbek D. The Hayman technique: A simple method to treat postpartum haemorrhage. BJOG 2007; 114(3): 362–5.

32. Cotzias C, Girling J. Uterine compression suture without hysterotomy: Why a non-absorbable suture should be avoided. J Obstet Gynaecol 2005; 25(2): 150–2.

33. Joshi VM, Shrivastava M. Partial ischemic necrosis of the uterus following a uterine brace compression suture. BJOG 2004; 111(3): 279–80.

34. Treloar EJ, Anderson RS, Andrews HS, Bailey JL. Uterine necrosis following B-Lynch suture for primary postpartum haemorrhage. BJOG 2006; 113(4): 486–8.

35. Reyftmann L, Nguyen A, Ristic V, Rouleau C, Mazet N, Dechaud H. Nécrose pariétale utérine partielle après capitonnage hémostatique selon la technique de Cho au cours d'une hémorragie du post-partum [Partial uterine wall necrosis following Cho hemostatic sutures for the treatment of postpartum hemorrhage]. Gynécol Obstét Fertil 2009; 37(6): 579–82.

36. Gottlieb AG, Pandipati S, Davis KM, Gibbs RS. Uterine necrosis: A complication of uterine compression sutures. Obstet Gynecol 2008; 112(2 Pt 2): 429–31.

37. Akoury H, Sherman C. Uterine wall partial thickness necrosis following combined B-Lynch and Cho square sutures for the treatment of primary postpartum hemorrhage. J Obstet Gynaecol Can 2008; 30(5): 421–4.

38. Amorim-Costa C, Mota R, Rebelo C, Silva PT. Uterine compression sutures for postpartum hemorrhage: Is routine postoperative cavity evaluation needed? Acta Obstet Gynecol Scand 2011; 90(7): 701–6.

39. Hwu YM, Chen CP, Chen HS, Su TH. Parallel vertical compression sutures: A technique to control bleeding from placenta praevia or accreta during caesarean section. BJOG 2005; 112(10): 1420–3.

40. Dawlatly B, Wong I, Khan K, Agnihotri S. Using the cervix to stop bleeding in a woman with placenta accreta: A case report. BJOG 2007; 114(4): 502–4.

41. Kayem G, Kurinczuk JJ, Alfirevic Z, Spark P, Brocklehurst P, Knight M. Specific second-line therapies for postpartum haemorrhage: A national cohort study. BJOG 2011; 118(7): 856–64.

42. Danso D, Reginald P. Combined B-lynch suture with intrauterine balloon catheter triumphs over massive postpartum haemorrhage. BJOG 2002; 109(8): 963.

43. Nelson WL, O'Brien JM. The uterine sandwich for persistent uterine atony: Combining the B-Lynch compression suture and an intrauterine Bakri balloon. Am J Obstet Gynecol 2007; 196(5): e9–10.

44. O'Leary JA. Uterine artery ligation in the control of postcesarean hemorrhage. J Reprod Med 1995; 40(3): 189–93.

45. Das BN, Biswas AK. Ligation of internal iliac arteries in pelvic haemorrhage. J Obstet Gynaecol Res 1998; 24(4): 251–4.

46. Boulleret C, Chahid T, Gallot D, Mofid R, Tran HD, Ravel A, et al. Hypogastric arterial selective and superselective embolization for severe postpartum hemorrhage: A retrospective review of 36 cases. Cardiovasc Intervent Radiol 2004; 27(4): 344–8.

47. Cheong JY, Kong TW, Son JH, Won JH, Yang JI, Kim HS. Outcome of pelvic arterial embolization for postpartum hemorrhage: A retrospective review of 117 cases. Obstet Gynecol Sci 2014; 57(1): 17–27.

48. National Institute for Health and Care Excellence. Caesarean Section: Guidance and Guidelines. 2011. http://guidance.nice.org.uk/CG132/Guidance/pdf/English.

49. Smaill F, Hofmeyr GJ. Antibiotic prophylaxis for cesarean section. Cochrane Database Syst Rev 2000; 2: CD000933.

50. Gates S, Anderson ER. Wound drainage for caesarean section. Cochrane Database Syst Rev 2013; 12: CD004549.

51. Kujovich JL. Hormones and pregnancy: Thromboembolic risks for women. Br J Haematol 2004; 126(4): 443–54.

52. Sultan AA, Tata LJ, West J, Fiaschi L, Fleming KM, Nelson-Piercy C, et al. Risk factors for first venous thromboembolism around pregnancy: A population-based cohort study from the United Kingdom. Blood 2013; 121(19): 3953–61.

53. Bain E, Wilson A, Tooher R, Gates S, Davis LJ, Middleton P. Prophylaxis for venous thromboembolic disease in pregnancy and the early postnatal period. Cochrane Database Syst Rev 2014; 2: CD001689.

54. Royal College of Obstetricians and Gynaecologists. Reducing the risk of thrombosis and embolism during pregnancy and the puerperium: Green-top Guideline No. 37a. 2015. http://www.rcog.org.uk/globalassets/documents/guidelines/gtg-37a.pdf.

55. National Institute for Health and Care Excellence. Venous thromboembolism in adults admitted to hospital: Reducing the risk. 2010. http://guidance.nice.org.uk/CG92/Guidance/pdf/English.

56. The Joint Commission and the American Medical Association-Convened Physician Consortium for Performance Improvement. 2013. Proceedings from the National Summit on Overuse. http://www jointcommission.org/assets/1/6/National_Summit_Overuse.pdf.

57. Holst LB, Petersen MW, Haase N, Perner A, Wetterslev J. Restrictive versus liberal transfusion strategy for red blood cell transfusion: Systematic review of randomised trials with meta-analysis and trial sequential analysis. BMJ 2015; 350: h1354.

58. Hebert PC, Carson JL. Transfusion threshold of 7 g per deciliter: The new normal. N Engl J Med 2014; 371(15): 1459–61.

59. Carson JL, Sieber F, Cook DR, Hoover DR, Noveck H, Chaitman BR, et al. Liberal versus restrictive blood transfusion strategy: 3-year survival and cause of death results from the FOCUS randomised controlled trial. Lancet 2015; 385(9974): 1183–9.

CHAPTER 9

Long-term complications after caesarean section

Eric Jauniaux and Davor Jurkovic

Introduction

Caesarean delivery is now a commonly performed operation and accounts for nearly one-third of all births in the United Kingdom and the United States. Although it is now overall a safe procedure, a caesarean section can be associated with a variety of immediate (see Chapter 8) and long-term complications. Considering the rapid increase in the number of caesarean sections worldwide (see Chapter 3), these complications have become an important and often unrecognized iatrogenic issue in obstetrics and gynaecology.

The mechanisms involved in tissue repair following injury following an accidental trauma or surgery differ among animal species and also vary depending on the type of affected tissue. Planaria, starfish, and some worms can regenerate most of their bodies, whereas many other species can only regenerate parts of specific tissues. Some tissues cannot be functionally repaired, as is the case for mammalian musculature and the mammalian central nervous system.

Tissue healing following an injury is accomplished through haemostasis, inflammation, proliferation, and remodelling. For a wound to heal effectively, these phases should be accomplished fully and in the right sequence. Scarring is considered abnormal when fibrosis is excessive or suboptimal. The modern caesarean section requires cutting and opening of the skin and underlying fat tissue, muscular sheet, peritoneum, and uterine muscle, including the myometrial–endometrial junction zone. All these layers need to go through the healing process afterwards, which will vary depending on the type of tissue involved.

The human skin is a composite material consisting of a collagen-rich fibrous network embedded in a ground substance matrix. The proteoglycan-rich matrix provides skin its viscous nature at low loads. The main fibrous constituents, collagen and elastin, provide structural stiffness and elasticity to the skin [1]. Surgical wounds alter the skin's fibrotic structure, thereby producing scar tissue with significant functional impairments. Cutaneous scar tissue demonstrates similar high-load stiffness, greatly reduced low-load compliance, and altered material directionality. Keloids and hypertrophic scars are generally characterized by abnormally proliferative scar tissue. Keloids are benign, fibroproliferative lesions that represent abnormal healing resulting in excessive fibrosis and can occur in all skin types but with a particularly high frequency in black women.

Adhesions are defined as abnormal fibrous connections between two anatomically different surfaces and are made of deposits of fibrous strands, which are a consequence of irritation by infection or surgical trauma. Peritoneal damage inflicted by surgical trauma or other insults evokes an inflammatory response, thereby promoting pro-coagulatory and anti-fibrinolytic reactions and a subsequent significant increase in fibrin formation

[2]. The balance between fibrin deposition and degradation is therefore critical in determining normal peritoneal healing or adhesion formation. Recent data suggest that the formation of adhesions is caused by the organization of a fibrin matrix; this process takes place during the coagulation process and is facilitated by suppression of fibrinolysis [3].

Muscles in general do not actually heal by regenerating muscle fibres but by forming 'foreign' substances, including collagen. The resulting scar tissue is weaker, less elastic, and more prone to injury than normal muscle tissue is. Myofibre disarray, tissue oedema, inflammation, and elastosis have all been observed in uterine wound healing after surgery [4]. Experiments in mice have indicated that differences in regenerative ability translate into histological,

proliferative, and functional differences in the biomechanical properties of the scarred myometrium after caesarean section [5]. These results could explain the wide individual variations observed in uterine healing after caesarean section.

The caesarean delivery scar leaves the patient susceptible to several peculiar abnormalities. Familiarity with the normal post-operative findings following caesarean section is necessary to recognize possible long-term complications, which are being encountered with increasing frequency. This chapter summarizes the current literature on the pathophysiology and long-term clinical consequences of caesarean section and presents the ultrasound diagnosis of uterine scar anomalies, pelvic adhesions, and secondary abnormalities of placentation.

Uterine complications after caesarean section

Early pregnancy failure after caesarean section

Human implantation relies on the interaction of the blastocyst trophoectoderm with the cells of the decidualized endometrium. A large number of regulatory molecules have been demonstrated to play functional roles in the process of normal decidualization, control of trophoblast adhesion, invasion, and directionality of penetration [6]. These findings suggest that the decidual defect following a uterine scar may have an adverse effect on early implantation by creating conditions for preferential attachment of the blastocyst to scar tissue and facilitating abnormally deep invasion of the extravillous trophoblast. A recent systematic review and meta-analysis of nearly 2 million pregnancies [7] have shown that, compared to those who had vaginal birth, women with a history of previous caesarean section are at higher risk of unexplained stillbirth. By contrast, there is no clear association between a history of previous caesarean section and the risk of miscarriage (see Box 9.1). These findings suggest that the caesarean scar is limited to a very small surface, with little impact on the rest of the endometrium lining

the uterine cavity and thus allowing for a normal implantation.

The aetiology behind the higher rates of unexplained stillbirth in subsequent pregnancies after caesarean delivery remains unknown but it could be explained by the increased prevalence of abruptio placentae, which may be in turn, a consequence of impaired placentation. A recent study of the uterine circulation in women with a previous caesarean section has shown that the uterine artery resistance is increased and the volume uterine blood flow is decreased as a fraction of maternal cardiac output, compared to that in women with a previous vaginal birth [8]. These data suggest a possible relationship between the presence of a poorly vascularized uterine scar area and an increase in the resistance to blood flow in the uterine circulation, with a secondary impact on placental implantation.

Placenta praevia and placenta abruptio after caesarean section

Over the last decade, several epidemiological studies have indicated that a caesarean birth is associated with increased risks of placenta praevia and

> ## Box 9.1 **Risks of long-term complications associated with caesarean delivery**
>
> ### Obstetric risks in subsequent pregnancy
>
> **Miscarriage:** Inconsistent results limited by lack of adjustment for confounding factors [1]
>
> **Unexplained stillbirth:** Odds ratio (OR), 1.47 (95% confidence interval (CI) 1.20–1.80) [1]
>
> ### Placenta praevia
>
> - Relative risk (RR) of 1.5 (95% CI, 1.30–1.80) [2]
> - Adjusted OR of 1.47 (95% CI, 1.41–1.52) [3]
> - Overall pooled random effects OR of 2.20 (95% CI, 1.96–2.46) [4]
> - OR of 1.47 (95% CI, 1.44–1.51) [5]
>
> ### Placenta abruptio
>
> - RR of 0.74 (95% CI, 1.20–1.50) [2]
> - Adjusted OR of 1.40 (95% CI, 1.41–1.52) [3]
> - OR of 1.38 (95% CI, 1.35–1.11) [5]
>
> ### Placenta accreta
>
> - ORs of 1.13 (95% CI, 1.10–1.20) for advancing maternal age, of 8.60 (95% CI, 3.50–21.1) for two or more
>
> caesarean sections, and of 51.40 (95% CI, 10.7–248.4) for placenta praevia [6]
> - OR of 4.9 (95% CI, 1.7–14.3) for placenta praevia after two caesarean sections, and 7.7 (95% CI, 2.4–24.9) for placenta praevia after three caesarean sections [7]
> - OR of 3.00 (95% CI 1.47–6.12) primary elective caesarean section and placenta praevia [8]
> - OR of 1.96 (95% CI 1.41–2.74) [5]
>
> ### Gynaecological risks after caesarean section
>
> - **Uterine scar defect/niche:** 49.6% on transvaginal ultrasound and 64.5% on gel instillation sonohysterography [9]
> - **Ectopic pregnancy:** No evidence of an association [1]
> - **Secondary infertility:** 9% lower subsequent pregnancy rate (RR, 0.91; 95% CI 0.87–0.95) and 11% lower birth rate (RR, 0.89; 95% CI, 0.87–0.92) [4]
> - **Endometriosis:** Hazard ratio of 1.8 (95% CI 1.70–1.90) [10]

abruption in the subsequent pregnancies [9–13]. The risk of placenta praevia is higher with increasing number of prior caesarean deliveries [9]. Following a single caesarean section, there is a 50% increase in the risk of placenta praevia and a 40% increase in the risk of placental abruption in a subsequent singleton pregnancy (see Box 9.1). Following two caesarean deliveries, the risk of placenta praevia is twofold greater than that following two vaginal deliveries [10]. A large cohort study comparing prior prelabour caesarean delivery and intrapartum caesarean delivery found that prior prelabour caesarean delivery is associated with a more than twofold increase in the risk of placenta praevia in the next pregnancy compared to a previous vaginal delivery [11]. By contrast, the 20% increased risk of placenta praevia associated with prior intrapartum caesarean delivery, compared to vaginal delivery, was not found to be significant.

A recent meta-analysis of 5 cohorts and 11 case-control studies published between 1990 and 2011 has indicated that, after a caesarean delivery, the calculated summary odds ratios (ORs) are 1.47 for placenta praevia, and 1.38 for placental abruption [13]. The increased incidence of placenta praevia after a previous caesarean section supports the concept of a biological dysfunction of the lower segment endometrium/superficial myometrium secondary to damage of the corresponding uterine area by previous lower segment caesarean section scar(s).

Placenta accreta after caesarean section

Pathophysiology of placenta accreta

The striking rise in frequency of placenta accreta in developed countries corresponds temporally to rising caesarean section rates. The first cases of placenta accreta were reported in 1937, within two decades after Munro Kerr (1868–1960) proposed substantial improvements in the surgical techniques for performing caesarean section (see Chapter 1). These changes made the operation safer than it had been before, thus ensuring that most mothers survived the surgical procedure and facilitating its use in clinical obstetric practice around the world.

Endometritis, manual removal of the placenta, previous myomectomy, hysteroscopic surgery, IVF procedures, endometrial resection, uterine artery embolization, chemotherapy, and radiotherapy all have been associated with an increased risk of placenta accreta. The risk was also found to be increased in women with major uterine congenital anomalies, adenomyosis, or submucous fibroids [14], and a recent survey has found that up to 18% of women presenting with a placenta accreta are nulliparous [12]. However, most of these factors are probably responsible for only a very small proportion of placenta accreta, given the rapid increase in the number of caesarean sections worldwide.

Several hypotheses have been proposed to explain why placenta accreta occurs. The oldest hypothesis is that a primary defect in trophoblast biology leads to excessive invasion of the uterine myometrium [14]. The other prevailing hypothesis is that a secondary defect of the utero-placental interface causes a failure of normal decidualization in the area of the uterine scar, allowing an abnormally deep trophoblastic infiltration. An abnormal vascularization resulting from the scarring process after surgery, with secondary localized hypoxia leading to both defective decidualization and excessive trophoblastic invasion, has recently been suggested to be another possible cause of placenta accreta [15]. The finding of leukocyte recruitment to the endometrium during the secretory phase following a caesarean section [16] supports the hypothesis that the abnormal decidualization and trophoblastic changes in the placental bed in the setting of placenta accreta is secondary to the abnormalities of the uterine scar and that individual wound healing characteristics may predispose to abnormal placentation.

Epidemiology of placenta accreta

Placenta accreta has only been described and studied by pathologists for less than a century [17]. There has been a substantial increase in the occurrence of placenta accreta over the last 50 years, with as much as a tenfold rise in its incidence in most Western countries. Large studies in the United States have indicated an overall incidence of placenta accreta of 1 : 333–533 deliveries [10]. A recent meta-analysis has shown a calculated summary OR of 1.96 for placenta accreta after one caesarean section [13]. A recent case-control study has shown that, compared with primary emergency caesarean section, primary elective caesarean section significantly increased the risk of placenta accreta in a subsequent pregnancy in the presence of placenta praevia [14]. Overall, placenta accreta remains a relatively uncommon obstetric pathology but has become a complication that an average obstetrician is likely to encounter more and more regularly compared to once or twice in a practice lifetime two decades ago. It is rapidly becoming recognized as a major cause of obstetric complications worldwide, including in low-income countries.

Placenta accreta complicates about 5% of pregnancies with placenta praevia, and large epidemiological studies have shown that the strongest risk factor for placenta praevia is a prior caesarean section [18]. The number of previous caesarean section increases the risk of placenta accreta. Among women with placenta praevia, 40% of those with two previous caesarean sections and 61% of those with three previous caesarean sections develop a placenta accreta [19]. This risk is independent of other maternal characteristics such as parity, BMI, tobacco use, and coexisting hypertension or diabetes [19]. It has been recently estimated that, if the caesarean section rate continue to rise as it has in recent years, by 2020 there will be an additional 6236 cases of placenta praevia, 4504 cases of placenta accreta, and 130 maternal deaths annually in the United States alone [18].

Clinical symptoms of placenta accreta

The term placenta accreta has been used in some cases to describe all types of abnormally adherent placentae, although it most specifically refers to invasion only in the superficial portion of the myometrium. The term 'placenta increta' is used to describe deep myometrial invasion of trophoblast villi, and 'placenta percreta' refers to accreta villi perforating through the full thickness of the myometrium and uterine serosa, with possible involvement of adjacent organs [14]. Placenta increta and placenta percreta are rare, representing less than 20% of cases of placenta accreta. Placenta accreta can also be classified as total, partial, or focal, depending on the amount of placental tissue involved. The symptoms of placenta accreta are usually those associated with placenta praevia, that is, chronic and often severe vaginal bleeding, which is often the only clinical symptom during the entire pregnancy. Placenta percreta may lead to other symptoms related to the pelvic organs involved, such as the bladder and/or the bowel. In the absence of a placenta praevia or invasion through the serosa, a woman with placenta accreta will likely be asymptomatic.

Severely deficient uterine scars with complete loss of myometrium could explain rare reports of placenta percreta leading to uterine rupture in the first half of pregnancy [20]. Although such an event is an extremely rare complication of placentation, the mechanism of uterine rupture due to a placenta percreta is likely to be similar to that of a tubal rupture in an ectopic placentation. These findings emphasize the role of the superficial myometrium in modulating uterine placentation.

Antenatal diagnosis of placenta accreta

The failure of the placenta to separate normally from the uterus during delivery in placenta accreta is typically accompanied by severe post-partum haemorrhage. Attempts to remove the adherent tissue may provoke further bleeding and a cascade of ongoing haemorrhage, shock, and coagulation disorders requiring complex clinical management. Thus, antenatal screening and diagnosis of placenta accreta in high-risk pregnancies is pivotal to ensure that delivery can be planned to occur in a tertiary care centre and be managed by a multidisciplinary team (see Chapter 6).

Most studies of placenta accreta have focused on identifying reliable ultrasound and other radiological markers of a defect in the deciduo-placental interface in order to facilitate antenatal detection and improve management at delivery [14]. Ultrasound has become the primary screening tool for the evaluation of women at risk of placenta accreta. Greyscale ultrasound features suggestive of placenta accreta include the loss of myometrial interface or retroplacental clear space, reduced myometrial

thickness, and chaotic intraplacental blood flow and intraplacental lacunae (Figure 9.1). In placenta percreta, the placenta is often seen bulging towards the bladder, and in some cases placental invasion into the bladder can be seen. A lot of attention has been focused on the presence or absence of the 'intraplacental lacunae' [14]. These sonolucent spaces contain slow-moving maternal blood on greyscale imaging and have been previously described as intraplacental 'lakes' [21]. When involving small area of the placenta, they have no clinical significance and are often are found in area of low villous tissue density, such as in the centre of the cotyledons or under the chorionic plate. In placenta accreta, the lacunae are often extensive, creating a 'moth-eaten' placental appearance (Figure 9.2).

The most common and most predictive sonographic finding associated with placenta accreta is the loss of myometrial interface, with enlargement of the underlying arcuate vasculature [22]. The addition of colour or power Doppler evaluation has been valuable in improving the diagnosis of placenta accreta [23–30]. Doppler features that suggest placenta accreta include chaotic intraplacental

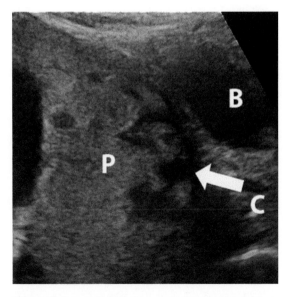

Figure 9.1 Transabdominal greyscale ultrasound longitudinal view of the lower uterine segment at 24 weeks of gestation in a case of placenta praevia major covering the cervix (C). The basal plate is missing (arrow) and the placenta (P) is bulging towards the bladder (B). The placental anatomy is distorted by large intervillous lakes or lacunae creating a 'moth-eaten' placental appearance.

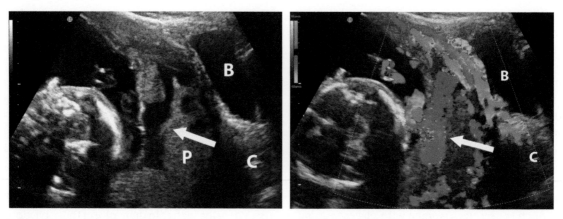

Figure 9.2 Transabdominal greyscale (left) and colour-mapping (right) ultrasound longitudinal view of the lower uterine segment at 20 weeks of gestation. The placenta (P) is praevia, covering the cervix (C). The basal plate is missing and the placenta is bulging towards the bladder (B) and extensively distorted by large intervillous lakes (arrow).

blood flow, the presence of increased blood flow in the retroplacental space and aberrant vessels crossing between placental surfaces (Figure 9.2). Overall, in at-risk women, greyscale ultrasound is quite sensitive (70%–90%), although this sensitivity is improved by colour ultrasound [30]. Table 9.1 displays the data of five large studies published since the year 2000 on the use of colour Doppler imaging in women presenting with a placenta praevia and an obstetric history of a previous caesarean section delivery. The sensitivity of ultrasound with colour Doppler imaging in the diagnosis of placenta accreta varied between 77% and 100%; thus, there may be an influence from confounding factors such as operator experience, and gestational age at first examination by a specialist. A recent meta-analysis of the prenatal diagnosis of invasive placentation has indicated that the overall sensitivity of ultrasound is 90.7% [31]. Interestingly, the negative predictive value ranged between 95% and 100% (Table 9.1); this result suggests that, in expert hands, ultrasound with colour Doppler imaging is very accurate at excluding placenta accreta (Figure 9.3). A recent prospective case study has shown that the sensitivity, negative predictive value, and accuracy of ultrasound used for routine prenatal diagnosis is 53.5%, 82.1%, and 64.8%, respectively, and thus lower than previously reported [32].

Table 9.1 Antenatal diagnosis of placenta praevia accreta with colour Doppler imaging

Authors	No. of cases	Sensitivity (%)	PPV (%)	NPV (%)
Chou et al. [1]	80	82.4	87.5	95.3
Twickler et al. [2]	215	100.0	72.0	100.0
Warshak et al. [3]	453	77.0	65.0	98.0
Esakoff et al. [4]	108	89.5	68.0	97.6
Chalubinski et al. [5]	232	91.4	80.0	98.4
Bowman et al. [6]	55	53.5	82.1	64.1

1. Chou MM, Ho ES, Lee YH. Prenatal diagnosis of placenta previa accreta by transabdominal color Doppler ultrasound. Ultrasound Obstet Gynecol. 2000; 15: 28–35.
2. Twickler DM, Lucas MJ, Balis AB, et al. Color flow mapping for myometrial invasion in women with a prior cesarean delivery. J Matern Fetal Med. 2000; 9: 330–5.
3. Warshak CR, Eskander R, Hull AD, et al. Accuracy of ultrasonography and magnetic resonance imaging in the diagnosis of placenta accreta. Obstet Gynecol. 2006; 108: 573–81.
4. Esakoff TF, Sparks TN, Kaimal AJ, Kim LH, Feldstein VA, Goldstein RB, et al. Diagnosis and morbidity of placenta accreta. Ultrasound Obstet Gynecol. 2011; 37: 324–7.
5. Chalubinski KM, Pils S, Klein K, Seemann R, Speiser P, Langer M, Ott J. Prenatal sonography can predict degree of placental invasion. Ultrasound Obstet Gynecol. 2013; 42: 518–24.
6. Bowman ZS, Eller AG, Kennedy AM, et al Accuracy of ultrasound for the prediction of placenta accreta. Am J Obstet Gynecol. 2014; 211: 177.e1–7.

NPV, negative predictive value; PPV, positive predictive value.

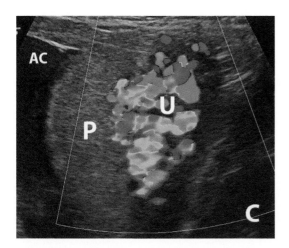

Figure 9.3 Transabdominal colour-mapping ultrasound longitudinal view of the lower uterine segment at 20 weeks of gestation in a case of anterior placenta after previous caesarean section and with a caesarean scar defect detected before pregnancy (see Figure 9.6). The placenta (P) has a normal appearance and the basal plate intact with normal uterine (U) circulation; AC, amniotic cavity; C, cervix.

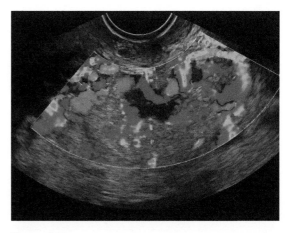

Figure 9.4 Transvaginal colour Doppler mapping of the image in Figure 9.2, showing chaotic intraplacental blood flow, the presence of altered blood flow in the retroplacental space, and aberrant vessels crossing between placental surfaces.

Disruption of the normal continuous colour flow appearance, corresponding to a gap in myometrial blood flow and the abnormal dilatation of the arcuate arteries, can be seen in many cases of placenta accreta. This gap represents the site of placental invasion into the myometrium and can be diagnosed from early in the first trimester of pregnancy [32–36]. A recent prospective study of nine cases has shown that the assessment of ongoing pregnancies implanted in caesarean scars is probably best performed between 7–9 weeks gestation [36]. Complete implantation within the myometrial defect, bulging of the trophoblast out of the uterine contour, and large placental lakes in the first trimester are the ultrasound findings that may predict a severe placenta accreta or percreta and a consequently poor outcome. Within this context, it should be possible to diagnose most cases of placenta accreta at the time of the 11–14 weeks ultrasound examination [37] and all cases at 20-22 weeks of gestation. In cases of a placenta preavia major covering the lower segment at that stage, a transvaginal scan (TVS) will help evaluate the utero-placental interface around the internal os of the uterine cervix (Figure 9.4). Another retrospective recent cohort study has indicated that only around 50% of cases of placenta accreta are suspected

before delivery [12]. This observation suggests that ultrasound screening for placenta accreta should be included in the training of ultrasonographers and obstetricians involved in the 12- and the 20-weeks screenings for fetal anomalies and that all women with a previous history of caesarean section and an anterior low/praevia placenta should be referred to a trained operator.

More recently, MRI has been introduced to evaluate placenta accreta. Some authors have suggested that MRI is better than ultrasound for defining areas of abnormal placentation and assessing the depth of myometrial invasion, particularly in cases of posterior placenta [38, 39]. A recent meta-analysis [40] of the prenatal diagnosis of invasive placentation has indicated that the overall sensitivity of MRI is 94.4% (Table 9.2). Large population-based studies are needed in order to assess whether MRI is truly better than ultrasound at predicting the depth and the topography of placental invasion. Overall, MRI can add information in cases of placenta percreta but the cost and limited access of MRI compared to ultrasound makes it impractical for screening for placenta accreta, in routine clinical practice.

Caesarean scar defect

A uterine caesarean section defect or 'niche' is a finding that has recently gained more attention

Table 9.2 Summary estimates of sensitivity, specificity, and diagnostic odds ratio of MRI for detection of presence, degree, and topography of placental invasion and for comparison between MRI and ultrasound for detection of invasive placentation

Parameter	Studies (n)	Total sample (n)	Sensitivity (%) (95% CI)	Specificity (%) (95% CI)	Diagnostic odds ratio (95% CI)
MRI					
Detection of invasive placentation	18*	1010	94.4 (86.0–97.9)	84.0 (76.0–89.8)	89.0 (22.80–348.10)
Depth of placental invasion	3†	62	92.9 (72.8–99.5)	97.6 (87.1–99.9)	44.2 (1.95–1001.00)
Topography of placental invasion	2†	428	99.6 (98.4–100.0)	95.0 (83.1–99.4)	803.0 (9.00–71,411.00)
Direct comparison, MRI vs ultrasound					
All studies	8*	255	—	—	—
MRI	—	—	90.2 (81.3–95.1)	88.2 (76.7–94.4)	68.8 (19.70–239.80)
Ultrasound	—	—	85.7 (77.2–91.4)	88.6 (73.0–95.7)	46.5 (13.40–161.00)
Only studies with blinding‡	4*	164	—	—	—
MRI	—	—	92.9 (82.4–97.3)	93.5 (82.2–97.8)	186.0 (40.00–864.50)
US	—	—	87.8 (75.8–94.3)	96.3 (74.4–99.6)	189.2 (15.80–2269.00)

CI, confidence interval.
*Computations based on hierarchical summary receiver–operating characteristics model.
†Computations based on DerSimonian–Laird random-effect model.
‡Studies in which radiologist was blinded to both US findings and final diagnosis.

Modified from D'Antonio F, Iacovella C, Palacios-Jaraquemada J, Bruno CH, Manzoli L, Bhide A., Prenatal Identification of invasive placentation using Magnetic Resonance Imaging (MRI): A systematic review and meta-analysis, 2014, Wiley

from obstetricians and gynaecologists. Most of the focus has been on identifying ultrasound criteria of caesarean scar defect during pregnancy that may indicate a higher risk of scar dehiscence and/or uterine rupture during trial of vaginal birth in subsequent pregnancies [41]. However, there is mounting evidence that gynaecological disorders such 'bleeding disorders' like postmenstrual spotting, 'pain/dysmenorrhoea', and 'secondary infertility' could be related to caesarean scar defect.

Ultrasound imaging including 3D imaging and sonohysterography has been increasingly used over the last decade to investigate uterine scars in non-pregnant women. Simple and multiple caesarean section scars can be accurately identified

with TVS (Figure 9.5). Caesarean scar defect is a tethering of the endometrium that can serve as a reservoir for intermenstrual blood and fluid and can be associated with clinical gynaecological symptoms such as postmenstrual spotting and dysmenorrhoea. Caesarean scar defect may range from a small defect of the superficial myometrium (Figure 9.6) to clear loss of substance with a direct communication between the endometrial cavity and the visceral serosa (Figures 9.7, 9.8). The relationship between the size of the caesarean scar defect and the clinical symptoms, uterine position, and number of previous caesarean sections has been evaluated in many different studies [42–47]. In women with a history of previous

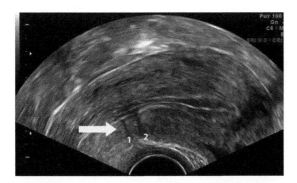

Figure 9.5 Transvaginal ultrasound view of the uterus in a non-pregnant woman with a history of two previous caesarean sections. Note the two small defects through the uterine wall at the junction between the lower and upper uterine segments (indicated by arrow and the numbers '1' and '2'), corresponding to the scars of the caesarean section incisions.

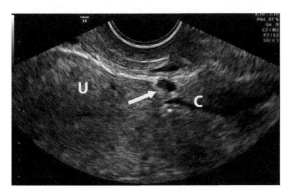

Figure 9.6 Transvaginal ultrasound view of the lower uterine (U) segment in a non-pregnant woman 1 year after an emergency caesarean section. Note the small scar defect (arrow) in the superficial myometrium at the junction between the lower segment and the cervix (C).

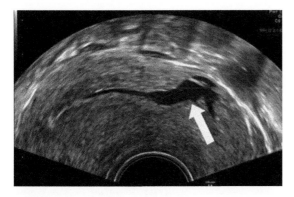

Figure 9.7 Transvaginal ultrasound view of the uterus in a non-pregnant woman with a history of a previous emergency caesarean section. There is a large caesarean scar defect creating a niche at the junction between lower and upper uterine segments (arrow).

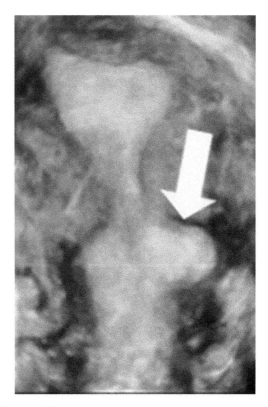

Figure 9.8 Transvaginal ultrasound 3D view of the uterus in a non-pregnant woman with a history of a previous emergency caesarean section, showing a large caesarean scar defect at the junction between the lower and upper uterine segments (arrow).

caesarean sections, the percentage with caesarean scar defects has been found to range between 20% and 65% on transvaginal ultrasound. A recent study using gel instillation sonohysterography 6–12 weeks after caesarean section has shown that spotting is more prevalent in women presenting with a "niche" and in women with a residual myometrial thickness that is <50% that of the adjacent myometrium [48].

The risk of scar deficiency/separation, where the defect involves the deep myometrium layers with intact serosa/visceral peritoneum (Figure 9.9), is increased in women with a retroflexed uterus, in those who have undergone multiple caesarean sections, and in women who underwent caesarean delivery in advanced labour [42–47]. A recent retrospective cohort study has shown that uterine scar dehiscence in a previous pregnancy is a potential risk factor for preterm delivery, low

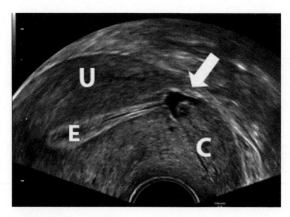

Figure 9.9 Transvaginal ultrasound view of the uterus (U) in a non-pregnant woman with a history of a previous emergency caesarean section. The caesarean scar defect (arrow) involves the entire myometrial thickness at the junction between the lower segment and the cervix (C) and connecting the endometrium (E) with the visceral serosa. Note acute uterine retroflexion creating a 90° angle between the upper and lower segments, suggesting adhesions.

birth weight, and peripartum hysterectomy in the following pregnancy [49]. Interestingly, in this study, previous uterine scar dehiscence does not increase the risk of uterine rupture, placenta accreta, or adverse perinatal outcomes such as low Apgar scores at 5 minutes, and perinatal mortality. A recent series of 14 women (20 pregnancies) with prior uterine rupture and 30 women (40 pregnancies) with prior uterine dehiscence has shown that these patients can have excellent outcomes in subsequent pregnancies if they are managed in a standardized manner, including undergoing caesarean delivery before the onset of labour or immediately at the onset of spontaneous preterm labour [50]. Theoretically, uterine scar surgical repair could prevent recurrent caesarean scar ectopic pregnancies [51] and also prevent placenta accreta and other obstetric complications in subsequent pregnancies, but this hypothesis remains unproven.

There is potential for the formation of abnormal vascular communications between arteries and veins during the healing process of a uterine scar [52]. A recent systematic review of studies reporting on hysteroscopic and laparoscopic caesarean scar defect resection has found that abnormal uterine bleeding improved in the vast majority of the patients after these interventions, ranging from 87% to 100% [53]. However, the methodological quality of the reviewed papers is considered to be

moderate to poor, and therefore the data from these papers are currently insufficient to support proposing microsurgical uterus reconstruction. Until surgical interventions are evaluated in a prospective trial, it will be impossible to evaluate the benefits and efficacy of surgical repair when a caesarean scar defect is observed.

Implantation of clinically detectable pregnancy into a scar (scar pregnancy) is very rare but is associated with severe maternal morbidity and significant mortality from very early in pregnancy. An accurate early prenatal diagnosis of this condition

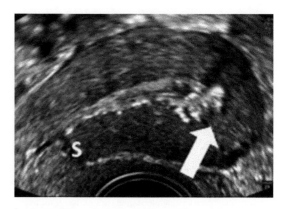

Figure 9.10 Transvaginal ultrasound 3D view of the uterus in a non-pregnant woman with a history of a previous emergency caesarean section showing a small uterine scar (S) and subendometrial fibrosis (arrow).

is pivotal to avoid catastrophic complications such as uterine rupture, massive vaginal bleeding, and placenta praevia/accreta, which might lead to hysterectomy [54].

Subendometrial fibrosis can also be observed after caesarean section (Figure 9.10), although the significance of this finding and its long-term impact on uterine function remains unknown.

Non-uterine complications following caesarean section

Most of the long-term complications related to caesarean section are related to the development of post-operative adhesions [53, 55]. The complications related to adhesions are diverse in nature and clinical consequences, varying from emergency reoperations for small bowel obstruction, to chronic pelvic pain and the need for fertility treatments. Adhesions can be indirectly diagnosed during pelvic ultrasound examination. The typical features include fusion of the uterine tissue with surrounding tissue, acute uterine retroflexion, and lack of uterine mobility (Figures 9.11, 9.12) and can be associated with a caesarean scar defect (Figures 9.9, 9.13) as well.

Adhesions are an inevitable consequence of intra-abdominal surgical tissue trauma and healing. A recent systematic review and meta-analysis has indicated that the incidence of small bowel obstruction after abdominal surgery was 9% and the incidence of small bowel obstruction due specifically to adhesions was 2% [56]. The authors concluded that the complications of post-operative

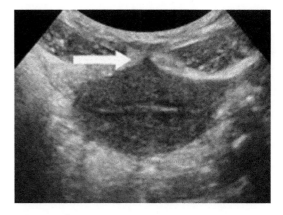

Figure 9.12 Transabdominal ultrasound view of the uterus in a non-pregnant woman with a history of a previous caesarean section, showing a fusion of the anterior uterine wall and the rectus sheet (arrow).

adhesion formation are frequent and have a large negative effect on patients' health.

With an increasing number of caesarean sections and repeat caesarean sections, clinicians have started to realize the importance of adhesions after caesarean delivery [57, 58]. Pelvic adhesions are

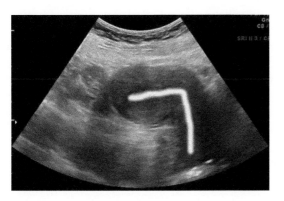

Figure 9.11 Transabdominal ultrasound view of the uterus in a non-pregnant woman with a history of a previous caesarean section. There is acute uterine retroflexion creating a 90° angle between the upper and lower segments, suggesting adhesions.

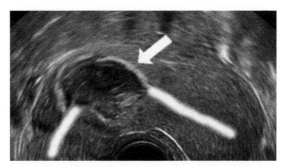

Figure 9.13 Transvaginal ultrasound view of the uterus in a non-pregnant woman with a history of a previous emergency caesarean section, showing a large caesarean scar defect (arrow); there is also acute uterine retroflexion creating a 90° angle between the upper and lower segments, suggesting adhesions.

present in more than a third of women with a history of caesarean section and are associated with chronic pelvic pain [58]. Adhesions in the vesico-uterine pouch are the most common, and post-operative wound infection increases the likelihood of adhesions developing in the anterior pelvic compartment (OR 11.7 (95% confidence interval, 3.5–39.5)). Multivariable logistic regression analysis has identified anterior abdominal wall adhesions and any adhesions present on ultrasound scan as independent predictors of chronic pelvic pain [58]. Adhesions develop more frequently and with increasing severity with each repeat caesarean and are associated with increasing maternal morbidity, such as bladder injury, in subsequent caesarean section deliveries, as well as increased delivery time [57].

It appears that adhesion formation may be reduced with closure of the peritoneum and double-layer closure of the uterine incision, although whether this reduction has clinical significance remains uncertain (see Chapter 4). Uterine adherence to the abdominal wall may increase morbidity at future caesarean section, as well as the need for hysterectomy. A recent study has shown a relation between depressed abdominal scars and intra-abdominal adhesions but no significant difference in the incidence of hyperpigmented and non-pigmented scars between women with or without adhesions [59]. Scar width is larger in patients with intra-abdominal adhesions than in patients without adhesions, whereas scar length does not differ in these two groups.

Ectopic pregnancies following caesarean section

Ectopic pregnancies affect up to 2.5% of pregnancies. The epidemiological risk factors for tubal ectopic pregnancy are well established and include tubal damage as a result of surgery or infection [60]. Around 98% of ectopic pregnancies are tubal, and current evidence supports the hypothesis that they are caused by a combination of retention of the blastocyst within the fallopian tube because of impaired embryo–tubal transport, and alterations in the tubal environment allowing premature implantation to occur. A recent systematic review

and meta-analysis found no evidence of an association between prior caesarean section and the occurrence of a subsequent ectopic pregnancy, but the studies included were of poor or variable quality and only a small number adjusted for potential confounding factors [61].

Secondary infertility following caesarean section

The possible link between caesarean delivery, post-operative pelvic adhesions, and tubal infertility has caused debates for decades but secondary infertility is not exclusively a consequence of caesarean delivery. A recent systematic review [56] has shown that the pregnancy rate after colorectal surgery in patients with inflammatory bowel disease was 50%, which was significantly lower than the pregnancy rate in medically treated patients (82%).

A recent meta-analysis has suggested that women who had undergone a caesarean section had a 9% lower subsequent pregnancy rate and 11% lower birth rate, compared with those who had vaginal delivery [62]. Residual bias in the adjusted results is likely, as no study was able to control for a number of important maternal characteristics, such as a history of infertility or maternal obesity. Similarly, a population-based study of 52,498 women has provided further corroboration of previous studies that have reported reduced childbearing subsequent to caesarean section in comparison with vaginal delivery [63]. However, the authors were unable to measure pre-pregnancy BMI, weight gain during pregnancy and prior infertility, which would have been reduced selection bias. Also, it is unclear whether it is more likely that women could not conceive or whether they actively chose to avoid further childbearing. Although, the impact of pathological and psychological factors may be quite different among women in low-income countries, caesarean section seems to be also associated with reduced subsequent fertility in sub-Saharan Africa [64]. However, most caesarean sections in low-income countries are emergency caesarean sections, and there is a need for more qualitative prospective studies to determine the relationship between caesarean section and secondary infertility.

Endometriosis following caesarean section

Caesarean section is known to be associated with an increased risk of chronic pelvic pain. Whether this association is due to pelvic adhesions or endometriosis is unknown. Caesarean section scar endometriosis is a rare but well-documented complication [65–67]. A recent prospective study has reported a hazard ratio of 1.8 for endometriosis in women with a previous caesarean section when they were compared with women with vaginal deliveries only. The risk of endometriosis increased over time, and one additional case of endometriosis was found for every 325 women undergoing caesarean section within 10 years [67]. The risk of caesarean section scar endometrioma is 0.1%. Further studies are needed to confirm these findings.

Key learning points

1. A history of caesarean is associated with an increased risk of unexplained stillbirth but not with an increased risk of first-trimester risk of miscarriage in subsequent pregnancies.
2. A history of caesarean section is associated with increased risks of placenta praevia and abruptio placentae in subsequent pregnancies, and the risk of placenta praevia increases as the number of prior caesarean deliveries increases.
3. The incidence of placenta accreta has increased in parallel with the increase in the frequency of caesarean section, indicating a direct causal effect.
4. Placenta accreta complicates about 5% of pregnancies with placenta praevia and one prior caesarean section. The strongest risk factor for placenta praevia, and therefore placenta accreta, is a prior caesarean section.
5. Ultrasound is the primary screening tool for the screening and diagnosis of placenta accreta, and the negative predictive value of colour Doppler imaging is close to 100%.
6. A caesarean section defect is a tethering of the endometrium that can be associated with gynaecological symptoms such as postmenstrual spotting, dysmenorrhoea, and caesarean scar ectopic pregnancies.
7. The risk of a caesarean section defect where the defect involves the deep myometrium layers is increased in women with a retroflexed uterus, in those who have undergone multiple caesarean sections, and after caesarean delivery in advanced labour.
8. There is currently no strong evidence of an association between prior caesarean section delivery and the occurrence of a subsequent ectopic pregnancy.
9. A prior caesarean section is associated with pelvic pains due to adhesions, as well as a lower subsequent pregnancy rate and lower birth rate, compared with vaginal birth. Adhesions increase maternal morbidity in subsequent caesarean section deliveries.
10. The risk of endometriosis may increase after caesarean section.

References

1. Corr DT, Hart DA. Biomechanics of scar tissue and uninjured skin. Adv Wound Care (New Rochelle) 2013; 2(2): 37–43.
2. Fometescu SG, Costache M, Coveney A, Oprescu SM, Serban D, Savlovschi C. Peritoneal fibrinolytic activity and adhesiogenesis. Chirurgia (Bucur) 2013; 108(3): 331–40.
3. Hellebrekers BW, Kooistra T. Pathogenesis of postoperative adhesion formation. Br J Surg 2011; 98(11): 1503–16.
4. Roeder HA, Cramer SF, Leppert PC. A look at uterine wound healing through a histopathological study of uterine scars. Reprod Sci 2012; 19(5): 463–73.
5. Buhimschi CS, Zhao G, Sora N, Madri JA, Buhimschi IA. Myometrial wound healing post-Cesarean delivery in the MRL/MpJ mouse model of uterine scarring. Am J Pathol 2010; 177(1): 197–207.
6. Knöfler M. Critical growth factors and signalling pathways controlling human trophoblast invasion. Int J Dev Biol 2010; 54(2–3): 269–80.
7. O'Neill SM, Kearney PM, Kenny LC, Khashan AS, Henriksen TB, Lutomski JE, et al. Caesarean delivery and subsequent stillbirth or miscarriage: Systematic review and meta-analysis. PLoS One 2013; 8(1): e54588.
8. Flo K, Widnes C, Vårtun Å, Acharya G. Blood flow to the scarred gravid uterus at 22–24 weeks of gestation. BJOG 2014; 121(2): 210–15.
9. Wu S, Kocherginsky M, Hibbard JU. Abnormal placentation: Twenty-year analysis. Am J Obstet Gynecol 2005; 192(5): 1458–61.
10. Getahun D, Oyelese Y, Salihu HM, Ananth CV. Previous cesarean delivery and risks of placenta previa and placental abruption. Obstet Gynecol 2006; 107(4): 771–8.
11. Downes KL, Hinkle SN, Sjaarda LA, Albert PS, Grantz KL. Previous prelabor or intrapartum cesarean delivery and risk of placenta previa. Am J Obstet Gynecol 2015; 212(5): 669.e1–6.
12. Bailit JL, Grobman WA, Rice MM, Reddy UM, Wapner RJ, Varner MW, et al. Morbidly adherent placent

treatments and outcome. Obstet Gynecol 2015; 125(3): 683–9.

13. Klar M, Michels KB. Cesarean section and placental disorders in subsequent pregnancies: A meta-analysis. J Perinat Med 2014; 42(5): 571–83.

14. Jauniaux E, Jurkovic D. Placenta accreta: Pathogenesis of a 20th century iatrogenic uterine disease. Placenta 2012; 33(4): 244–51.

15. Wehrum MJ, Buhimschi IA, Salafia C, Thung S, Bahtiyar MO, Werner EF, et al. Accreta complicating complete placenta previa is characterized by reduced systemic levels of vascular endothelial growth factor and by epithelial-to-mesenchymal transition of the invasive trophoblast. Am J Obstet Gynecol 2011; 204(5): 411.e1–11.

16. Ben-Nagi J, Walker A, Jurkovic D, Yazbek J, Aplin JD. Effect of cesarean delivery on the endometrium. Int J Gynaecol Obstet 2009; 106(1): 30–4.

17. Irving C, Hertig AT. A study of placenta accreta. Surg Gynec Obstet 1937; 64: 178–200.

18. Solheim KN, Esakoff TF, Little SE, Cheng YW, Sparks TN, Caughey AB. The effect of cesarean delivery rates on the future incidence of placenta previa, placenta accreta, and maternal mortality. J Matern Fetal Neonatal Med 2011; 24(11): 1341–6.

19. Bowman ZS, Eller AG, Bardsley TR, Greene T, Varner MW, Silver RM. Risk factors for placenta accreta: A large prospective cohort. Am J Perinatol 2014; 31(9): 799–804.

20. Kamara M, Henderson JJ, Doherty DA, Dickinson JE, Pennell CE. The risk of placenta accreta following primary elective caesarean delivery: A case-control study. BJOG 2013; 120(7): 879–86.

21. Yang JI, Lim YK, Kim HS, Chang KH, Lee JP, Ryu HS. Sonographic findings of placental lacunae and the prediction of adherent placenta in women with placenta previa totalis and prior Cesarean section. Ultrasound Obstet Gynecol 2006; 28(2): 178–82.

22. Jauniaux E, Toplis PJ, Nicolaides KH. Sonographic diagnosis of a non-previa placenta accreta. Ultrasound Obstet Gynecol 1996; 7(1): 58–60.

23. Twickler DM, Lucas MJ, Balis AB, Santos-Ramos R, Martin L, Malone S, et al. Color flow mapping for myometrial invasion in women with a prior cesarean delivery. J Matern Fetal Med 2000; 9(6): 330–5.

24. Chou MM, Ho ES, Lee YH. Prenatal diagnosis of placenta previa accreta by transabdominal color Doppler ultrasound. Ultrasound Obstet Gynecol 2000; 15(1): 28–35.

25. Warshak CR, Eskander R, Hull AD, Scioscia AL, Mattrey RF, Benirschke K, Resnik R. Accuracy of ultrasonography and magnetic resonance imaging in the diagnosis of placenta accreta. Obstet Gynecol 2006; 108(3 Pt 1): 573–81.

26. Wong HS, Cheung YK, Strand L, Carryer P, Parker S, Tait J, et al. Specific sonographic features of placenta accreta: Tissue interface disruption on gray-scale imaging and evidence of vessels crossing interface-disruption sites on Doppler imaging. Ultrasound Obstet Gynecol 2007; 29(2): 239–40.

27. Woodring TC, Klauser CK, Bofill JA, Martin RW, Morrison JC. Prediction of placenta accreta by ultrasonography and color Doppler imaging. J Matern Fetal Neonatal Med 2011; 24(1): 118–21.

28. Esakoff TF, Sparks TN, Kaimal AJ, Kim LH, Feldstein VA, Goldstein RB, et al. Diagnosis and morbidity of placenta accreta. Ultrasound Obstet Gynecol 2011; 37(3): 324–7.

29. Chalubinski KM, Pils S, Klein K, Seemann R, Speiser P, Langer M, et al. Prenatal sonography can predict degree of placental invasion. Ultrasound Obstet Gynecol 2013; 42(5): 518–24.

30. Comstock CH, Bronsteen RA. The antenatal diagnosis of placenta accreta. BJOG 2014; 121(2): 171–81.

31. D'Antonio F, Iacovella C, Bhide A. Prenatal identification of invasive placentation using ultrasound: Systematic review and meta-analysis. Ultrasound Obstet Gynecol 2013; 42(5): 509–17.

32. Bowman ZS, Eller AG, Kennedy AM, Richards DS, Winter TC III, Woodward PJ, et al. Accuracy of ultrasound for the prediction of placenta accreta. Am J Obstet Gynecol 2014; 211(2): 177.e1–7.

33. Shih JC, Cheng WF, Shyu MK, Lee CN, Hsieh FJ. Power Doppler evidence of placenta accreta appearing in the first trimester. Ultrasound Obstet Gynecol 2002; 19(6): 623–5.

34. Comstock CH, Lee W, Vettraino IM, Bronsteen RA. The early sonographic appearance of placenta accreta. J Ultrasound Med 2003; 22(1): 19–23.

35. Ben Nagi J, Ofili-Yebovi D, Marsh M, Jurkovic D. First-trimester cesarean scar pregnancy evolving into placenta previa/accreta at term. J Ultrasound Med 2005; 24(11): 1569–73.

36. Zosmer N, Fuller J, Shaikh H, Johns J, Ross JA. The natural history of early first trimester pregnancies implanted in Caesarean scars: A prospective study. Ultrasound Obstet Gynecol 2015; 46(3): 367–75.

37. Stirnemann JJ, Mousty E, Chalouhi G, Salomon LJ, Bernard JP, Ville Y. Screening for placenta accreta at 11–14 weeks of gestation. Am J Obstet Gynecol 2011; 205(6): 547.e1–6.

38. McLean LA, Heilbrun ME, Eller AG, Kennedy AM, Woodward PJ. Assessing the role of magnetic resonance imaging in the management of gravid patients at risk for placenta accreta. Acad Radiol 2011; 18(9): 1175–80.

39. Elhawary TM, Dabees NL, Youssef MA. Diagnostic value of ultrasonography and magnetic resonance

imaging in pregnant women at risk for placenta accreta. J Matern Fetal Neonatal Med 2013; 26(14): 1443–9.

40. D'Antonio F, Iacovella C, Palacios-Jaraquemada J, Bruno CH, Manzoli L, BhideA. Prenatal identification of invasive placentation using magnetic resonance imaging (MRI): A systematic review and meta-analysis. Ultrasound Obstet Gynecol 2014; 44(1): 8–16.

41. Jastrow N, Chaillet N, Roberge S, Morency AM, Lacasse Y, Bujold E. Sonographic lower uterine segment thickness and risk of uterine scar defect: a systematic review. J Obstet Gynaecol Can 2010; 32(4): 321–7.

42. Ofili-Yebovi D, Ben-Nagi J, Sawyer E, Yazbek J, Lee C, Gonzalez J, Jurkovic D. Deficient lower-segment Cesarean section scars: Prevalence and risk factors. Ultrasound Obstet Gynecol 2008; 31(1): 72–7.

43. Wang CB, Chiu WW, Lee CY, Sun YL, Lin YH, Tseng CJ. Cesarean scar defect: Correlation between Cesarean section number, defect size, clinical symptoms and uterine position. Ultrasound Obstet Gynecol 2009; 34(1): 85–9.

44. Chang WC, Chang DY, Huang SC, Shih JC, Hsu WC, Chen SY, et al. Use of three-dimensional ultrasonography in the evaluation of uterine perfusion and healing after laparoscopic myomectomy. Fertil Steril 2009; 92(3): 1110–15.

45. Osser OV, Jokubkiene L, Valentin L. High prevalence of defects in Cesarean section scars at transvaginal ultrasound examination. Ultrasound Obstet Gynecol 2009; 34(1): 90–7.

46. Osser OV, Valentin L. Clinical importance of appearance of cesarean hysterotomy scar at transvaginal ultrasonography in nonpregnant women. Obstet Gynecol 2011; 117(3): 525–32.

47. Roberge S, Boutin A, Chaillet N, Moore L, Jastrow N, Demers S, et al. Systematic review of cesarean scar assessment in the nonpregnant state: Imaging techniques and uterine scar defect. Am J Perinatol 2012; 29(6): 465–71.

48. Van der Voet LF, Bij de Vaate AM, Veersema S, Brölmann HA, Huirne JAF. Long-term complications of caesarean section. The niche in the scar: A prospective cohort study on niche prevalence and its relation to abnormal uterine bleeding. BJOG 2014; 121(2): 236–44.

49. Baron J, Weintraub AY, Eshkoli T, Hershkovitz R, Sheiner E. The consequences of previous uterine scar dehiscence and cesarean delivery on subsequent births. Int J Gynaecol Obstet 2014; 126(2): 120–2.

50. Fox NS, Gerber RS, Mourad M, Saltzman DH, Klauser CK, Gupta S, et al., Pregnancy outcomes in patients with prior uterine rupture or dehiscence. Obstet Gynecol 2014; 123(4): 785–9.

51. Ben Nagi J, Ofili-Yebovi D, Sawyer E, Aplin J, Jurkovic D. Successful treatment of a recurrent Cesarean scar ectopic pregnancy by surgical repair of the uterine defect. Ultrasound Obstet Gynecol 2006; 28(6): 855–6.

52. Rygh AB, Greve OJ, Fjetland L, Berland JM, Eggebø TM. Arteriovenous malformation as a consequence of a scar pregnancy. Acta Obstet Gynecol Scand 2009; 88(7): 853–5.

53. Van der Voet LF, Vervoort AJ, Veersema S, BijdeVaate AJ, Brölmann HAM, Huirne HAF. Minimally invasive therapy for gynaecological symptoms related to a niche in the caesarean scar: A systematic review. BJOG 2014; 121(2): 145–56.

54. Qian ZD, Guo QY, Huang LL. Identifying risk factors for recurrent cesarean scar pregnancy: A case-control study. Fertil Steril 2014; 120(1): 129–34.

55. Practice Committee of American Society for Reproductive Medicine in collaboration with Society of Reproductive Surgeons. Pathogenesis, consequences, and control of peritoneal adhesions in gynecologic surgery: A committee opinion. Fertil Steril 2013; 99(6): 1550–5.

56. Ten Broek RP, Issa Y, Van Santbrink EJ, Bouvy ND, Kruitwagen RF, Jeekel J, et al. Burden of adhesions in abdominal and pelvic surgery: Systematic review and meta-analysis. BMJ 2013; 347: f5588.

57. Lyell DJ. Adhesions and perioperative complications of repeat cesarean delivery. Am J Obstet Gynecol 2011; 205(6): S11–18.

58. Moro F, Mavrelos D, Pateman K, Holland T, Hoo WL, Jurkovic D. Prevalence of pelvic adhesions on ultrasound examination in women with a history of cesarean section. Ultrasound Obstet Gynecol 2015; 45(2): 223–8.

59. Kahyaoglu I, Kayikcioglu F, Kinay T, Mollamahmutoglu L. Abdominal scar characteristics: Do they predict intraabdominal adhesions with repeat cesarean deliveries? J Obstet Gynaecol Res 2014; 40(6): 1643–8.

60. Shaw JL, Dey SK, Critchley HO, Horne AW. Current knowledge of the aetiology of human tubal ectopic pregnancy. Hum Reprod Update 2010; 16(4): 432–44.

61. O'Neill SM, Khashan AS, Kenny LC, Greene RA, Henriksen TB, Lutomski JE, et al. Caesarean section and subsequent ectopic pregnancy: A systematic review and meta-analysis. BJOG 2013; 120(6): 671–80.

62. Gurol-Urganci I, Bou-Antoun S, Lim CP, Cromwell DA, Mahmood TA, Templeton A, et al. Impact of Caesarean section on subsequent fertility: A systematic review and meta-analysis. Hum Reprod 2013; 28(7): 1943–52.

63. Kjerulff KH, Zhu J, Weisman CS, Ananth CV. First birth Caesarean section and subsequent fertility: A

population-based study in the USA, 2000–2008. Hum Reprod 2013; 28(12): 3349–57.

64. Collin SM, Marshall T, Filippi V. Caesarean section and subsequent fertility in sub-Saharan Africa. BJOG 2006; 113(3): 276–83.

65. Taff L, Jones S. Cesarean scar endometriosis. A report of two cases. J Reprod Med 2002; 47(1): 50–2.

66. Kaloo P, Reid G, Wong F. Caesarean section scar endometriosis: Two cases of recurrent disease and a literature review. Aust N Z J Obstet Gynaecol 2002; 42(2): 218–20.

67. Andolf E, Thorsell M, Källén K. Caesarean section and risk for endometriosis: A prospective cohort study of Swedish registries. BJOG 2013; 120(9): 1061–5.

CHAPTER 10

Perinatal outcome of neonates born by caesarean section

Emily Robertson and Tom Lissauer

Introduction

For many years it was assumed that, once pregnancy had reached 'term', that is, from 37 weeks of gestation onwards, delivery by caesarian section would not have any additional neonatal consequences compared to vaginal delivery. However, neonates delivered by caesarean section are at increased risk of respiratory complications from higher rates of respiratory distress syndrome, transient tachypnoea of the newborn and pneumothorax, compared to those delivered vaginally (see Figure 10.1). Recent evidence has also shown a clear neonatal advantage in waiting to deliver at 39 weeks, whenever possible, to reduce the risk of neonatal respiratory morbidity. The mode of delivery has been proposed to affect not only short-term outcomes but also long-term development and health. Caesarean delivery impacts not only on the physiological changes of the infant's respiratory system at birth but also on endocrine, metabolic, gastrointestinal, and even haematological systems. This chapter aims to provide an evidence-based summary of the potential neonatal complications and outcomes of caesarean section delivery on the neonate. This information should aid clinical decision-making and counselling of parents.

Effect of mode of delivery on neonatal outcomes

Caesarean delivery of term infants with cephalic presentation

While emergency caesarean delivery at term of infants with cephalic presentation may protect an individual baby from perinatal asphyxia and intrapartum fetal death, it is associated with increased neonatal morbidity and mortality compared to vaginal delivery. This is even the case in infants of low intrapartum risk women a study in the United States found the neonatal mortality rate for caesarean delivery to be 1.77 deaths per 1000 live births, which is 2.9 times the rate of 0.62 for vaginal births [1]. Increased neonatal morbidity comes largely from an increased risk of respiratory complications, particularly transient tachypnoea of the newborn, and respiratory distress syndrome. There is also increased extended admission to neonatal intensive care, and increased neonatal mortality up to hospital discharge, following both elective and emergency caesarean delivery [2].

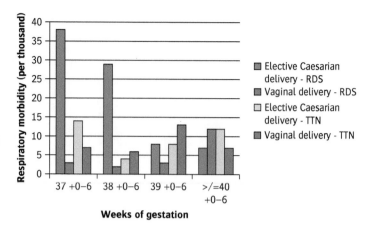

Figure 10.1 Respiratory morbidity following elective lower segment caesarean section compared to that following vaginal delivery at 37–40 weeks. There is a marked increase in neonatal respiratory morbidity following elective caesarean section for each week before 39 weeks; RDS, respiratory distress syndrome; TTN, transient tachypnoea of the newborn.

Zanardo V, Simbi AK, Franzoi M, Soldà G, Salvadori A, Trevisanuto D. Neonatal respiratory morbidity risk and mode of delivery at term: influence of timing of elective caesarean delivery, 2004, Wiley

Caesarean delivery of term infants with breech presentation

Studies of term infants with breech presentation show an outcome that differs from that for infants with cephalic presentation: planned caesarean delivery for infants with breech presentation not only reduce intrapartum death but also reduces neonatal morbidity and mortality, compared to vaginal delivery [2, 3]. This observation has led to recommendations for caesarean delivery to be offered for all infants with breech presentation at term. However, the greatest risk reduction is in countries with low national perinatal mortality rates [3]; thus, vaginal breech delivery may still be appropriate management in some settings [4].

Term infants delivered following repeat caesarean section

Outcomes of infants delivered following repeat caesarean section have been assessed in small cohort studies, a number of which showed repeat elective caesarean to be associated with a higher rate of respiratory morbidity, a higher rate of admission to the neonatal intensive care unit, and a longer length of hospital stay, as compared with vaginal birth after caesarean [5]. However, a systematic review has not supported an increase in neonatal mortality or serious morbidity following repeat caesarean section versus following a planned vaginal birth after caesarean section [6].

Gestational age of term infants for caesarean delivery

The timing of caesarean delivery plays an important role in the outcome even of term infants. Elective caesarean section prior to onset of labour is associated with a higher risk for neonatal respiratory morbidity, compared to caesarean after labour commences [7] There is increasing evidence that outcomes differ by the week of gestation; delivery between 39+0 and 39+6 of gestation has a lower risk of respiratory complications than delivery between weeks 37 + 0 and 38 + 6 [7–9]. Therefore, current guidance by the Royal College of Obstetricians and Gynaecologists (RCOG) in the United Kingdom and the American College of Obstetricians and Gynecologists (ACOG) is to wait until week 39 of pregnancy to perform an elective caesarean section, unless otherwise medically indicated [10].

Caesarean delivery of preterm and low-birth-weight infants

Evidence regarding the impact of mode of delivery on preterm infants and low-birth-weight infants is limited [11]. Analysis of data from 1990 through 2004 in the United States showed a dramatic increase in caesarean delivery rates for preterm infants, increasing by as much as 50% in the 24–27-week group [12]. At the same time, a reduction in perinatal death was noted; this reduction has been mainly attributed to a reduction in the number of stillbirths [12]. Data analysis and observation from cohort studies do not support an association between improved neonatal outcomes and caesarean delivery of preterm infants, particularly for moderately preterm or near-term infants (32–36 weeks) [13–15]. Indeed, a number of studies observed an increased risk of neonatal mortality and morbidity with preterm caesarean delivery [13–15], with the exception of infants with non-vertex presentation [16]. To date, there has been insufficient evidence for a conclusive Cochrane review [11] but evidence from small randomized controlled trials (RCTs) showed no significant difference between preterm infants delivered by caesarean section and those who underwent vaginal delivery, with respect to perinatal death, birth asphyxia, birth injury, low Apgar score at 5 minutes, neonatal seizures, or respiratory distress syndrome [11]. This evidence is in contrast to that provided by a systematic review of non-RCTs for breech preterm infants; this review showed a significant reduction in mortality with caesarean delivery as compared to vaginal delivery [17]. We can therefore only conclude that, in the absence of additional complications or indications, delivery by caesarean section does not improve the neonatal outcomes of preterm infants, with the exception of those infants with non-vertex presentation. Further research in this area is required.

Caesarean section for extreme preterm delivery

Despite caesarean section rates being highest in this group, the effect of mode of delivery on the survival of extremely preterm infants is also unclear. A population-based study of infants delivered at less than 28 weeks gestation in the United States from 1995 and 2005 showed a steady mortality rate of 33%–34% despite an increase in caesarean delivery rate from 43% to 54% [18]. Although a number of studies have shown improvements in neonatal mortality and a reduction in risk of intraventricular haemorrhage with caesarean delivery of extremely preterm infants, other evidence has been contradictory and,

as a result, the World Association of Perinatal Medicine do not recommend routine caesarean delivery in this group [19].

Caesarean delivery of infants of multiple pregnancies

Multiple pregnancies are associated with increased fetal and neonatal mortality, and infants from multiple pregnancies have a higher incidence of cerebral palsy than those from singleton pregnancies. In addition, there are increased risks of obstetric and fetal complications with multiple pregnancies; such risks are likely to influence both the choice of mode of delivery and the outcomes of the infants.

Cohort studies looking at the impact of elective caesarean section on term or near-term twins showed that it was associated with a reduction in the risk of poor perinatal outcomes, particularly for the second twin [20–22]. However, results of a systematic review comparing planned caesarean versus planned vaginal delivery found no difference in perinatal outcomes, including perinatal or neonatal death or serious neonatal morbidity. This review only included the results of one RCT, which was the only one available at the time of analysis, but the findings have subsequently been supported by findings of the Twin Birth Study [23, 24], a large RCT which assessed twins delivered at 32–38 weeks gestation and where the first twin was in cephalic presentation [24]. For non-cephalically presenting twins, the evidence is insufficient to draw a definite conclusion but so far suggests no difference in outcomes of vaginal versus caesarean birth [25]. There is however evidence, as with singletons, that the timing of caesarean delivery for uncomplicated twin pregnancies is important, with twins delivered during weeks 36 and 37 of pregnancy being exposed to a higher risk for respiratory morbidity than those delivered between 39 and 40 weeks [26].

Caesarean section is often the mode of delivery of choice for triplets. Evidence for outcomes of triplets according to mode of delivery is limited to retrospective case-control studies, but these have failed to demonstrate that outcomes are improved by caesarean compared to vaginal delivery [27–29].

Neonatal respiratory morbidity following caesarean section

Respiratory extrauterine adaptation following caesarean section

Respiratory adaptation to extrauterine life is influenced by an infant's mode of delivery. Caesarean delivery is associated with retained fetal lung fluid and relatively impaired lung function during the first hours of life. One possible explanation for this may be the absence of mechanical pressure on the thorax to squeeze lung fluid from the respiratory tract, as this pressure would normally be experienced by infants delivered vaginally. However, animal studies and an improved understanding of the pathophysiology of respiratory disorders in neonates have shown that clearance of fetal lung fluid is largely dependent on reabsorption of alveolar fluid via sodium channels in the lung epithelium. This mechanism is thought to be influenced by the level of circulating catecholamines in the newborn. Newborns delivered by caesarean section have lower concentrations of circulating catecholamines than newborns delivered vaginally [30], particularly following delivery without prior labour, and the low catecholamine level is thought to be the main cause of delay in early fetal lung fluid clearance.

Transient tachypnoea of the newborn following caesarean section

Transient tachypnoea of the newborn is commonly associated with delivery by caesarean section (see Figures 10.2, 10.3). First described by Avery et al. [31], it causes respiratory distress as a result of retention of fetal lung fluid and aberrant lung adaptation to extrauterine life. The risk is increased after both emergency and elective caesarean sections, [32]. Although self-limiting, it is not a benign condition and can be associated with significant morbidity [33], including hypoxaemia, pulmonary air leaks, and persistent pulmonary hypertension of the newborn. The risk of transient tachypnoea of the newborn is markedly reduced by delaying delivery until 39 weeks of gestation.

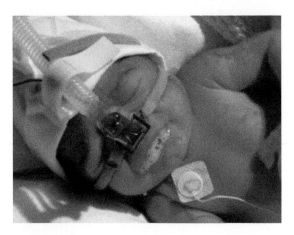

Figure 10.2 Lung liquid in infant requiring continuous positive airway pressure following delivery by elective caesarean section.

Lissauer T, Fanaroff AA, Miall L, Fanaroff J. Neonatology at a Glance., 2015, Wiley

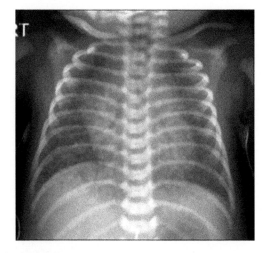

Figure 10.3 Chest X-ray in transient tachypnoea of the newborn showing fluid in the horizontal fissure and some streaky infiltrates with hyperinflation.

(Courtesy of Dr Berlin).

Respiratory distress syndrome following caesarean section

Respiratory distress syndrome is caused by surfactant deficiency, which results in early and often severe respiratory distress (Figure 10.4). The risk of respiratory distress syndrome is inversely

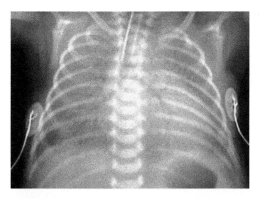

Figure 10.4 Chest X-ray of an infant aged 4 hours and with respiratory distress syndrome. The diffuse, uniform granular (ground glass) appearance of the lungs can be seen, as well as an air bronchogram (i.e. the outline of air-filled large airways against opaque lungs). In addition, lung volume is reduced, and the heart border is indistinct as the lung fields are opaque (termed 'white-out'). A tracheal tube is in place.

Lissauer T, Fanaroff AA, Miall L, Fanaroff J From Neonatology at a Glance., 2015, Wiley

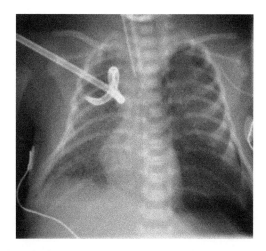

Figure 10.5 Chest X-ray showing a left pneumothorax and mediastinal shift to the right, as shown by the displacement of the trachea and tracheal tube and heart to the right side. There is a right chest tube (pigtail chest tube) which has been inserted to drain a pneumothorax on the right side.

Lissauer T, Fanaroff AA, Miall L, Fanaroff J Neonatology at a Glance., 2015, Wiley

related to gestational age and is a common complication of preterm delivery; however, caesarean delivery may independently predispose infants to respiratory distress syndrome, even at term [34, 35]. The timing of elective caesarean delivery at term can have a significant impact on the risk of severe respiratory distress syndrome, with one study demonstrating the risk of requiring mechanical ventilation for surfactant deficiency to be 120 times greater in neonates born by elective caesarean section at 37–38 weeks gestation than in those born by elective caesarean section at 39–41 weeks gestation [35]. Surfactant deficiency is therefore an important differential diagnosis of respiratory complications even in term infants delivered by caesarean section, particularly when symptoms of respiratory distress are severe.

Pneumothorax following caesarean section

Delivery by caesarean section may be associated with neonatal pneumothorax (Figure 10.5). One cohort study found that the risk of neonatal pneumothorax in infants born at term or preterm (30–36 weeks) by caesarean delivery was significantly greater than in those delivered vaginally [36]. For infants delivered by elective caesarean delivery at term, there appears to be a progressive reduction in the incidence of pneumothorax with each week beyond 37 weeks gestation [37].

Antenatal steroids in caesarean delivery

Antenatal corticosteroids have been shown to significantly reduce the risk of respiratory distress syndrome in preterm infants (relative risk, 0.69; confidence interval (CI), 0.58–0.81). In addition, their use in preterm infants is associated with an overall reduction in neonatal death, intraventricular haemorrhage, necrotizing enterocolitis, respiratory support, intensive care admissions, and systemic infections in the first 48 hours of life [38]. Antenatal corticosteroids are therefore recommended for all women at risk of preterm labour at up to 34 + 6 weeks gestation. Evidence is now also increasing for the use of corticosteroids in elective term deliveries. A Cochrane review identified one RCT which showed that corticosteroid use was associated with a significant reduction in the risk of admission to neonatal intensive care for respiratory morbidity, although this study did not show a reduced incidence of respiratory distress syndrome, transient tachypnoea of the newborn, or the need for mechanical ventilation, or a reduction in the length of stay in the neonatal intensive care unit [39]. Therefore, even though the RCOG recommends antenatal corticosteroids for women planning for an elective caesarean before 39 weeks, corticosteroids do not provide protection from all respiratory complications of elective caesarean delivery; the ACOG do not recommend antenatal corticosteroids beyond 34 weeks gestation.

Early care of the newborn following caesarean delivery

Neonatal resuscitation following caesarean delivery

Emergency caesarean delivery is frequently associated with fetal compromise, so staff skilled in neonatal resuscitation should be present. Preterm deliveries require the presence of the paediatric team, as well as special preparation of resuscitation equipment, such as appropriately sized masks, laryngoscopes, tracheal tubes, and additional items for thermal support, such as plastic wrapping. The need for paediatricians to attend planned (or elective) caesarean deliveries is debated. Non-emergency caesarean section at term has an increased risk of requiring bag-and-mask ventilation, from 3.8% following normal vaginal delivery to 5.1% and 7.4% under spinal and epidural anaesthesia, respectively [40], but the requirement for intubation is not increased and is only 0.04% [41–43]. Therefore, the recommendation of the 2010 International Consensus on Cardiopulmonary Resuscitation is, 'When an infant without antenatally identified risk factors is delivered at term by Caesarean section under regional anaesthesia, a provider capable of performing bag–mask ventilation should be present at the delivery. It is not necessary for a provider skilled in neonatal intubation to be present at that delivery.' In addition, the gestation at caesarean section also impacts on the likely need for neonatal resuscitation, with a significant reduction in need for resuscitation by waiting until 39 weeks gestation for elective caesarean delivery [44].

Delayed cord clamping following caesarean delivery

Delayed umbilical cord clamping for at least 1 minute is now recommended for all births unless the neonate requires resuscitation [45]. Term infants benefit from placental transfusion of blood; those who have undergone such transfusion have higher haemoglobin concentrations in the first 2 days of life and improved iron stores at 6 months than those who have not [46]. Evidence is less reliable for preterm infants than for term infants, but studies suggest they also benefit, showing a reduction in the need for transfusion for anaemia or hypotension, a reduced risk of intraventicular haemorrhage, and a reduced risk of necrotizing enterocolitis [47]. Studies have not looked directly at the impact of delayed cord clamping in caesarean section, but data from caesarean births have been included in several studies [46, 47]. However, as caesarean section is known to be associated with reduced placental transfusion and lower haematocrit, haemoglobin, and erythrocyte levels in the infant [48], it is likely that the benefits of delayed cord clamping may be even greater for infants born by caesarean section than for those delivered vaginally.

If the neonate requires resuscitation, immediate cord clamping is currently recommended in order to be able to provide resuscitation without delay, as this objective clearly takes priority over all others. However, in order to allow resuscitation to be performed with the umbilical cord intact, a small portable resuscitation table has been developed which can be placed directly alongside the mother, even for caesarean deliveries. Outcome studies of the use of this device are awaited [49].

Contraindications to delayed cord clamping with caesarean delivery have not been identified. No significant differences have been found between early and late cord clamping for maternal outcomes of post-partum haemorrhage, use of uterotonic drugs, or early post-partum maternal haemoglobin levels [46]. They have also not been identified for neonatal mortality, Apgar score at 5 minutes, or admission to specialist neonatal care [46]. However, late cord clamping is associated with an increased risk of jaundice requiring phototherapy, so availability and access to treatment for jaundice is important when implementing a policy of delayed cord clamping [46].

Skin-to-skin contact, thermal support, and feeding of newborns following caesarean delivery

Skin-to-skin contact involves placing the naked newborn prone on the mother's bare chest with a hat and dry warm blanket across their back. Advantages of early skin-to-skin contact after delivery for the neonate include cardiorespiratory stability, increased blood glucose, maintenance of normothermia, decreased infant crying, and improved breastfeeding outcomes. It is also likely to improve attachment and bonding between mother and baby [50]. The World Health Organization recommends immediate skin-to-skin contact for all infants who do not require resuscitation [51]. Caesarean delivery often results in separation of mother and baby, but with simple changes in practice this separation can be minimized or prevented [52–55]. Provided mother and baby are clinically stable, newborns delivered by caesarean section under regional anaesthesia should receive early skin-to-skin contact.

In preterm infants, skin-to-skin contact has also been shown to be an effective intervention in the prevention of hypothermia [56]. Infants delivered by caesarean have lower skin temperatures after birth, compared to infants delivered vaginally [57]. The aberrant metabolic adaptation and low levels of catecholamine associated with caesarean delivery may explain the reduced thermogenesis and hence reduced body temperature in infants delivered by caesarean. In practice, infants who receive early skin-to-skin contact following caesarean delivery do not develop hypothermia [58].

Caesarean delivery is associated with decreased rates of exclusive breastfeeding compared to vaginal delivery. Initiation of early breastfeeding in the delivery room and rates of breastfeeding at discharge through to 6 months are higher in newborns delivered vaginally than in those delivered by either elective or emergency caesarean section [59]. Caesarean delivery is associated with suboptimal feeding behaviour in the neonate. There is delayed onset of lactation in the mother [60], a lag in the volumes of milk transferred to the infant, and an increase in the time taken for the neonate to regain birth weight [61]. Simple interventions such as early skin-to-skin contact and breastfeeding support, particularly during the first 72 hours, assist in preventing both difficulty in initiating or early discontinuation of breastfeeding [60].

Long-term outcomes associated with caesarean section

Respiratory outcomes associated with caesarean section

Childhood respiratory disorders may be increased in individuals delivered by caesarean section. A meta-analysis of 23 studies showed a 20% increase in the subsequent risk of asthma in children who had been delivered by caesarean section [62]. A retrospective cohort study of 212,068 singleton term births in Western Australia found infants under 12 months of age who were delivered by elective caesarean section were 17% more likely to have multiple hospitalizations for bronchiolitis than

those delivered vaginally [63]. The large Norwegian Mother and Child Cohort Study found a positive association between asthma at 36 months and delivery by caesarean section, with a relative risk of 1.17 (see Box 10.1) for elective and emergency caesarean section groups [64]. Developing a respiratory disorder during the neonatal period is associated with an increased risk of asthma in childhood, and the increased respiratory morbidity following caesarean section may explain the link [65]. Another explanation that has been proposed is the impact of caesarean section on the development of the immune system [66].

Box 10.1 Long-term outcomes following caesarean section delivery

- Asthma: relative risk, 1.17 (95% confidence interval (CI), 1.03–1.32) [1] and odds ratio, 1.18 (95% CI, 1.05–1.32) [2, 3]
- Food allergy/food atopy: OR, 1.32 (95% CI, 1.12–1.55) [2, 3]
- Allergic rhinitis: OR, 1.23 (95% CI, 1.12–1.35) [2, 3]
- Coeliac disease: OR, 1.8 (95% CI, 1.13–2.88) [4]

1. Magnus MC, Håberg SE, Stigum H, Nafstad P, London SJ, Vangen S, et al. Delivery by cesarean section and early childhood respiratory symptoms and disorders: The Norwegian Mother and Child Cohort Study. Am J Epidemiol 2011; 174(11): 1275–85.
2. Bager P, Wohlfahrt J, Westergaard T. Caesarean delivery and risk of atopy and allergic disesase: Meta-analyses. Clinical and Experimental Allergy 2008; 38(4): 634–42.
3. Cho CE, Norman M. Cesarean section and development of the immune system in the offspring. Am J Obstet Gynecol 2013; 208(4): 249–54.
4. Decker E, Engelmann G, Findeisen A, Gerner P, Laass M, Ney D, et al. Cesarean delivery is associated with celiac disease but not inflammatory bowel disease in children. Pediatrics 2010; 125(6): e1433–40.

Immune system outcomes associated with caesarean section

In addition to asthma, caesarean delivery has been linked to an increased risk in developing immune diseases. The incidence of allergic rhinitis and/ or food allergy, in particular IgE-mediated sensitization to food allergens, has been shown to be increased in infants delivered by caesarean section [66]. A systematic review of 26 studies showed increased risk of food allergy/food atopy (odds ratio (OR), 1.32; 6 studies), allergic rhinitis (OR, 1.23; 7 studies), asthma (OR, 1.18; 13 studies), and hospitalization for asthma (OR, 1.21; 7 studies) [67, 68]. A small multicentre case-control study investigating associations between enteric inflammatory diseases in children and caesarean delivery found children with coeliac disease were more likely to have been delivered by caesarean section than controls (OR, 1.8) [69] and a meta-analysis of observational studies showed a 20% increased risk of childhood-onset type 1 diabetes mellitus after caesarean section delivery [70].

Neurodevelopmental outcomes associated with caesarean section

A term infant's mode of delivery does not impact on long-term developmental or neurological outcomes [71–74]. Even a comparison of term and breech singleton infants delivered by planned caesarean section and those delivered vaginally in the International Randomized Term Breech Trial of over 900 children showed no difference in neurodevelopment outcome at 2 years of age [71]. Childhood IQ was also shown to not be affected when caesarean sections were performed following maternal request, as shown in a cohort study of term singletons conducted in China [72].

One might expect that caesarean delivery would confer some protection from outcomes associated with neurological damage, such as cerebral palsy. However, mode of delivery has not been shown to reduce the risk of abnormal neurological development or cerebral palsy [73]. A meta-analysis of 13 studies, which included a total of 3810 children with cerebral palsy and 1.7 million controls, did not demonstrate an overall increase or decrease in the risk of cerebral palsy with caesarean delivery (OR, 1.29; 95% CI, 0.92–1.79), whether the delivery was elective or emergency [74]. Notably, despite a fivefold increase in caesarean delivery rate and the widespread use of fetal monitoring over the last 30 years, rates of cerebral palsy have not decreased in developed countries. This result does not appear to be explained by the increased survival of neurologically impaired preterm infants, as many have postulated [75]. Analysis of cerebral palsy rates of term infants shows no change over 30 years (Figure 10.6). In addition, the number of low-birth-weight infants delivered by caesarean section for fetal distress is insufficient to impact on overall outcomes [75].

When considering elective caesarean delivery, the procedure itself may not impact on the long-term neurological outcome of the infant, but the timing of delivery is important. Extreme preterm infants are recognized to have significantly increased risk for developmental delay [76], but even infants born late preterm (34–36 weeks gestation) have been shown to have poorer neurodevelopmental

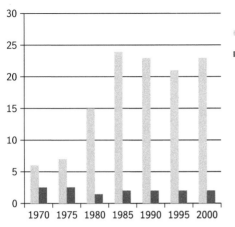

Figure 10.6 Cerebral palsy prevalence (black bars) in term infants in 9 developed countries. Dark grey bars indicate the caesarean section rate.

Sweden, Australia, Canada, Scotland, Denmark, England, United States, Norway, and Ireland. Clark SL, Hankins GDV., Temporal and demographic trends in cerebral palsy – Fact and fiction, 2003, Wiley

outcomes, compared to term infants [77]. One population study assessed gestation of birth and risk of special educational needs. While the incidence of special educational needs is highest in extremely preterm infants, it is markedly higher in those born moderately preterm and even near term, as compared to those born at 39–41 weeks gestation (Figure 10.7) [78]. Therefore, deciding to perform an elective caesarean section before 39 weeks gestation may be placing the infant at increased risk not only of respiratory morbidity but also of poor neurodevelopmental outcome.

Other conditions (malignancies, dentition, metabolic syndrome) and caesarean section

The evidence for the impact of caesarean delivery on malignancies, dentition, and metabolic syndrome is contradictory. An increased risk of childhood

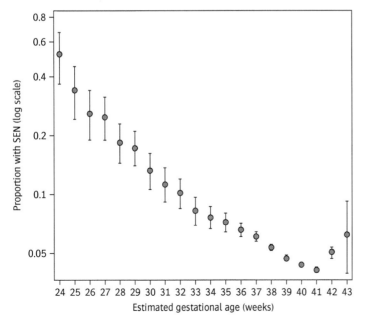

Figure 10.7 Prevalence of special educational need by gestation at delivery of schoolchildren in Scotland. This graph shows that the proportion of infants delivered who will go on to have special educational needs increases not just in the case of extreme prematurity but with each week before full term at 39–41 weeks gestation; SEN, special educational need.

Gestational age at delivery and special educational need: retrospective cohort study of 407,503 schoolchildren., MacKay DF, Smith GC, Dobbie R, Pell JP., PLoS Med., 8;7(6), 2010 doi: 10.1371/journal.pmed.1000289. http://www.ncbi.nlm.nih.gov/pmc/articles/PMC2882432/

cancer has been proposed as a potential long-term complication of caesarean delivery. Studies previously reported an association with both childhood myeloid leukaemia [79] and non-seminomatous testicular cancer [80], but a recent large population study found no association with or increased risk of childhood cancer in children born by caesarean section [81].

An effect on childhood dentition has also been investigated. One study showed an association between caesarean delivery and impaired development of dentition in a group of low-birth-weight infants [82]. However, the authors acknowledge the confounding impact that low birth weight may have on the choice of delivery mode, and other studies have not supported this finding [83, 84].

Lastly, implication of caesarean delivery in the development of the metabolic syndrome has been suggested. An association between caesarean delivery and BMI in the offspring is unclear, and investigation is complicated by significant confounding factors such as maternal BMI and infant feeding choices. Measurements of central adiposity in 3-year-olds concluded no association with mode of delivery [85], and additional aspects of the metabolic syndrome, such as dyslipidaemia and insulin resistance have not been studied. Conclusions are therefore difficult to draw without further research into these outcomes.

Key learning points

1. Elective caesarean delivery has only been shown to improve short-term neonatal outcomes for term infants of breech presentation.
2. Evidence for the impact of caesarean delivery on the outcomes of preterm infants is controversial, but current evidence suggests no difference in outcomes of preterm infants delivered vaginally or by caesarean section, except for those with breech presentation.
3. Elective caesarean for multiple pregnancies alone does not appear to improve neonatal outcomes.
4. Unless otherwise medically indicated, elective delivery at term should be postponed until week 39 of pregnancy
5. Delivery by caesarean section increases the risk of respiratory complications of the newborn, which can result in significant neonatal morbidity in both the short term and the long term.
6. Delaying elective caesarean delivery until 39 weeks gestation reduces the risk of complications from transient tachypnea of the newborn, respiratory distress syndrome, and air leaks (pneumothorax).
7. Caesarean delivery is associated with an increased risk of requiring neonatal resuscitation. A person skilled in neonatal resuscitation should be present at all non-elective caesarean deliveries.
8. As with vaginal delivery, delayed cord clamping should be performed at caesarean delivery, provided the infant does not require resuscitation.
9. Early skin-to-skin contact should be offered to all newborns delivered by caesarean section under regional anaesthesia, provided mother and baby are clinically stable. Additional breastfeeding support, particularly in the first 72 hours, should be offered following caesarean delivery, to ensure successful initiation and continuation of breastfeeding.
10. Caesarean delivery may be associated with an increased risk of childhood diseases, including asthma, allergic rhinitis, food allergy, type 1 diabetes mellitus, and coeliac disease. Further research into the long-term impact of caesarean delivery is required.

References

1. MacDorman MF, Declercq E, Menacker F, Malloy MH. Infant and neonatal mortality for primary cesarean and vaginal births to women with "no indicated risk," United States, 1998–2001 birth cohorts. Birth 2006; 33(3): 175–82.
2. Villar J, Carroli G, Zavaleta N, Donner A, Wojdyla D, Faundes A, et al. Maternal and neonatal individual risks and benefits associated with caesarean delivery: Multicentre prospective study. BMJ 2007; 335: 1025–36.
3. Hofmeyr GJ, Hannah ME. Planned caesarean section for term breech delivery. Cochrane Database Syst Rev 2003; 3: CD000166.
4. Goffinet F, Carayol M, Foidart JM, Alexander S, Uzan S, Subtil D, et al. PREMODA Study Group. Is planned vaginal delivery for breech presentation at term still an option? Results of an observational prospective survey in France and Belgium. Am J Obstet Gynecol 2006; 194(4): 1002–11.
5. Kamath BD, Todd JK, Glazner JE, Lezotte D, Lynch AM. Neonatal outcomes after elective cesarean delivery. Obstet Gynecol 2009; 113(6): 1231–8.
6. Dodd JM, Crowther CA, Huertas E, Guise JM, Horey D. Planned elective repeat caesarean section versus planned vaginal birth for women with a previous caesarean birth. Cochrane Database of Syst Rev 2013; 12: CD004224.

7. Morrison JJ, Rennie JM, Milton PJ. Neonatal respiratory morbidity and mode of delivery: Influence of timing of elective caesarean rate. Br J Obstet Gynaecol 1995; 102(2): 101–6.

8. Zanardo V, Simbi AK, Franzoi M, Soldà G, Salvadori A, Trevisanuto D. Neonatal respiratory morbidity risk and mode of delivery at term: Influence of timing of elective caesarean delivery. Acta Paediatr 2004; 93(5): 643–7.

9. Tita AT, Landon MB, Spong CY, Lai Y, Leveno KJ, Varner MW, et al. Timing of elective repeat cesarean delivery at term and neonatal outcomes. N Engl J Med 2009; 360(2): 111–20.

10. American College of Obstetricians and Gynecologists. ACOG committee opinion no. 559: Cesarean delivery on maternal request. Obstet Gynecol 2013; 121(4): 904–7.

11. Alfirevic Z, Milan SJ, Livio S. Caesarean section versus vaginal delivery for preterm birth in singletons. Cochrane Database Syst Rev 2013; 9: CD000078.

12. Ananth CV, Vintzileos AM. Trends in cesarean delivery at preterm gestation and association with perinatal mortality. Am J Obstet Gynaecol 2011; 204(6): 505. e1–8.

13. Werner EF, Savitz DA, Janevic TM, Ehsanipoor RM, Thung SF, Funai EF, et al. Mode of delivery and neonatal outcomes in preterm, small-for-gestational-age newborns. Obstet Gynecol 2012; 120(3): 560–4.

14. Werner EF, Han CS, Savitz DA, Goldshore M, Lipkind HS. Health outcomes for vaginal compared with cesarean delivery of appropriately grown preterm neonates. Obstet Gynecol 2013; 121(6): 1195–200.

15. Malloy MH. Impact of cesarean section on intermediate and late preterm births: United States, 2000–2003. Birth 2009; 36(1): 26–33.

16. Lodha A, Zhu Q, Lee SK, Shah PS. Neonatal outcomes of preterm infants in breech presentation according to mode of birth in Canadian NICUs. Postgrad Med J 2011; 87(1025): 175–9.

17. Bergenhenegouwen LA, Meertens LJ, Schaaf J, Nijhuis JG, Mol BW, Kok M, et al. Vaginal delivery versus caesarean section in preterm breech delivery: A systematic review. Eur J Obstet Gynecol Reprod Biol 2014; 172: 1–6.

18. Batton B, Burnett C, Verhulst S, Batton D. Extremely preterm infant mortality rates and cesarean deliveries in the United States. Obstet Gynecol 2011; 118(1): 43–8.

19. Skupski DW, Greenough A, Donn SM, Arabin B, Bancalari E, Vladareanu R. Delivery mode for the extremely premature fetus: A statement of the prematurity working group of the World Association of Perinatal Medicine. J Perinat Med 2009; 37(6): 583–6.

20. Smith GC, Shah I, White IR, Pell JP, Dobbie R. Mode of delivery and the risk of delivery-related perinatal death among twins at term: A retrospective cohort study of 8073 births. BJOG 2005; 112(8): 1139–44.

21. Armson BA, O'Connell C, Persad V, Joseph KS, Young DC, Baskett TF. Determinants of perinatal mortality and serious neonatal morbidity in the second twin. Obstet Gynecol 2006; 108(3 Pt 1): 556–64.

22. Hoffmann E, Oldenburg A, Rode L, Tabor A, Rasmussen S, Skibsted L. Twin births: Cesarean section or vaginal delivery? Acta Obstet Gynecol Scand 2012; 91(4): 463–9.

23. Hofmeyr GJ, Barrett JF, Crowther CA. Planned caesarean section for women with a twin pregnancy. Cochrane Database Syst Rev 2011; 12: CD006553.

24. Barrett JF, Hannah ME, Hutton EK, Willan AR, Allen AC, Armson BA, et al. A randomized trial of planned cesarean or vaginal delivery for twin pregnancy. N Engl J Me 2013; 369(14): 1295–305.

25. Steins Bisschop CN, Vogelvang TE, May AM, Schuitemaker NW. Mode of delivery in non-cephalic presenting twins: A systematic review. Arch Gynecol Obstet 2012; 286(1): 237–47.

26. Chasen ST, Madden A, Chervenak FA. Cesarean delivery of twins and neonatal respiratory disorders. Am J Obstet Gynecol 1999; 181(5 Pt 1): 1052–6

27. Wildschut HI, Van Roosmalen J, Van Leeuwen E, Keirse MJ. Planned abdominal compared with planned vaginal birth in triplet pregnancies. Br J Obstet Gynaecol 1995; 102(4): 292–6.

28. Dommergues M, Mahieu-Caputo D, Mandelbrot L, Huon C, Moriette G, Dumez Y. Delivery of uncomplicated triplet pregnancies: Is the vaginal route safer? A case-control study. Am J Obstet Gynecol 1995; 172(2 Pt 1): 513–17.

29. Ziadeh SM. Perinatal outcome in 41 sets of triplets in Jordan. Birth 2000; 27(3): 185–8.

30. Faxelius G, Hägnevik K, Lagercrantz H, Lundell B, Irestedt L. Catecholeamine surge and lung function after delivery. Arch Dis Child 1983; 58(4): 262–6.

31. Avery MR, Gatewood OB, Brumley G. Transient tachypnoea of newborn: Possible delayed resorption of fluid at birth. Am J Dis Child 1966; 111(4): 380–5.

32. Dani C, Reali MF, Bertini G, Wiechmann L, Spagnolo A, Tangucci M, et al. Risk factors for the development of respiratory distress syndrome and transient tachypnoea in newborn infants. Eur Respir J 1999; 14(1): 155–9.

33. Riskin A, Abend-Weinger M, Riskin-Mashiah S, Kugelman A, Bader D. Cesarean section, gestational age, and transient tachypnea of the newborn: Timing is the key. Am J Perinatol 2005; 22(7): 377–382.

34. Gerten KA, Coonrod DV, Bay RC, Chambliss LR. Cesarean delivery and respiratory distress syndrome: Does labour make a difference? Am J Obstet Gynecol 2005; 193(3 Pt 2): 1061–4.

35. Madar J, Richmond S, Hey E. Surfactant-deficient respiratory distress after elective delivery at 'term'. Acta Ped 1999; 88(11): 1244–8.

36. Benterud T, Sandvik L, Lindemann R. Cesarean section is associated with more frequent pneumothorax and respiratory problems in the neonate. Acta Obstet Gynecol Scand 2009; 88(3): 359–61.

37. Zanardo V, Padovani E, Pittini C, Doglioni N, Ferrante A, Trevisanuto D. The influence of timing of elective cesarean section on risk of neonatal pneumothorax. J Pediatr 2007; 150(3): 252–5.

38. Roberts D, Dalziel SR. Antenatal corticosteroids for accelerating fetal lung maturation for women at risk of preterm birth. Cochrane Database Syst Rev 2006; 3: CD004454.

39. Sotiriadis A, Makrydimas G, Papatheodorou S, Ioannidis JPA. Corticosteroids for preventing neonatal respiratory morbidity after elective caesarean section at term. Cochrane Database Syst Rev 2009; 4: CD006614.

40. Atherton N, Parsons SJ, Mansfield P. Attendance of paediatricians at elective Caesarean sections performed under regional anaesthesia: Is it warranted? J Paediatr Child Health 2006; 42(6): 332–6.

41. Ozlu F, Yapicioglu H, Ulu B, Buyukkurt S, Unlugenc H. Do all deliveries with elective caesarean section need paediatrician attendance? J Matern Fetal Neonatal Med 2012; 25(12): 2766–8.

42. Gordon A, McKechnie EJ, Jeffery H. Pediatric presence at cesarean section: Justified or not? Am J Obstet Gynecol 2005; 193(3 Pt 1): 599–605.

43. Parsons SJ, Sonneveld S, Nolan T. Is a paediatrician needed at all Caesarean sections? J Paediatr Child Health 1998; 34(3): 241–4.

44. Zanardo V, Simbi KA, Vedovato S, Trevisanuto D. The influence of timing of elective caesarean section on neonatal resuscitation risk. Pediatr Crit Care Med 2004; 5(6): 566–70.

45. World Health Organization. WHO Recommendations for the Prevention and Treatment of Postpartum Haemorrhage. Geneva: World Health Organization, 2012.

46. McDonald SJ, Middleton P, Dowswell T, Morris PS. Effect of timing of umbilical cord clamping of term infants on maternal and neonatal outcomes. Cochrane Database Syst Rev 2013; 7: CD004074.

47. Rabe H, Diaz-Rossello JL, Duley L, Dowswell T. Effect of timing of umbilical cord clamping and other strategies to influence placental transfusion at preterm birth on maternal and infant outcomes. Cochrane Database Syst Rev 2012; 8: CD003248.

48. Zhou YB, Li HT, Zhu LP, Liu JM. Impact of cesarean section on placental transfusion and iron-related hematological indices in term neonates: A systematic review and meta-analysis. Placenta 2014; 35(1): 1–8.

49. Hutchon DJ. Immediate or early cord clamping vs delayed clamping. J Obstet Gynaecol 2012; 32(8): 724–9.

50. Moore ER, Anderson GC, Bergman N, Dowswell T. Early skin-to-skin contact for mothers and their healthy newborn infants. Cochrane Database of Syst Rev 2012; 5: CD003519.

51. World Health Organization. Kangaroo Mother Care: A Practical Guide. Geneva: World Health Organization, 2003.

52. Zwelling E, Phillips CR. Family-centered maternity care in the new millennium: Is it real or is it imagined? J Perinat Neonatal Nurs 2001; 15(3): 1–12.

53. Miesnik SR, Reale BJ. A review of issues surrounding medically elective cesarean delivery. J Obstet Gynecol Neonatal Nurs 2007; 36(6): 605–15.

54. Nolan A, Lawrence C. A pilot study of a nursing intervention protocol to minimize maternal-infant separation after Cesarean birth. J Obstet Gynecol Neonatal Nurs 2009; 38(4): 430–42.

55. Hung KJ, Berg O. Early skin-to-skin after caesarean to improve breastfeeding. MCN AM J Matern Child Nurs 2011; 36(5): 318–24.

56. McCall EM, Alderdice F, Halliday HL, Jenkins JG, Vohra S. Interventions to prevent hypothermia at birth in preterm and/or low birthweight infants. Cochrane Database Syst Rev 2010; 3: CD004210.

57. Christensson K, Siles C, Cabrera T, Belaustequi A, de la Fuente P, Lagercrantz H, et al. Lower body temperatures in infants delivered by caesarean section than in vaginally delivered infants. Acta Paediatr 1993; 82(2): 128–31.

58. Gouchon S, Gregori D, Picotto A, Patrucco G, Nangeroni M, Di Giulio P. Skin-to-skin contact after cesarean delivery: An experimental study. Nurs Res 2010; 59(2): 78–84.

59. Zanardo V, Svegliado G, Cavallin F, Giustardi A, Cosmi E, Litta P, et al. Elective cesarean delivery: Does it have a negative effect on breastfeeding? Birth 2010; 37(4): 275–9.

60. Dewey KG, Nommsen-Rivers LA, Heinig MJ, Cohen RJ. Risk factors for suboptimal infant breastfeeding behavior, delayed onset of lactation, and excess neonatal weight loss. Pediatrics 2003; 112(3 Pt 1): 607–19.

61. Evans KC, Evans RG, Royal R, Esterman AJ, James SL Effect of caesarean section on breast milk transfer to the normal term newborn over the first week of life. Arch Dis Child Fetal Neonatal Ed 2003; 88(5): F380–2.

62. Thavagnanam S, Fleming J, Bromley A, Shields MD, Cardwell CR. A meta-analysis of the association between cesarean section and childhood asthma. Clin Exp Allergy 2008; 38(4): 629–33.

63. Moore HC, de Klerk N, Holt P, Richmond PC, Lehmann D. Hospitalisation for bronchiolitis in infants is

more common after elective caesarean delivery. Arch Dis Child 2012; 97(5): 410–14.

64. Magnus MC, Håberg SE, Stigum H, Nafstad P, London SJ, Vangen S, et al. Delivery by cesarean section and early childhood respiratory symptoms and disorders: The Norwegian Mother and Child Cohort Study. Am J Epidemiol 2011; 174(11): 1275–85.

65. Smith GC, Wood AM, White IR, Pell JP, Cameron AD, Dobbie R. Neonatal respiratory morbidity at term and the risk of childhood asthma. Arch Dis Child 2004; 89(10): 956–60.

66. Koplin J, Allen K, Gurrin L, Osborne N, Tang ML, Dharmage S. Is caesarean delivery associated with sensitization to food allergens and IgE-mediated food allergy? A systematic review. Pediatric Allergy and Immunology 2008; 19(8): 682–7.

67. Bager P, Wohlfahrt J, Westergaard T. Caesarean delivery and risk of atopy and allergic disesase: Meta-analyses. Clinical and Experimental Allergy 2008; 38(4): 634–42.

68. Cho CE, Norman M. Cesarean section and development of the immune system in the offspring. Am J Obstet Gynecol 2013; 208(4): 249–54.

69. Decker E, Engelmann G, Findeisen A, Gerner P, Laass M, Ney D, et al. Cesarean delivery is associated with celiac disease but not inflammatory bowel disease in children. Pediatrics 2010; 125(6): e1433–40.

70. Cardwell CR, Stene LC, Joner G, Cinek O, Svensson J, Goldacre MJ, et al. Caesarean section is associated with an increased risk of childhood-onset type 1 diabetes mellitus: A meta-analysis of observational studies. Diabetologia 2008; 51(5): 726–35.

71. Whyte H, Hannah ME, Saigal S, Hannah WJ, Hewson S, Amankwah K, et al. Outcomes of children at 2 years after planned cesarean birth versus planned vaginal birth for breech presentation at term: The International Randomized Term Breech Trial. Am J Obstet Gynecol 2004; 191(3): 864–71.

72. Li HT, Ye RW, Pei LJ, Ren AG, Zheng XY, Liu JM. Cesarean delivery on maternal request and childhood intelligence: a cohort study. Chin Med J (Engl) 2011; 124(23): 3982–7.

73. Scheller JM, Nelson KB. Does cesarean delivery prevent cerebral palsy or other neurologic problems of childhood? Obstet Gynecol 1994; 83(4): 624–30.

74. O'Callaghan M, MacLennan A. Cesarean delivery and cerebral palsy: a systematic review and meta-analysis. Obstet Gynecol 2013; 122(6): 1169–75.

75. Clark SL, Hankins GDV. Temporal and demographic trends in cerebral palsy: Fact and fiction. Am J Obstet Gynecol 2003; 188(3): 628–33.

76. Wood NS, Marlow N, Costeloe K, Gibson AT, Wilkinson AR. Neurologic and developmental disability after extremely preterm birth. N Engl J Med 2000; 343: 378–84.

77. Woythaler MA, McCormick MC, Smith VC. Late preterm infants have worse 24 month neurodevelopmental outcomes than term infants. Paediatrics 2011; 127(3): e622–9.

78. MacKay DF, Smith GC, Dobbie R, Pell JP. Gestational age at delivery and special educational need: Retrospective cohort study of 407,503 schoolchildren. PLoS Med 2010; 7(6): e1000289.

79. Cnattingius S, Zack M, Ekbom A, Gunnarskog J, Linet M, Adami HO. Prenatal and neonatal risk factors for childhood myeloid leukemia. Cancer Epidemiol Biomarkers Prev 1995; 4(5): 441–5.

80. Cook MB, Graubard BI, Rubertone MV, Erickson RL, McGlynn KA. Perinatal factors and the risk of testicular germ cell tumors. Int J Cancer 2008; 122(11): 2600–6.

81. Momen NC, Olsen J, Gissler M, Cnattingius S, Li J. Delivery by caesarean section and childhood cancer: A nationwide follow-up study in three countries. BJOG 2014; 121(11): 1343–50.

82. Velló M, Martínez-Costa C, Catalá M, Fons J, Brines J, Guijarro-Martínez R. Prenatal and neonatal risk factors for the development of enamel defects in low birth weight children. Oral Dis 2010; 16(3): 257–62.

83. Eli I, Sarnat H, Talmi E. Effect of the birth process on the neonatal line in primary tooth enamel. Pediatr Dent 1989; 11(3): 220–3.

84. Zanolli C, Bondioli L, Manni F, Rossi P, Macchiarelli R. Gestation length, mode of delivery, and neonatal line-thickness variation. Hum Biol 2011; 83(6): 695–713.

85. Huh SY, Rifas-Shiman SL, Zera CA, Edwards JW, Oken E, Weiss ST, et al. Delivery by caesarean section and risk of obesity in preschool age children: A prospective cohort study. Arch Dis Child 2012; 97(7): 610–16.

CHAPTER 11
Trial of labour after caesarean

Emily S. Miller and William A. Grobman

Introduction

Rates of caesarean section vary dramatically across the globe, ranging from less than 5% of all births in many African countries to 60% in some regions in China and more than 80% in private hospitals of Brazil (see Chapter 3). The ideal rate of caesarean delivery for any given population is unknown, but the World Health Organization recommends that caesarean section rates around the world should not be higher than 10% to 15% [1, 2]. To achieve a caesarean section rate within this range, the number of both primary and repeat caesarean deliveries must be reduced in many areas of the world.

Repeat caesarean birth is the largest single indication for caesarean section, contributing to nearly 40% of caesareans annually in the United States [3]. One reason for the increase in repeat caesareans is a steady decline in the number of women undergoing a trial of labour after caesarean (TOLAC).

A number of reasons for this decline, including both medical and non-medical factors, have been posited. Patient preferences regarding route of delivery after a prior caesarean section involve a complex relationship of both the patient's risk assessment as well as her personal evaluation of various outcomes, such as having vaginal delivery. Factors shown to influence a woman's desire to attempt TOLAC include familial obligations, level of involvement of a woman's partner, and the strength of her wish to experience vaginal delivery [4–6].

In terms of provider effect on TOLAC utilization, litigation risk has been cited as a reason for performing repeat caesarean, with many providers reporting litigation as a direct influence on cessation of offering TOLAC [7, 8]. Corroborating this observation is evidence that malpractice caps are associated with increased utilization of TOLAC and, correspondingly, decreased caesarean section rates [8].

Finally, systems and organizational issues can lead to TOLAC being more limited. For example, in 1999 the American College of Obstetricians and Gynecologists (ACOG) stated that a physician capable of an emergency caesarean must be 'immediately available' for women in active labour undergoing TOLAC [9]. Hospitals that felt they could not reliably meet this criterion stopped offering TOLAC to their patients, and the number of hospitals that supported TOLAC declined by 30% [10, 11].

Understanding optimal patient selection and obstetric management of TOLAC may help safely reduce rates of caesarean section. This chapter reviews the various issues around vaginal birth after a previous caesarean delivery.

Risks of TOLAC

The decision to undergo TOLAC involves a balance of maternal and neonatal risks, which are, at times, in conflict with each other. A systematic review by Guise et al. estimated the excess maternal and fetal risks associated with route of delivery after one prior caesarean. They concluded that, compared to TOLAC, repeat caesarean would avert 83 perinatal deaths per 100,000 women but would result in 9 additional maternal deaths [12]. Future risks must also be taken into account, as multiple caesareans are associated with increases in both maternal and neonatal risks in subsequent pregnancies [13].

Maternal morbidity in TOLAC

Women with a successful TOLAC have less morbidity than women who undergo elective repeat caesarean section [14–17]. However, women who require repeat caesarean section in labour have more morbidity [14–16, 18] than those who undergo elective repeat caesarean section. Thus, predicting the chance of a vaginal birth after caesarean (VBAC) if TOLAC were undertaken is intrinsically related to risks of morbidity.

Observational studies comparing women undergoing TOLAC versus women undergoing a planned repeat caesarean have been used to guide the assessment of these risks. The largest of these studies included women with a prior caesarean at 19 academic medical centres; 17,898 of these women underwent TOLAC, and 15,801 of them underwent a planned caesarean [15]. In this and other studies, the frequency of maternal and neonatal adverse outcomes associated with either approach to delivery was low. Maternal risks that must be considered include haemorrhage, infection, operative injury, uterine rupture, hysterectomy, and maternal death. Table 11.1 provides an overview of the published risks, which are discussed in more detail in this section.

Haemorrhage in TOLAC

There are conflicting data as to whether haemorrhage is more common with TOLAC or after planned repeat caesarean. Landon and colleagues demonstrated an increased risk of blood transfusion in their TOLAC cohort (1.7% vs 1.0%; adjusted odds ratio (aOR), 1.7; 95% confidence interval (CI), 1.4–2.1). [15]. However, a meta-analysis pooling results from five studies that assessed blood transfusion demonstrated no difference between the two approaches to delivery [19]. Notably, any increased risk of transfusion for women undergoing TOLAC is predominantly associated with women who require a caesarean in labour, and thus assessment of the chance of achieving VBAC remains an integral aspect of counselling [15, 20, 21].

Infection in TOLAC

The women in the MFMU cohort who underwent TOLAC more commonly experienced endometritis, compared to the women who underwent elective repeat caesarean (2.9% vs 1.8%; aOR, 1.6; 95% CI, 1.4–1.9) [15]. This risk is predominantly driven by the risk of endometritis in women who require repeat caesarean in labour. As with haemorrhage, however, the data are conflicting and some investigators have identified increased risks of endometritis in women undergoing elective caesarean [16, 21].

Operative Injury in TOLAC

Reports of operative injury often include injury to the urinary system and bowel and, in some studies, laceration of the uterine artery [15, 17, 22, 23]. Results from studies are inconsistent with regard to whether operative injury is more frequent among women undergoing TOLAC or planned repeat caesarean. Nevertheless, as with other adverse outcomes, any identified increased risk is predominantly due to women requiring repeat caesarean in labour, as women with a successful TOLAC have low rates of operative injury [17].

Uterine rupture or dehiscence in TOLAC

One risk of TOLAC is uterine rupture—a disruption of the myometrium and the serosa, with associated maternal or neonatal morbidity. Uterine dehiscence, on the other hand, is considered to have occurred when there is a disruption of the prior uterine incision but no adverse maternal or

Table 11.1 Maternal risks by route of delivery in women with a prior caesarean

Maternal morbidity

	Blanchette (26)		Gregory (18)		Hibbard (14)		Landon (15)		Loebel (25)	
	TOLAC (n=754)	Elective Cesarean (n=727)	TOLAC (n=11,480)	Elective Cesarean (n=29,970)	TOLAC (n=1324)	Elective Cesarean (n=431)	TOLAC (n=17,898)	Elective Cesarean (n=15,801)	TOLAC (n=927)	Elective Cesarean (n=481)
Transfusion	3 (0.4%)	2 (0.3%)	63 (0.55%)	153 (0.51%)	11 (0.8%)	6 (1.4%)	304 (1.7%)*	158 (1.0%)	12 (1.3%)	3 (0.6%)
Endometritis	11 (1.5%)	9 (1.2%)	—	—	108 (8.2%)	38 (8.8%)	517 (2.9%)*	285 (1.8%)	—	—
Operative Injury	2 (0.3%)	3 (0.4%)	—	—	—	—	64 (0.4%)	52 (0.3%)	4 (0.4%)	2 (0.4%)
Uterine Rupture	12 (1.6%)*	0 (0.0%)	78 (0.68%)	38 (0.013%)	10 (0.8%)	0 (0.0%)	124 (0.7%)*	0 (0.0%)	4 (0.4%)	2 (0.4%)
Hysterectomy	2 (0.3%)	0 (0.0%)	0 (0.0%)	2 (0.007%)	6 (0.5%)	0 (0.0%)	41 (0.2%)	47 (0.3%)	—	—
Maternal Death	0 (0.0%)	0 (0.0%)	0 (0.0%)	2 (0.007%)	0 (0.0%)	0 (0.0%)	3 (0.02%)	7 (0.04%)	0 (0.0%)	0 (0.0%)

	Macones (16)		Tan (22)		Wen (21)	
	TOLAC (n=13,706)	Elective Cesarean (n=11,299)	TOLAC (n=768)	Elective Cesarean (n=232)	TOLAC (n=128,960)	Elective Cesarean (n=179,795)
Transfusion	96 (0.7%)*	136 (1.2%)	36 (4.7%)	17 (7.3%)	245 (0.19%)*	268 (0.15%)
Endometritis	1288 (9.4%)*	1469 (13.0%)	—	—	487 (0.38%)*	837 (0.47%)
Operative Injury	178 (1.3%)	113 (1.0%)	6 (0.9%)	0 (0.0%)	—	—
Uterine Rupture	134 (0.9%)*	1 (0.004%)	2 (0.3%)	0 (0.0%)	843 (0.65%)*	453 (0.25%)
Hysterectomy	—	—	2 (0.3%)	2 (0.9%)	245 (0.19%)*	268 (0.15%)
Maternal Death	—	—	0 (0.0%)	0 (0.0%)	2 (0.002%)	10 (0.006%)

*Denotes a statistically significant difference.

perinatal sequelae. While the vast majority of uterine ruptures occur in labour, uterine rupture also can occur even in women who are planning for elective repeat caesarean section, as a rupture can occur prior to or in early labour.

The factor most associated with uterine rupture risk is the type of uterine scar. Women with prior low transverse scars have a risk of rupture of less than 1%, whereas women with prior classical caesarean section scars have a uterine rupture risk that is much higher [14–16, 18, 21, 23, 24].

Hysterectomy in TOLAC

While uterine rupture is a risk factor for a hysterectomy, elective repeat caesarean delivery is associated with an increased risk, compared to successful TOLAC. Thus, overall, TOLAC does not appear to increase the risk of hysterectomy, compared to elective repeat caesarean [13, 15, 21–24].

Maternal Death in TOLAC

For all women with a prior caesarean, the frequency of maternal mortality is reported to be 10.1 per 100,000 women [25]. One large study showed that maternal mortality in women undergoing TOLAC was not different from that in women undergoing planned repeat caesarean [15]. However, a review of multiple cohorts demonstrated that there was a small but statistically significant increase in mortality rates in women undergoing elective repeat caesarean delivery, as compared to those undergoing TOLAC (0.013% vs 0.004%; relative risk (RR), 0.33; 95% CI, 0.13–0.88) [25].

Neonatal morbidity in TOLAC

Discussing neonatal morbidities according to route of delivery is a critical part of patient counselling. Outcomes that have been examined in observational studies include Apgar scores, neonatal intensive care unit (NICU) admission, hypoxic ischaemic encephalopathy (HIE), and perinatal death. An overview of the published risks can be found in Table 11.2.

Apgar scores in newborns following delivery by TOLAC

Five-minute Apgar scores are often reported as a proxy for evidence of perinatal depression, although they are poor predictors of the risk of future neurologic compromise. The existing literature has not consistently demonstrated a difference in mean Apgar scores or the risk of a low Apgar score (e.g. less than 4 at 5 minutes) in newborns of women who have undergone TOLAC compared to those who have undergone planned repeat caesarean [25].

NICU admission following delivery by TOLAC

Most studies comparing women undergoing TOLAC to those who have undergone elective repeat caesarean do not demonstrate a difference in the frequency of NICU admission [22, 23, 25–27]. In one study that identified a statistically significant difference in NICU admission by route of delivery, it was found that women who underwent elective repeat caesarean had an increased frequency of NICU admissions (9.3% vs 4.9%, $P = 0.025$) [29]. This increase was predominantly related to either an increased frequency of hypoglycaemia or the need for supplemental oxygen.

HIE in newborns following delivery by TOLAC

HIE is defined as a perinatal asphyxial event leading to both short-term and long-term neurologic morbidity. Landon and colleagues demonstrated that HIE occurs in 6.2% of cases of uterine rupture [15]. However, given how infrequent uterine rupture is, the overall difference in the frequency of HIE in neonates of women undergoing TOLAC compared to those having elective caesarean is small (0.1% vs 0.0%, $P < 0.001$) [15]. Furthermore, when women in the elective caesarean group who desired repeat caesarean but presented in labour were included in the analysis, rates of HIE in the caesarean group were 0.013% [29]. While Richardson et al. did not study HIE directly, they used umbilical cord arterial pH as a surrogate marker for asphyxia and found that the point estimate for the odds of pH <7.0 among women who underwent TOLAC was higher than that for women who underwent repeat caesarean (0.5% vs 0.1%; odds ratio (OR), 0.3; 95% CI, 0.1–1.8) [27]. This difference, however, was not statistically significant.

Perinatal death following delivery by TOLAC

Perinatal death is defined as fetal death beyond 20 weeks gestation, or neonatal death at less than 28 days of life. In the Landon et al. study, when uterine

Table 11.2 Neonatal risks by route of delivery in women with a prior caesarean

Neonatal morbidity

	Blanchette (23)		Bujold (84)		Kamath (29)		Landon (15)	
	TOLAC (n=755)	Elective Cesarean (n=737)	TOLAC (n=6,718)	Elective Cesarean (1,862)	TOLAC (n=343)	Elective Cesarean (n=329)	TOLAC (n=15,338)	Elective Cesarean (n=15,014)
5 Minute Apgar < 7	12 (1.6%)	11 (1.5%)	–	–	–	–	–	–
NICU Admission	36 (4.8%)	31 (4.2%)	–	–	16 (4.9%)*	32 (9.3%)	–	–
HIE/Asphyxia	–	–	–	–	–	–	12 (0.08%)*	0 (0.0%)
Perinatal Death	2 (0.2%)	0 (0%)	4 (0.06%)	2 (0.11%)	–	–	47 (0.3%)*	20 (0.1%)

	Richardson (28)		Smith (45)		Tan (22)	
	TOLAC (n=2,646)	Elective Cesarean (n=843)	TOLAC (n=15,515)	Elective Cesarean (n=9,014)	TOLAC (n=768)	Elective Cesarean (n=232)
5 Minute Apgar < 7	26 (1%)	13 (1.5%)	–	–	6 (0.8%)	0 (0%)
NICU Admission	220 (8.3%)	74 (8.8%)	–	–	51 (6.6%)	14 (6.0%)
HIE/Asphyxia	–	–	–	–	–	–
Perinatal Death	3 (0.11%)	0 (0%)	20 (0.13%)	1 (0.01%)	3 (0.4%)	0 (0%)

*Denotes a statistically significant difference.

rupture occurred, the frequency of perinatal death was 1.8% [15]. When all women with a prior caesarean were included, the perinatal mortality rates were 0.29% in the TOLAC cohort and 0.13% in the repeat caesarean group. It should be noted that the study by Landon et al. excluded women who desired elective caesarean if they presented in spontaneous labour. When these women were included in the analysis, the frequency of perinatal death in the elective caesarean cohort rose [29]. In addition, these data are observational and subject to limitation. For example, it is not clear that all perinatal deaths associated with TOLAC were a result of the procedure itself. Women with an intrauterine fetal demise diagnosed antenatally are often encouraged to undergo TOLAC, and this dynamic may inflate the published frequency of perinatal mortality associated with TOLAC.

Maternal and neonatal risks in subsequent pregnancies after TOLAC

The risks documented above are estimates only for the index pregnancy (i.e. the pregnancy in which the decision is made to have TOLAC or a planned repeat caesarean). Importantly, each additional caesarean magnifies both maternal and perinatal risks in subsequent pregnancies. One major reason for the increase in maternal risk is the risk of abnormal placentation, such as placenta praevia and placenta accreta. These types of placentation increase the risks of transfusion, operative injury, hysterectomy, and even maternal death [30].

Neonatal risks also increase with each additional caesarean. The increased frequency of placenta praevia leads to a decrease in the median gestational age at delivery, with a corresponding increase in the chance of prematurity [30].

Repeat pregnancy after uterine rupture is another concern. While cases are limited, women with a prior uterine rupture who labour have a 4%–33% risk of recurrent uterine rupture, depending on the location of the prior rupture [31, 32]. Thus, if a woman does become pregnant after a uterine rupture, repeat caesarean should be performed before labour ensues, with consideration towards delivery at 37 weeks to reduce the risk of recurrent rupture [9].

Predictors of VBAC

The frequency of VBAC for women who undertake TOLAC has ranged in most studies from 60%–80% [15–18, 33–35]. As previously noted, repeat caesarean in labour is responsible for the majority of the morbidity associated with TOLAC. Therefore, determining the individual likelihood of VBAC gives insight into whether the risk for morbidity associated with TOLAC for a woman is greater than that associated with repeat caesarean [36, 37]. A myriad of factors have been shown to influence the chance of VBAC and may be used to help with individualized counselling (Table 11.3).

Demographic characteristics and VBAC

Various demographic characteristics have been examined for their association with VBAC. In the United States, race and ethnicity have been shown to be to be associated with VBAC. Specifically, women of Hispanic and African-American race/ethnicity are more likely to undergo TOLAC but are over 30% less likely to have a VBAC, compared with white women [38, 39]. Maternal age is associated with route of delivery as well—younger women undergoing TOLAC are more likely to experience a VBAC than older women are [17, 40, 41]. In addition, maternal BMI is also predictive of VBAC, with an increase in BMI being associated with an increased risk of requiring a caesarean in labour [42, 43]. Similarly, weight gain in pregnancy is negatively associated with the chance of VBAC, as women who gain more than 40 pounds are less likely to achieve vaginal delivery than women who gain less than 40 pounds [43].

Table 11.3 Predictors of successful vaginal birth after caesarean section

Increased chance of VBAC
Younger maternal age
Prior vaginal birth
Prior caesarean section for malpresentation, multiple gestation, placenta praevia, or non-reassuring fetal status
Spontaneous labour
Lower chance of VBAC
Increase in BMI and/or weight gain during pregnancy
Prior caesarean section for arrest disorders of labour
Maternal co-morbidities (diabetes, asthma, thyroid disease, seizure disorder, hypertension, renal disease, and/or connective tissue disease)
Birth weight larger than that in the index pregnancy
Labour induction

VBAC, vaginal birth after caesarean section.

Factors from the medical history associated with VBAC

A prior vaginal delivery has been strongly associated with an increased chance of VBAC in many prior studies [38, 41, 44–46]. The sequence of the prior vaginal delivery also seems to be important, as a prior VBAC affords a higher likelihood of VBAC than a prior vaginal delivery before a prior caesarean delivery does. The chance of VBAC also rises with each successive VBAC achieved [47].

The indication for the prior caesarean affects the chance of VBAC. Non-recurrent indications (i.e. malpresentation or non-reassuring fetal status) are associated with a higher chance of VBAC, compared to arrest disorders of labour [38, 41, 45, 48, 49]. Similarly, women with a prior caesarean in the setting of a multiple gestation have a higher chance of VBAC in a singleton pregnancy, compared to those with a prior caesarean of a singleton gestation (86% vs 73%; OR, 2.2; 95% CI, 1.7–2.8) [50].

Women with maternal diseases (including diabetes, asthma, thyroid disease, seizure disorder, hypertension, renal disease, and/or connective

tissue disease) have a decreased chance of VBAC [38, 40, 45].

There are conflicting reports about the chance of VBAC with more than one prior uterine incision. While Macones et al. [51] have demonstrated that women with more than one prior caesarean had similar vaginal delivery rates, compared to women who had only one prior caesarean, Landon et al. [52] have shown a slightly decreased chance of VBAC for women with multiple prior caesareans ($P < 0.001$).

Factors related to the current pregnancy associated with VBAC

Studies that have evaluated the relationship between fetal size and VBAC have used birth weight, not estimated fetal weight, for their analyses. This approach may limit the clinical applicability of the findings with regard to prediction. Nevertheless, high birth weight is associated with a low likelihood of VBAC [38]. Similarly, if the prior indication for caesarean was labour dystocia, having a larger fetal size, in comparison to that in the prior pregnancy, reduces the chance of a VBAC [53, 54]. The adverse impact of fetal size may be mitigated by having had a prior vaginal delivery. In one study, VBAC rates in women with a prior vaginal delivery were not affected by fetal size [55].

While women with a multifetal gestation are less likely to choose TOLAC, those that do proceed have a similar chance of VBAC as those with singletons [56, 57].

Most studies that have analysed labour induction have compared induction to spontaneous labour; thus, it remains uncertain whether labour induction decreases the chance of VBAC, compared to the clinical alternative of expectant management. However, the literature has consistently shown that women that require an induction of labour have a decreased chance of VBAC, compared to women who experience spontaneous labour. This fact is particularly true when women with an unfavourable cervix are induced [12, 54, 58].

Some studies have demonstrated a decreased risk of VBAC when delivery occurs after the estimated due date, but others have demonstrated this change only among women with a gestational age greater than 41 weeks [59, 60]. Importantly, success rates even among those who delivered after their due date are relatively high (approximately 65%).

Predictors of success models for VBAC

While the above-listed factors are all related to VBAC, they are not, when considered individually, able to accurately predict VBAC. Thus, models have been developed using combinations of factors to predict VBAC [40, 48, 61–64]. One of these models, designed for women with a term pregnancy and one prior low transverse caesarean, incorporates variables known only at the first prenatal visit and can inform counselling early in prenatal care [40]. A second model is available that can be used to incorporate information available only as pregnancy progresses (e.g. labour induction) [63]. Both models have been externally validated in populations other than in which they were developed and are available online at http://www.bsc.gwu.edu/mfmu/vagbirth.html [64, 65].

Uterine rupture in TOLAC

Demographic factors associated with uterine rupture in TOLAC

One of the risks of TOLAC is uterine rupture, which carries with it both potential maternal and neonatal morbidity. Various characteristics can be used to assess this risk (Table 11.4). However, even understanding these associations offers limited ability to accurately predict uterine rupture [66, 67].

Demographic factors have been evaluated as risk factors for uterine rupture. White race (in the United States), increasing maternal age, and obesity all have been associated with an increased risk of uterine rupture [16, 42, 43, 66, 68].

Studies examining the association of prior vaginal delivery with uterine rupture have consistently shown that having a prior vaginal delivery lowers the chance of uterine rupture (ORs ranging from 0.2–0.6) [51, 67, 69]. Similarly, a prior VBAC seems to be protective for uterine rupture [51].

Short inter-delivery intervals have been associated with an increased chance of uterine rupture [51, 69, 70].

One study that examined the relationship between post-partum febrile morbidity and uterine rupture showed a four-fold increase in the odds of uterine rupture in women who experienced post-partum fever after their prior caesarean [71].

Table 11.4 Factors associated with increased risks of uterine rupture in a trial of labour after caesarean

Demographic factors
Advanced maternal age
High BMI
Factors from the medical history
No prior vaginal delivery
Shorter inter-delivery interval
Prior endometritis
Previous classical uterine incision
Factors from current pregnancy
Induction of labour

One study reported that women with Mullerian anomalies were at higher risk of uterine rupture than those without such anomalies were [72]. However, in this study, women with Mullerian anomalies also were more likely to undergo induction of labour than those without Mullerian anomalies were; this factor may have confounded the results. More recent evidence suggests that, if labour induction is adjusted for, women with Mullerian anomalies are not at any increased risk of uterine rupture [73].

Surgical factors associated with uterine rupture in TOLAC

The majority of caesareans occur via a low transverse uterine incision. A low vertical incision is a vertical incision only in the non-contractile lower aspect of the uterus. A classical incision is a vertical incision that extends beyond the limits of the lower uterine segment. The type of the prior uterine scar is strongly associated with the chance of uterine rupture and thus it is important to attempt to know the type of prior uterine incision.

The existing data, although limited, do not support a difference in the rate of uterine rupture when comparing a low transverse incision to a low vertical incision [74, 75]. On the other hand, labour in the presence of a classical incision results in a significantly increased frequency of uterine rupture. Frequencies of uterine rupture ranging from 0.75% with a low transverse incision to more than 5% with classical or T-incisions have been reported [29, 76]. Given the high risk of uterine rupture associated with a prior classical uterine incision, this type of incision is considered a contraindication to a planned TOLAC.

Sometimes, despite best efforts, the operative report from the prior caesarean cannot be obtained. In this circumstance, there does not appear to be an increased risk of uterine rupture when TOLAC is undertaken [77]. The lack of an identified difference reflects the fact that the majority of unknown incisions are most likely low transverse type. Therefore, unless there is a high suspicion, based on clinical information, of a prior classical incision, the inability to document the type of prior scar is not a contraindication to TOLAC.

Uterine closure can be performed in either one or two layers. Closure in one layer is associated with a decrease in operative time and blood loss at the initial caesarean, but some have questioned whether a one-layer closure could affect the chance of uterine rupture in future pregnancies [78]. Studies examining the association between uterine rupture and the uterine closure have yielded conflicting results. For example, in one study in which predominantly a chromic locking suture hysterotomy closure was reported, there was an increased risk of rupture with one-layer closure [79]. By contrast, in a study

in which a Vicryl unlocking stitch was utilized, no impact of single-layer uterine closure on subsequent uterine rupture was observed [80]. It is possible, then, that it is the suture type and technique, and not the number of layers closed, that is associated with the risk of uterine rupture. To date, there are insufficient data to definitively determine the relationship between surgical technique in a prior caesarean and chance of rupture in a subsequent TOLAC.

Many studies have attempted to assess the risk of uterine rupture with more than one prior caesarean. Some have reported rates of uterine rupture as high as 3.7% in women with two prior caesareans and no prior vaginal delivery [81]. Macones et al. [52] noted that the risk of rupture was marginally higher for women with two prior caesareans than for those with one prior caesarean (1.8% vs 0.9%; aOR, 2.3; 95% CI, 1.37–3.85). However, Landon et al. [51] did not find any difference when comparing the frequency of rupture in women who had undergone two or more caesareans with that in women who had undergone only one prior caesarean (0.9% vs 0.7%, p = 0.37). Accordingly, ACOG suggests that TOLAC in women with two prior caesareans is an option [9].

Current pregnancy factors associated with uterine rupture in TOLAC

There are inconsistent results about the relationship between birth weight and the risk of rupture. One study demonstrated an increased risk of uterine rupture in women who delivered a neonate with a birth weight over 4000 grams (2.8% vs 1.2%, $P \le 0.001$) [55]. This finding, however, has not been reproduced in other studies [51, 74, 82]. Also, birth weight is not known until after delivery, and there is not good evidence that estimated fetal weight is associated with uterine rupture. Accordingly, there is not a strong evidence base to suggest that estimated fetal weight can be used to predict the risk of uterine rupture during TOLAC.

The majority of reported studies, including the two largest, do not demonstrate an increased risk of rupture when a twin gestation is present [56, 57, 83, 84].

The frequency of uterine rupture is approximately twofold higher when TOLAC is the result of induction than when it is the result of spontaneous labour [15, 16, 38, 40, 85, 86]. However, the increased absolute risk is less than 1%. Notably, this increased risk has not been demonstrated to exist among women who have had a prior vaginal delivery [58], and it remains unknown whether the risk of rupture related to labour induction is higher than that related to expectant management.

The type of induction agent used may affect the risk of rupture. Early studies of prostaglandins (prostaglandin E_1 or prostaglandin E_2) demonstrated that induction via prostaglandin was associated with a three- to fivefold increased risk of uterine rupture, compared to spontaneous labour [38, 85, 86]. It remains unclear if this risk is shared equally among the prostaglandin types. In addition, it may be that it is not the use of prostaglandin but rather the type of induction in which a prostaglandin is required (i.e. in the presence of an unfavourable cervix). Nevertheless, based on the existing data, ACOG states that misoprostol should not be used in patients with a prior caesarean [9]. Transcervical Foley catheter placement does not appear to be associated with an increased risk of uterine rupture and can be used as an alternative [86, 88, 89] cervical ripening agent.

Oxytocin is often used to either induce or augment labour in women undergoing TOLAC. As with other induction agents, there are conflicting data on its association with uterine rupture. Landon et al. reported that, when oxytocin alone is used to induce labour, the risk of rupture is 1.1%, compared to a 0.4% risk in spontaneous labour (aOR 3.01; 95% CI, 1.66–5.46) [15]. A similar increase in risk occurred with the use of oxytocin for augmentation (0.9% vs 0.4%; aOR, 2.42; 95% CI, 1.49–3.93). This increase has not been shown in all studies [16]. Two studies have attempted to quantify a dose-response effect of oxytocin on rates of uterine rupture [90, 91]. These authors identified an association between high doses of oxytocin and increased rates of uterine rupture, although a specific threshold at which the risk increases has not been clearly identified.

Predictors of uterine rupture models in TOLAC

Researchers have attempted to develop an accurate prediction model that could be derived from the aforementioned risk factors that would help to guide clinical decision-making [44, 66–68]. Unfortunately, none of these models have the ability to accurately predict rupture. Thus, one important aspect of patient counselling is the unpredictability of this uncommon event.

Signs and symptoms of uterine rupture

The most common sign of uterine rupture is an abnormal fetal heart-rate tracing. Specific patterns reported include bradycardia, prolonged variable decelerations, or late decelerations [92, 93]. Other signs and symptoms of uterine rupture include vaginal bleeding, loss of fetal station, and/or severe abdominal pain. There had been concern that use of an epidural could mask this latter symptom and thereby delay the diagnosis. However, investigators have shown that women who experience rupture often will still feel pain and may request frequent re-dosing of their epidural when rupture occurs [94]. Thus, epidural analgesia should not be withheld from women undergoing TOLAC and who desire this form of pain control.

Antenatal management of uterine rupture in TOLAC

Antenatal counselling regarding route of delivery requires a discussion of complications related to TOLAC as well as complications related to repeat caesarean. It is important to include both risks in the current pregnancy and risks to future pregnancies associated with the chosen approach to delivery.

Counselling on short-term risks includes an assessment of the chance of VBAC and the risk of adverse outcomes based on individual characteristics. A VBAC success calculator is available online at https://mfmunetwork.bsc.gwu.edu/PublicBSC/MFMU/VGBirthCalc/vagbirth.html and can help inform discussions about the approach to delivery. As pregnancy evolves, other factors can be added into the calculator to assist decision-making. An accurate uterine rupture prediction model has not been established. However, information about factors associated with uterine rupture, such as the type of prior uterine scar, can be used to counsel a woman about her risk.

The ultimate decision regarding route of delivery must be made by both a woman and her healthcare provider, based on the patient's individual preferences. The counselling should be documented in the medical records. As there is no clear superiority of TOLAC versus repeat caesarean, ACOG considers global mandates for or against TOLAC to be inappropriate [9].

The only data on outcomes of external cephalic version in women with a prior caesarean are from case series; however, these all report version rates similar to those of women without a prior caesarean [95]. Additionally, there were no cases of uterine rupture in the 192 reported attempts at external cephalic version in these case series.

Intrapartum management of uterine rupture in TOLAC

Because the most common sign of uterine rupture is a change in the fetal heart-rate tracing, continuous fetal monitoring once labour is diagnosed has been recommended [9]. External monitoring is sufficient if an adequate tracing can be obtained.

Women undergoing TOLAC can be induced; however, the potential decreased chance of VBAC success and the potential increased risk of rupture, when compared to that for spontaneous labour, should be noted. Similarly, labour augmentation with oxytocin can be used; however, the slightly increased risk of uterine rupture reported in some studies should be noted [15, 16]. The amount of oxytocin used should be monitored, as the amount of oxytocin used has been associated with the risk of uterine rupture [91].

The use of epidural analgesia by women undergoing TOLAC does not affect their chance of VBAC or the risk of uterine rupture [38, 48, 51, 68, 82, 94]. As noted before, there is no good evidence that use of epidural analgesia will delay the diagnosis of uterine rupture. Thus, ACOG recommends maternal request as a sufficient indication for epidural analgesia in labour in all women, including those undergoing TOLAC [9].

When a uterine rupture is suspected, delivery should be accomplished expeditiously. The timing of delivery required to avoid adverse perinatal outcomes is poorly understood, but limited data suggests that delivery within 18 minutes of suspected rupture is optimal in order to minimize adverse neonatal outcomes [96]. When uterine rupture occurs, the uterine defect often can be repaired. However, in approximately 10%–20% of cases, hysterectomy is required to achieve haemostasis [17].

There are no data supporting routine scar inspection by palpation in asymptomatic women who have had a VBAC [9]. However, if there is clinical suspicion of rupture, such as signs of maternal hypovolaemia or excessive vaginal bleeding, exploration is warranted.

Second-trimester TOLAC

The use of prostaglandin E_1 in the second trimester in women with a prior caesarean is not associated with an increased risk of uterine rupture, compared with the use of other induction agents [97]. The frequency of uterine rupture among women undergoing induction with prostaglandin E_1 in the second trimester has been reported to be 0.3%–0.4% in women with one prior caesarean—a range comparable to that of women in spontaneous labour at term [98].

The rate of failed induction in women with a prior caesarean and who are undergoing second-trimester labour induction is similar to that in women without a prior caesarean and who are undergoing second-trimester labour induction, as is the time to delivery interval. Use of mifepristone before misoprostol shortens the interval to delivery and improves vaginal delivery rates in second-trimester inductions in women without a prior caesarean [98]. While data in women with a prior caesarean are limited, use of mifepristone in these women has not been shown to be contraindicated.

Intrauterine fetal demise and TOLAC

TOLAC is appropriate in women with intrauterine fetal demise and a prior low transverse caesarean section, as these situations require an explicit focus on maternal outcomes. Prostaglandin E_1 should be avoided in the third trimester, given its association with an increased risk of uterine rupture.

Key learning points

1. Encouraging TOLAC is one way to curtail the rising rates of caesarean across the globe.
2. Women undergoing TOLAC must have access to expeditious delivery, if it is required.
3. Women who have a successful TOLAC have less morbidity, compared to women who undergo elective repeat caesarean, while women who require repeat caesarean in labour have more morbidity than women who undergo elective repeat caesarean.
4. Multiple patient-level factors can be used to estimate the chance of achieving a VBAC. One example of such a calculator is available online at https://mfmunetwork.bsc.gwu.edu/PublicBSC/MFMU/VGBirthCalc/vagbirth.html.
5. The risk of uterine rupture associated with TOLAC in women with one prior low transverse caesarean in spontaneous labour is less than 1%.
6. If uterine rupture occurs, there is a 10% risk of serious neonatal sequelae, including death or permanent neurologic damage.
7. The most common signs and symptoms of uterine rupture include an abnormal fetal heart-rate tracing, vaginal bleeding, loss of station, or severe maternal abdominal pain. If uterine rupture is suspected, delivery must occur expeditiously.
8. Contraindications to TOLAC include a prior classical caesarean incision, or any contraindication to a vaginal birth (e.g. placenta praevia).
9. Given the increased risk of rupture, misoprostol should not be used in the third trimester in women undergoing TOLAC. Oxytocin for induction or augmentation may slightly increase the chance of uterine rupture but can be used if monitored closely.
10. Women undergoing TOLAC should have continuous fetal monitoring in labour.

References

1. Gibbons L, Belizan JM, Lauer JA, Betran AP, Merialdi M, Althabe F. Inequities in the use of cesarean section deliveries in the world. Am J Obstet Gynecol 2012; 206(4): 331.e1–19.
2. World Health Organization. Appropriate technology for birth. Lancet 1985; 2(8452): 436–7.
3. Menacker F and Hamilton BE. Recent trends in cesarean delivery in the United States. NCHS Data Brief 2010; 35: 1–8.
4. Eden KB, Hashima JN, Osterweil P, Nygren P, Guise JM. Childbirth preferences after Cesarean birth: A review of the evidence. Birth 2004; 31(1): 49–60.
5. Moffat MA, Bell JS, Porter MA, Lawton S, Hundley V, Danielian P, et al. Decision making about mode of delivery among pregnant women who have previously had a caesarean section: A qualitative study. Br J Obstet Gynaecol 2007; 114(1): 86–93.
6. Cleary-Goldman J, Cornelisse L, Simpson LL, Robinson JN. Previous cesarean delivery: Understanding and satisfaction with mode of delivery in a subsequent pregnancy in patients participating in a formal vaginal birth after cesarean counseling program. Am J Perinatal 2005; 22(4): 217–21.
7. Coleman VH, Erickson K, Schulkin J, Zinberg S, Sachs BP. Vaginal birth after cesarean delivery: Practice patterns of obstetrician-gynecologists. J Reprod Med 2005; 50(4): 261–6.
8. Yang YT, Mello MM, Subramanian SV, Studdert DM. Relationship between malpractice litigation pressure and rates of cesarean section and vaginal birth after cesarean section. Med Care 2009; 47(2): 234–42.
9. American College of Obstetricians and Gynecologists. ACOG Practice Bulletin No.115: Vaginal birth after previous cesarean delivery. Obstet Gynecol 2010; 116(2 Pt 1): 450–63.
10. Shihady IR, Broussard P, Bolton LB, Fink A, Fridman M, Fridman R, et al. Vaginal birth after cesarean: Do California hospital policies follow national guidelines? J Reprod Med 2007; 52(5): 349–58.
11. Roberts RG, Deutchman M, King VJ, Fryer GE, Miyoshi TJ. Changing policies on vaginal birth after cesarean: Impact on access. Birth 2007; 34(4): 316–22.
12. Guise JM, Denman MA, Emeis C, Marshall N, Walker M, Fu R, et al. Vaginal birth after cesarean: New insights on maternal and neonatal outcomes. Obstet Gynecol 2010; 115(6): 1627–78.
13. Miller ES, Hahn K, Grobman WA. Consequences of a primary elective cesarean delivery across the reproductive life. Obstet Gynecol 2013; 121(4): 789–97.
14. Hibbard JU, Ismail MA, Wang Y, Te C, Karrison T. Failed vaginal birth after a cesarean section: How risky is it? I. Maternal morbidity . Am J Obstet Gynecol 2001; 184(7): 1365–71.
15. Landon MB, Hauth JC, Leveno KJ, Spong CY, Leindecker S, Varner MW, et al. Maternal and perinatal outcomes associated with a trial of labor after prior cesarean delivery. N Engl J Med 2004; 351(25): 2581–9.
16. Macones GA, Peipert J, Nelson DB, Odibo A, Stevens EJ, Stamilio DM, et al. Maternal complications with vaginal birth after cesarean delivery: A multicenter study. Am J Obstet Gynecol 2005; 193(5): 1656–62.
17. McMahon MJ, Luther ER, Bowes WA Jr, Olshan AF. Comparisons of a trial of labor with an elective second cesarean section. N Engl J Med 1996; 335(10): 689–95.

18. Gregory KD, Korst LM, Cane P, Platt LD, Kahn K. Vaginal birth after cesarean and uterine rupture rates in California. Obstet Gynecol 1999; 94(6): 985–89.

19. Rossi AC, D'Addario V. Maternal morbidity following a trial of labor after cesarean section vs elective repeat cesarean delivery: A systematic review with metaanalysis. Am J Obstet Gynecol 2008; 199(3): 224–31.

20. El-Sayed YY, Watkins MM, Fix M, Druzin ML, Pullen KM, Caughey AB. Perinatal outcomes after successful and failed trials of laborafter cesarean delivery. Am J Obstet Gynecol 2007; 196(6): 583.e1–5.

21. Wen SW, Rusen ID, Walker M, Liston R, Kramer MS, Baskett T, et al. Comparison of maternal mortality and morbidity between trial of labor and elective cesarean section among women with previous cesarean delivery. Am J Obstet Gynecol 2004; 191(4): 1263–9.

22. Tan PC, Subramaniam RN, Omar SZ. Labour and perinatal outcome in women at term with one previous lower-segment caesarean: A review of 1000 consecutive cases. Aust N Z J Obstet Gynaecol 2007; 47(1): 31–6.

23. Blanchette H, Blanchette M, McCabe J, Vincent S. Is vaginal birth after cesarean safe? Experience at a community hospital. Am J Obstet Gynecol 2001; 184(7): 1478–84.

24. Fitzpatrick KE, Kurinczuk JJ, Alfirevic Z, Spark P, Brocklehurst P, Knight M. Uterine rupture by intended mode of delivery in the UK: A national case-control study. PLoS Med 2012; 9(3): e1001184.

25. Guise JM, Eden K, Emeis C, Denman MA, Marshall N, Fu RR, et al. Vaginal birth after cesarean: New insights. Evid Rep Technol Assess 2010; 191: 1–397.

26. Menacker F, MacDorman MF, Declercq E. Neonatal mortality risk for repeat cesarean compared to vaginal birth after cesarean (VBAC) deliveries in the United States, 1998–2002 birth cohorts. Matern Child Health J 2010; 14(2): 147–54.

27. Richardson BS, Czikk MJ, daSilva O, Natale R. The impact of labor at term on measures of neonatal outcome. Am J Obstet Gynecol 2005; 192(1): 219–26.

28. Kamath BD, Todd TK, Glazner JE, Lezontte D, Lynch AM. Neonatal outcomes after elective cesarean delivery. Obstet Gynecol 2009; 113(6): 1231–8.

29. Spong CY, MB, Gibert S, Rouse DJ, Leveno KJ, Varner MW, et al. Risk of uterine rupture and adverse perinatal outcome at term after cesarean delivery. Obstet Gynecol 2007; 110(4): 801–7.

30. Grobman WA, Gersnoviez R, Landon MB, Spong CY, Leveno KJ, Rouse DJ, et al. Pregnancy outcomes for women with placenta previa in relation to the number of prior cesarean deliveries. Obstet Gynecol 2007; 110(6): 1249–55.

31. Al Qahtani NH, Hajeri FA. Pregnancy outcome and fertility after complete uterine rupture: A report of 20 pregnancies and a review of literature. Arch Gynecol Obstet 2011; 284(5): 1123–6.

32. Usta IM, Hamdi MA, Musa AA, Nassar AH. Pregnancy outcome in patients with previous uterine rupture. Acta Obstet Gynecol Scand 2007; 86(2): 172–6.

33. Flamm BL, Newman LA, Thomas SJ, Fallon D, Yoshida MM. Vaginal birth after cesarean delivery: Results of a 5-year multicenter collaborative study. Obstet Gynecol 1990; 76(5): 750–754.

34. Miller DA, Diaz FG, Paul RH. Vaginal birth after cesarean: A 10-year experience. Obstet Gynecol 1994; 84(2): 255–8.

35. Tessmer-Tuck JA, El-Nashar SA, Racek AR, Lohse CM, Famuyide AO, Wick MJ. Predicting vaginal birth after cesarean section: A cohort study. Gynecol Obstet Invest 2014; 77(2): 121–6.

36. Cahill AG, Stamilio DM, Odibo AO, Peipert JF, Ratcliffe SJ, Stevens EJ, et al. Is vaginal birth after cesarean (VBAC) or elective repeat cesarean safer in women with a prior vaginal delivery? Am J Obstet Gynecol 2006; 195(4): 1143–7.

37. Grobman WA, Lai Y, Landon MB, Spong CY, Leveno KJ, Rouse DJ, et al. Can a prediction model for vaginal birth after cesarean also predict the probability of morbidity related to a trial of labor? Am J Obstet Gynecol 2009; 200(1): 56.e1–6.

38. Landon MB, Leindecker S, Spong CY, Hauth JC, Bloom S, Varner MW, et al. The MFMU cesarean registry: Factors affecting the success of trial of labor after previous cesarean delivery. Am J Obstet Gynecol 2005; 193(3): 1016–23.

39. Cahill AG, Stamilio DM, Odibo AO, Peipert J, Stevens E, Macones GA. Racial disparity in the success and complications of vaginal birth after cesarean delivery. Obstet Gynecol 2008; 111(3): 654–8.

40. Grobman WA, Lai Y, Landon MB, Spong CY, Leveno KJ, Rouse DJ, et al. Development of a nomogram for prediction of vaginal birth after cesarean delivery. Obstet Gynecol 2007; 109(4): 806–12.

41. Knight HE, Gurol-Urganci I, Van der Meulen JH, Mahmood TA, Richmond DH, Dougall A, et al. Vaginal birth after caesarean section: A cohort study investigating factors associated with its uptake and success. BJOG 2014; 121(2): 183–92.

42. Hibbard JU, Gilbert S, Landon MB, Hauth JC, Leveno KJ, Spong CY. Trial of labor or repeat cesarean delivery in women with morbid obesity and previous cesarean delivery. Obstet Gynecol 2006; 108(1): 125–33.

43. Juhasz G, Gyamfi C, Gyamfi P, Tocce K, Stone JL. Effect of body mass index and excessive weight gain on success of vaginal birth after cesarean delivery. Obstet Gynecol 2005; 106(4): 741–6.

44. Smith GC, White IR, Pell JP, Dobbie R. Predicting cesarean section and uterine rupture among women

attempting vaginal birth after prior cesarean section. PLoS Med 2005; 2(9): 871–8.

45. Gyamfi C, Juhasz G, Gyamfi P, Stone JL. Increased success of trial of labor after previous vaginal birth after cesarean. Obstet Gynecol 2004; 104(4): 715–19.

46. Macones GA, Hausman N, Edelstein R, Stamilio DM, Marder SJ. Predicting outcomes of trials of labor in women attempting vaginal birth after cesarean delivery: A comparison of multivariate methods with neural networks. Am J Obstet Gynecol 2001; 184(3): 409–13.

47. Mercer BM, Gilbert S, Landon MB, Spong CY, Leveno KJ, Rouse DJ, et al. Labor outcomes with increasing number of prior vaginal births after cesarean delivery. Obstet Gynecol 2008; 111(2 Pt 2): 285–91.

48. Gonen R, Tamir A, Degani S, Ohel G. Variables associated with successful vaginal birth after one cesarean section: A proposed vaginal birth after cesarean score. Am J Perinatol 2004; 21(8): 447–53.

49. Spaans WA, Sluijs MB, Van Roosmalen J, Bleker OP. Risk factors at caesarean section and failure of subsequent trial of labor. Eur J Obstet Gynecol Reprod Biol 2002; 100(2): 163–6.

50. Varner MW, Thom E, Spong CY, Landon MB, Leveno KJ, Rouse DJ. Trial of labor after one previous cesarean delivery for multifetal gestation. Obstet Gynecol 2007; 110(4): 814–19.

51. Landon MB, Spong CY, Thom E, Hauth JC, Bloom SL, Varner MW, et al. Risk of uterine rupture with a trial of labor in women with multiple and single prior cesarean delivery. Obstet Gynecol 2006; 108(1): 12–20.

52. Macones GA, Cahill A, Pare E, Stamilio DM, Ratcliffe S, Stevens E, et al. Obstetric outcomes in women with two prior cesarean deliveries: Is vaginal birth after cesarean delivery a viable option? Am J Obstet Gynecol 2005; 192(4): 1223–9.

53. Peaceman AM, Gersnoviez R, Landon MB, Spong CY, Leveno KJ, Varner MW, et al. The MFMU Cesarean Registry: Impact of fetal size on trial of labor success for patients with previous cesarean for dystocia. Am J Obstet Gynecol 2006; 195(4): 1127–31.

54. Schoorel EN, Van Kuijk SM, Melman S, Nijhuis JG, Smits LJ, Aardenburg R, et al. Vaginal birth after a caesarean section: The development of a Western European population-based prediction model for deliveries at term. BJOG 2014; 121(2): 194–201.

55. Elkousy MA, Sammel M, Stevens E, Peipert JF, Macones G. The effect of birth weight on vaginal birth after cesarean delivery success rates. Am J Obstet Gynecol 2003; 188(3): 824–30.

56. Cahill A, Stamilio DM, Pare E, Peipert JP, Stevens EJ, Nelson DB, et al. Vaginal birth after cesarean (VBAC) attempt in twin pregnancies: Is it safe? Am J Obstet Gynecol 2005; 193(3): 1050–5.

57. Sansregret A, Bujold E, Gauthier RJ. Twin delivery after a previous caesarean: Twelve-year experience. J Obstet Gynaecol Can 2003; 25(4): 294–8.

58. Grobman WA, Gilbert S, Landon MB, Spong CY, Leveno KJ, Rouse DJ, et al. Outcomes of induction of labor after one prior cesarean. Obstet Gynecol 2007; 109(2 Pt 1): 262–9.

59. Zelop CM, Shipp TD, Cohen A, Repke JT, Lieberman E. Trial of labor after 40 weeks' gestation in women with a prior cesarean. Obstet Gynecol 2001; 97(3): 391–3.

60. Coassolo KM, Stamilio DM, Pare E, Peipert JF, Stevens E, Nelson DB, et al. Safety and efficacy of vaginal birth after cesarean attempts at or beyond 40 weeks of gestation. Obstet Gynecol 2005; 106(4): 700–6.

61. Hashima JN, Guise JM. Vaginal birth after cesarean: A prenatal scoring tool. Am J Obstet Gynecol 2007; 196(5): e22–3.

62. Srinivas SK, Stamilio DM, Stevens EJ, Odibo AO, Peipert JF, Macones GA. Predicting failure of a vaginal birth attempt after cesarean delivery. Obstet Gynecol 2007; 109(4): 800–5.

63. Grobman WA, Lai Y, Landon MB, Spong CY, Leveno KJ, Rouse DJ. Does information available at admission for delivery improve prediction of vaginal birth after cesarean? Am J Perinatol 2009; 26(10): 693–701.

64. Costantine MM, Fox KA, Pacheco LD, Mateus J, Hankins GD, Grobman WA, et al. Does information available at delivery improve the accuracy of predicting vaginal birth after cesarean? Validation of the published models in an independent patient cohort. Am J Perinatol 2011; 28(4): 293–8.

65. Schoorel E, Melman S, Van Kuijk S, Grobman W, Kwee A, Mol B, et al. Predicting successful intended vaginal delivery after previous caesarean section: External validation of two predictive models in a Dutch nationwide registration-based cohort with a high intended vaginal delivery rate. BJOG 2014; 121(7): 840–47.

66. Macones GA, Cahill AG, Stamilio DM, Odibo A, Peipert J, Stevens EJ. Can uterine rupture in patients attempting vaginal birth after cesarean delivery be predicted? Am J Obstet Gynecol 2006; 195(4): 1148–52.

67. Grobman WA, Lai Y, Landon MB, Spong CY, Leveno KJ, Rouse DJ. Prediction of uterine rupture associated with attempted vaginal birth after cesarean delivery. Am J Obstet Gynecol 2008; 199(1): 30.e1–5.

68. Shipp TD, Zelop C, Repke JT, Cohen A, Caughey AB, Lieberman E. The association of maternal age and symptomatic uterine rupture during a trial of labor after prior cesarean delivery. Obstet Gynecol 2002; 99(4): 585–8.

69. Zelop CM, Shipp TD, Repke JT, Cohen A, Lieberman E. Effect of previous vaginal delivery on the risk of

uterine rupture during a subsequent trial of labor. Am J Obstet Gynecol 2000; 183(5): 1184–6.

70. Bujold E, Mehta SH, Bujold C, Gauthier RJ. Interdelivery interval and uterine rupture. Am J Obstet Gynecol 2002; 187(5): 1199–202.

71. Shipp TD, Zelop C, Cohen A, Repke JT, Lieberman E. Post-cesarean delivery fever and uterine rupture in a subsequent trial of labor. Obstet Gynecol 2003; 101(1): 136–9.

72. Ravasia DJ, Brain PH, Pollard JK. Incidence of uterine rupture among women with mullerian duct anomalies who attempt vaginal birth after cesarean delivery. Am J Obstet Gynecol 1999; 181(4): 877–81.

73. Erez O, Dukler D, Novack L, Rozen A, Zolotnik L, Bashiri A, et al. Trial of labor and vaginal birth after cesarean section in patients with uterine Mullerian anomalies: A population-based study. Am J Obstet Gynecol 2007; 196(6): 537.e1–11.

74. Shipp TD, Zelop CM, Repke JT, Cohen A, Caughey AB, Lieberman E. Intrapartum uterine rupture and dehiscence in patients with prior lower uterine segment vertical and transverse incisions. Obstet Gynecol 1999; 94(5): 735–40.

75. Martin JN, Perry KG, Roberts WE, Meydrech EF. The case for trial of labor in the patient with a prior low-segment vertical cesarean incision. Am J Obstet Gynecol 1997; 117(1): 144–8.

76. de Costa C. Vaginal birth after classical caesarean section. Aust N Z J Obstet Gynaecol 2005; 45(3): 182–6.

77. Leung AS, Farmer RM, Leung EK, Medearis AL, Paul RH. Risk factors associated with uterine rupture during trial of labor after cesarean delivery: A case-control study. Am J Obstet Gynecol 1993; 168(5): 1358–63.

78. Dodd, JM, Anderson ER, Gates S. Surgical techniques for uterine incision and uterine closure at the time of caesarean section. Cochrane Database Syst Rev 2008; 3: CD004732.

79. Bujold E, Bujold C, Hamilton EF, Harel F, Gauthier RJ. The impact of a single-layer or double-layer closure on uterine rupture. Am J Obstet Gynecol 2002; 186(6): 1326–30.

80. Durnwald C, Mercer B. Uterine rupture, perioperative and perinatal morbidity after single-layer and double-layer closure at cesarean delivery. Am J Obstet Gynecol 2003; 189(4): 925–9.

81. Caughey AB, Shipp TD, Repke JT, Zelop CM, Cohen A, Lieberman E. Rate of uterine rupture during a trial of labor in women with one or two prior cesarean deliveries. Am J Obstet Gynecol 1999; 181(4): 872–6.

82. Bujold E, Gauthier RJ. Neonatal morbidity associated with uterine rupture: What are the risk factors? Am J Obstet Gynecol 2002; 186(2): 311–14.

83. Varner MW, Thom E, Spong CY, Landon MB, Leveno KJ, Rouse DJ. Trial of labor after one previous cesarean delivery for multifetal gestation. Obstet Gynecol 2007; 110(4): 814–19.

84. Miller DA, Mullin P, Hou D, Paul RH. Vaginal birth after cesarean section in twin gestation. Am J Obstet Gynecol 1996; 175(1): 194–8.

85. Lydon-Rochelle M, Holt VL, Easterling TR, Martin DP. Risk of uterine rupture during labor among women with a prior cesarean delivery. N Engl J Med 2001; 345(1): 3–8.

86. Ravasia DJ, Wood SL, Pollard JK. Uterine rupture during induced trial of labor among women with previous cesarean delivery. Am J Obstet Gynecol 2000; 183(5): 1176–9.

87. Zelop CM, Shipp TD, Repke JT, Cohen A, Caughey AB, Liberman E. Uterine rupture during induced or augmented labor in gravid women with one prior cesarean delivery. Am J Obstet Gynecol 1999; 181(4): 882–6.

88. Ben-Aroya Z, Hallak M, Segal D, Friger M, Katz M, Mazor M. Ripening of the uterine cervix in a post-cesarean parturient: Prostaglandin E2 versus Foley catheter. J Matern Fetal Neonatal Med 2002; 12(1): 42–5.

89. Bujold E, Blackwell SC, Hendler I, Berman S, Sorokin Y, Gauthier RJ. Modified Bishop's score and induction of labor in patients with a previous cesarean delivery. Am J Obstet Gynecol 2004; 191(5): 1644–8.

90. Goetzl L, Shipp TD, Cohen A, Zelop CM, Repke JT, Lieberman E. Oxytocin dose and the risk of uterine rupture in a trial of labor after cesarean. Obstet Gynecol 2001; 97(3): 381–4.

91. Cahill AG, Waterman BM, Stamilio DM, Odibo AO, Allsworth JE, Evanoff B, et al. Higher maximum doses of oxytocin are associated with an unacceptably high risk for uterine rupture in patients attempting vaginal birth after cesarean delivery. Am J Obstet Gynecol 2008; 199(1): 32.e1–5.

92. Craver Pryor E, Mertz HL, Beaver BW, Koontz G, Martinez-Borges A, Smith JG, et al. Intrapartum predictors of uterine rupture. Am J Perinatol 2007; 24(5): 317–21.

93. Leung AS, Leung E, Paul RH. Uterine rupture after previous cesarean delivery: Maternal and fetal consequences. Am J Obstet Gynecol 1993; 169(4): 945–50.

94. Cahill AG, Odibo AO, Allsworth JE, Macones GA. Frequent epidural dosing as a marker for impending uterine rupture in patients who attempt vaginal birth after cesarean delivery. Am J Obstet Gynecol 2010; 202(4): 355.e1–5.

95. Abenhaim HA, Varin J, Boucher M. External cephalic version among women with a previous cesarean

delivery: Report on 36 cases and review of the literature. J Perinat Med 2009; 37(2): 156–60.

96. Holmgren C, Scott JR, Porter TF, Esplin MS, Bardsley T. Uterine rupture with attempted vaginal birth after cesarean delivery: Decision-to-delivery time and neonatal outcome. Obstet Gynecol 2012; 119(4): 725–31.

97. Hammond C. Recent advances in second-trimester abortion: An evidence-based review. Am J Obstet Gynecol 2009; 200(4): 347–56.

98. Berghella V, Airoldi J, O'Neill AM, Einhorn K, Hoffman M. Misoprostol for second trimester pregnancy termination in women with prior caesarean: A systematic review. BJOG 2009; 116(9): 1151–7.

CHAPTER 12
Caesarean delivery and human evolution

Michel Odent and Eric Jauniaux

Introduction

Epidemiological studies on the mode of delivery clearly indicate that, in the near future, the majority of humanity will be born via the surgical abdominal route. All projections of birth statistics since the middle of the twentieth century have paved the way to this kind of prediction and, in many parts of the world, caesarean section delivery rates have reached or are over 50% of all births (see Chapter 3). At such an unprecedented turning point in the history of our species, we are faced with the inevitable question: should we expect an acceleration of human evolution in relation to changes in our mode of birth?

Until now, experts in human evolution have been exploring the past, and the authoritative experts have been mainly palaeontologists, palaeoanthropologists, archaeologists, and geneticists. 'Neo-Darwinism' is 'the modern synthesis' or blending of Darwinian evolutionary theory with Mendelian genetics inheritance laws and became a new school of thought from the beginning of the twentieth century [1]. Neo-Darwinism has concentrated on genes as the fundamental entities in biology. Genetic mutation is considered to be the ultimate source of variation within populations, and natural selection has been considered the main evolutionary force which could produce adaptation. Evolution of the species is understood to be a very slow process, measured by mutation rates. Within this restrictive theoretical framework, there was a lack of curiosity for the possible fast and spectacular transformations of species. Modern techniques of genetics and molecular biology have provided us with a detailed understanding of the genes that define the molecular composition of any organism, as well as the ability to transfer genes from one species to another, and have challenged 'Neo-Darwinism' as an evolutionary theory.

Epigenetics is a new science that studies heritable phenotypes resulting from changes in a chromosome without alterations in the DNA sequence. Epigenetic changes have been observed to occur in response to environmental exposure, in both humans and animals. The 'microbiome' or 'microbiota' is a new concept which refers to the ecological community of communal, symbiotic, and pathogenic microorganisms that literally share our body space [2]. Recent advances that allow us to collect more data on DNA sequences and metabolites have increased our understanding of connections between the gut microbiota and metabolism at a whole-organ level. These revolutionary concepts, supported by a decade of new scientific data, have led to a new phase in our understanding of the evolution of living organisms and a rising interest in possible transformations of the species *Homo sapiens* in the near future. Rapid transformations under the effects of environmental factors are well documented among mammals in general. It is now established that it does not take a long time for the process of domestication of mammals to modify brain structures and behaviours. For example, after only 120 years of domestication, a brain size reduction of about 20% has been observed in mink [3].

The advent of epigenetics as a science has also stimulated studies exploring the transgenerational effects of external modifications of DNA that turn genes 'on' or 'off', in particular during fetal life and the perinatal period. It now appears that epigenetic markers (the 'epigenome') may be, to a certain extent, transmitted to subsequent generations. Understanding one of the mechanisms through which acquired traits can be transmitted to the following generations is an important step in our understanding of the transformation of species and their adaptation to environmental factors. Such an understanding gives us a new perspective in looking at the history of evolutionary biology and should help us to interpret old findings that

have been left unexplained or unexplored, such as the evolution of epigenetic regulation along the human lineage. A recent study of full DNA methylation maps of Neanderthals (a hominin species that lived between 600,000 and 45,000 years ago) and Denisovans (a hominin species that lived about 40,000 years ago) finds substantial changes that may explain the phenotypic differences between the two hominin species and provides new insight into the epigenetic landscape of our closest evolutionary relatives [4].

The period surrounding human birth is the phase of modern life that has been the most dramatically changed during the past decades. This initial and short phase of human life is deemed critical in the formation of individuals by a great variety of developing disciplines (such as ethology, epidemiology, hormonology, epigenetics, immunology, and modern bacteriology). The present chapter reviews and discusses the possible impact of caesarean section on the evolution in humans of the encephalization quotient (EQ), the microbiome, and the maternofetal endocrinology system.

Caesarean section and EQ

EQ is a measure of the relative size of the brain as defined by the ratio between actual and predicted brain mass for a given animal according to its body weight. The main characteristic of *Homo sapiens* is an extremely high EQ, compared with all other land and sea mammals (Figure 12.1). Since our ancestors separated from the other members of the higher primate family (about six million years ago) the size of the brain in the genus *Homo* has been gradually increasing. It is commonplace to claim that the evolutionary process adopted a combination of solutions to make birth possible, up to the time when the birth canal became an 'evolutionary bottleneck', so that the development of the human brain had reached its limits. With the advent of the caesarean section, this bottleneck has suddenly disappeared. In other words, a tendency towards an increased head circumference can suddenly be transmitted to the following generations.

It is therefore plausible that the average EQ of the modern human will increase in the future (Figure 12.2). Within this context, it is possible that we have reached a landmark in the evolution of the human brain size.

It is the development of neocortical structures that is responsible for the gradual increased brain volume throughout the process of evolution of *Homo sapiens*. This fact is important when considering the capacity to give birth. The concept of neocortical inhibition is crucial for interpreting the specifically human difficulties during the birth process as an involuntary process under the control of archaic brain structures. It is easy to interpret the solution that the evolutionary process found to overcome the human handicap in the perinatal period. One can observe that, when a woman gives birth without any pharmacological assistance, her neocortical activity is significantly reduced. A

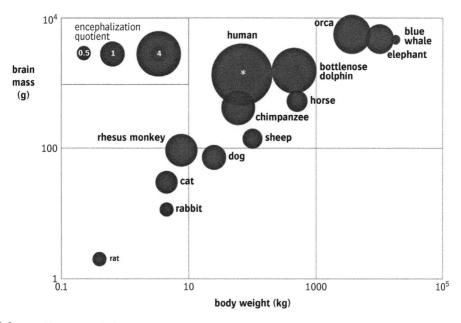

Figure 12.1 Animal brain versus body mass.

From www.theinformationdiet.blogspot.co.uk/2011/12/encephalization-quotient-is-metric.html

labouring woman tends to forget what is happening around her and she tends to forget what she learned and what her plans are. She can behave in a way that usually would be considered unacceptable regarding a civilized woman (e.g. screaming, swearing, being impolite) and she can find herself in the most unexpected primitive postures. This obvious reduction of neocortical control makes human birth possible by increasing the similarities between humans and other mammals. It implies that a labouring

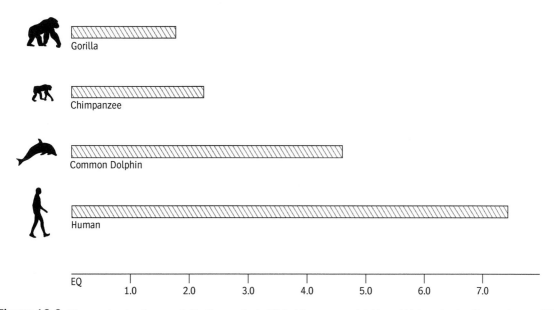

Figure 12.2 Diagram showing the encephalization quotients (EQs) of the common dolphin and higher primates. Humans have an EQ over 7, which is more than double that of other primates.

woman needs to be protected against all stimulants of her neocortex, including language, light, feeling observed, and attention-stimulating situations.

Mode of delivery, and evolution of the EQ

Maternal stature remains strongly associated with perinatal mortality in many populations, and obstructed labour has become a major cause of obstetric complications. The difficult birth process of humans, often described as the 'obstetric dilemma', is commonly assumed to reflect antagonistic selective pressures favouring neonatal encephalization and the effect of maternal bipedal locomotion on pelvic architecture by the assumption of an upright, bipedal posture [5]. Both maternal pelvic dimensions and fetal growth patterns are sensitive to ecological factors such as diet and the thermal environment but the change resulting from these factors is a slow process happening over thousands of years. Secular trends in body size may therefore exacerbate or decrease the 'obstetric dilemma'. For example, the emergence of agriculture may have exacerbated the dilemma by decreasing maternal stature and increasing neonatal growth and adiposity due to dietary shifts [5]. Similarly, the iatrogenic impact of surgical (non-vaginal) deliveries on the EQ may have a direct effect on the human obstetrical riddle by allowing babies to survive who would not have survived before caesarean delivery became available. These evolutionary changes may happen at a speed never seen before and raise the question on how to balance the evolutionary advantage of bigger babies with larger brains against the presence of a narrow pelvis that is difficult for a fetus to get through during labour. Within this context, we must also raise the question about our future capacity to give birth vaginally at all.

Will it be more and more difficult to neutralize the effects of neocortical activity during the involuntary process of parturition? In this case, one solution might be to renew the bases of pharmacological assistance by developing drugs that electively reduce neocortical activity. The other more probable solution will be to continue to increase the rate of caesarean section, in which case we may be at the start of a self-perpetuating evolutionary process—that is, an increased need for caesarean section being induced by increasing rates of caesarean section?

Caesarean delivery and the microbiome

Studies of the diversity of the human microbiome started with the 'father of microbiology' Antonie van Leewenhoek (1632–1723), who, as early as the 1680s, had compared his oral and faecal microbiota [2]. He noted the striking differences in microbes between these two habitats and also between samples from individuals in states of health and disease in both of these sites. The development of molecular-based techniques, particularly PCR amplification of the 16S ribosomal RNA gene, and in computerized data acquisition and analytical techniques, our previously limited view of human–microbe interactions, strictly as pathogens causing infectious diseases, has undergone rapid and dramatic expansion over the past two decades. These new techniques have increased the detection of different microorganisms, the number of known species, and our understanding of bacterial communities and the essential role of the microbiota as commensals and symbionts integral to immune and metabolic health. In the current scientific context, one may present *Homo sapiens* as an ecosystem, with a constant interaction between the trillions of cells that are the products of our genes (the 'host') and the 10–100 trillions of microorganisms (the 'microbiota') that colonize the body, mainly our skin, oral mucosa and saliva, conjunctiva, and gastrointestinal tract.

The suite of genes provided by microorganisms, or the microbiota, living in and on the human body is known as the human microbiome. Average adults possess ten times more microbial cells than human cells and the bacterial genes comprising our microbiome outnumber human genes by more than 100-fold [2, 6]. The genes expressed by these microorganisms constitute the microbiome and may participate in diverse functions that are essential to the host, including modulation of inflammation and immunity. By far, the most important predominant populations of microorganisms are found in the colon. The gut microbiome represents around 80% of the human immune system and is essential for digestion and for the regulation of energy metabolism. The recent mapping of the human gut microbiota in both health and disease states has shown the complexity of the system and have revealed that, rather than a constellation of individual species, a healthy microbiota comprises an interdependent network of microbes. In brief, 'normobiosis' characterizes a composition of the gut 'ecosystem' in which microorganisms with potential health benefits predominate in number over potentially harmful ones, in contrast to 'dysbiosis', in which one or a few potentially harmful microorganisms are dominant, thus creating a disease-prone situation. In particular, some changes in the microbiota's composition, especially increases in bifidobacteria, are now regarded as a marker of intestinal health. By contrast, changes in the gut microbiota composition are classically considered as one of the many factors involved in the pathogenesis of either inflammatory bowel disease or irritable bowel syndrome. The gut microbiota composition (especially the number of bifidobacteria) may contribute to modulate metabolic processes associated with obesity and type 2 diabetes. Colon cancer is another pathology for which a possible role of gut microbiota composition has been hypothesized.

Perinatal transfer of the maternal microbiota

The maternal skin microbiome, the oral flora, and the breast milk microbiome have also an important role in the development of the human immune system. The physiological changes that occur during pregnancy may disrupt this balanced ecosystem and predispose women to harbouring potentially pathogenic microbiota. The vaginal microbiome in humans is unique and differs from that of any other species, including nonhuman primates. In particular, the vaginal concentration of glycogen and lactic acid, as well as of *Lactobacillus* spp., is greatly reduced in nonhuman primates compared with humans. In situations where the vaginal microbiota of pregnant women is not dominated by lactobacilli, there is an increased association with infection-related preterm birth, and maternal and neonatal morbidity.

The initial development and maturation of the neonatal microbiome is largely determined by maternal–offspring exchanges of microbiota. There is emerging evidence to support the role of first microbial contacts in promoting and maintaining a balanced immune response in early life. Early colonization may permanently influence microbiota composition and function, with ramifications for health, and recent findings have suggested that microbial contact begins prior to birth and is shaped by the maternal microbiota [6]. Microbial colonization of the newborn occurs during a critical time window for immune and gastrointestinal development, particularly mucosal immune protection [7]. Postnatal maturation of immune regulation seems to be largely driven by exposure to microbes, and the gastrointestinal tract is the largest source of maternal microbial exposure (Figure 12.3). Among infants born vaginally, several bifidobacterium strains transmit from the mother and colonize the infant's intestine shortly after birth [8]; this finding supports the hypothesis that the mother's intestine is the primary source for newborn intestinal microbiota. These data also suggest that the initial faecal inoculum of microbiota results from the proximity of the birth canal and anus. Secondary sources of inocula include mouths and skin of kin, animals, and objects, as well as the human milk microbiome.

The observation that microbiota in infants delivered vaginally is different from that in infants delivered by caesarean suggests that the newborn microbiome is acquired at or immediately after birth. Novel findings in microbiology question the long-standing paradigm that a healthy pregnancy implies a sterile uterus [9, 10]. Metagenomic sequencing has elucidated a rich placental microbiome in normal term

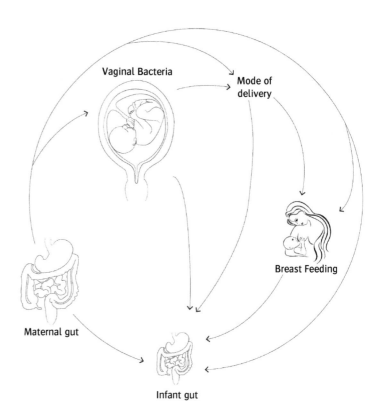

Figure 12.3 Diagram showing the interactions of human perinatal microbiota.

pregnancies; this microbiome likely provides important metabolic and immune contributions to the growing fetus [10]. It now seems that the placenta is frequently colonized with bacteria, and a placental microbiome has been identified. Thus, infants may incorporate an initial microbiome before birth and receive copious supplementation of maternal microbes during vaginal birth and breastfeeding. The very low-birth-weight infant is at great risk for marked dysbiosis of the gut microbiome via multiple factors, including physiological immaturity and prenatal/postnatal influences that disrupt the development of a normal gut flora [11]. Recent clinical studies show that intestinal dysbiosis or microbial imbalance precedes late-onset neonatal sepsis and necrotizing enterocolitis in intensive care nurseries [12]. Epidemiologic evidence has also linked late-onset neonatal sepsis and necrotizing enterocolitis in long-term psychomotor disabilities of very low-birth-weight infants.

Infant colonization sets the stage for the adult microbiome (Figure 12.4). The intestinal flora of the children born by caesarean section contains less bifidobacteria [18–21] than infants delivered vaginally and is similar to the intestinal flora found in diabetic individuals. Dysbiosis of the microbiome in childhood and adults has been associated with the development of both type 1 and type 2 diabetes mellitus, obesity, eczema, inflammatory bowel disorders, and colorectal cancer. The maternal gut microbiome and therefore the neonatal microbiome acquired at birth can be modulated during pregnancy by dietary changes and weight gain, antibiotic use, or disease such as diabetes [6, 13–16]. The development of the neonatal microbiome and in particular the gut microbiota diversity and delayed colonization are also influenced by the mode of delivery [16–23] and maternal breastfeeding [17, 22–24]. Given the rising prevalence of maternal obesity and increasing rate of caesarean delivery, we may soon observe radical changes in

Maternal Microbiome

Neonatal Microbiome

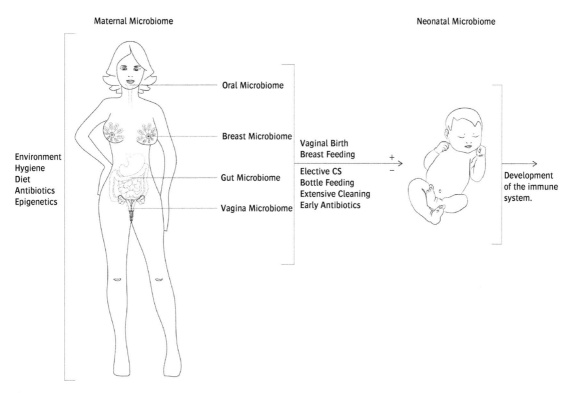

Oral Microbiome

Breast Microbiome

Gut Microbiome

Vagina Microbiome

Environment
Hygiene
Diet
Antibiotics
Epigenetics

Vaginal Birth
Breast Feeding

Elective CS
Bottle Feeding
Extensive Cleaning
Early Antibiotics

+

−

Development
of the immune
system.

Figure 12.4 Diagram showing the impact of different artificial perinatal interventions on the microbiome of the newborn.

the way human microbiomes are established from birth. At a time when the immune system is compared to a sensory organ that needs specific stimulations during critical periods of development, we expect significant changes in the comparative prevalence of pathological conditions, even if, later on in life, dietary intake influences the structure and activity of the human microbiome [13].

Microbiome and the newborn immune system

Th1-type cytokines tend to produce the pro-inflammatory responses responsible for killing intracellular parasites and for perpetuating autoimmune responses, whereas Th2-type cytokines are associated with the promotion of IgE and eosinophilic responses in atopy and an anti-inflammatory response. The fetus can switch on an immune response early in pregnancy, and because pregnancy is chiefly a Th2 situation, babies tend to be born

with Th2-biased immune responses. These responses can be switched off rapidly postnatally under the influence of microbiological exposure or can be enhanced by early exposure to allergens. The low levels of Th1-associated chemokines are related to lower total microbiota diversity and are associated with a lower total microbial diversity and delayed colonization by species from the Bacteroidetes phylum [21]. It is also hypothesized that babies with allergies and those who go on to develop full-blown allergies may have been born with a generally weak Th1 response. Recent data comparing infants born vaginally and by caesarean section, followed up from the age of 1 week until the age of 2 years, has shown that there is a reduced Th1 response among those born by caesarean section [21]. By contrast, breast milk stimulates the proliferation of a well-balanced and diverse microbiota, which initially influences a switch from an intrauterine Th2 predominant to a Th1/Th2 balanced response and with activation of T-regulatory cells by breast milk-stimulated specific organisms (bifidobacteria, lactobacilli, and bacteroides) [24].

The dysregulation of these tight interactions between host and microbiota can be responsible for important health childhood disorders, including inflammation and sepsis. Low microbial diversity in infancy is also observed to precede onset of allergic disease. The concept of dysregulation of the immune system is first evocative of allergic diseases. It is interesting to note that all studies of atopic diseases and asthma included in the Primal Health Research Database (http://www.primalhealthresearch.com) indicate similar outcomes, with caesarean section as a risk factor [25–28]. These data suggest that a caesarean delivery is a risk factor for asthma and allergic diseases and have changed our perspective in terms of cause and effect of vaginal versus caesarean birth. Caesarean-born babies are also often exposed to antibiotics in the perinatal period, and pre- and perinatal exposure to antibiotics has been shown to be independent risk factors for asthma and allergic diseases, as well as for serious infection in infancy by antibiotic-resistant bacteria [28–32]. It has also been suggested that the mode of delivery can influence the risks of developing autoimmune diseases such as inflammatory bowel disease. However, a recent systematic review and meta-analysis of observational studies observed no significant difference in the risk of inflammatory bowel disease in offspring delivered by caesarean section compared with those born vaginally [33].

Studies using new DNA sequencing methods confirm previous findings that early environmental exposures, for example caesarean delivery, are associated with an increased risk of childhood-onset type 1 diabetes [33, 34], as well as obesity in both childhood and adulthood [35–40]. Subjects born by caesarean section had a higher risk for increased peripheral and central adiposity during young adult age, compared to those born by vaginal delivery [38]. However, overall caesarean delivery including non-medically indicated maternal request caesarean delivery, compared with vaginal delivery, increases childhood overweight risk only modestly [39]. There is a well-defined association between alterations of the gut microbiome and adult obesity and type 2 diabetes [30, 31, 41, 42].

Those who are obese and have low microbiota diversity are characterized by more marked overall adiposity, insulin resistance, and dyslipidaemia than those with high microbiota diversity are, and gain more weight over time [15]. There are many possible confounding factors for the link between caesarean section and childhood obesity and/or diabetes, in particular maternal BMI, weight gain during pregnancy, and birth weight, but also breastfeeding and maternal diet during and after pregnancy. Similarly, the possible association between caesarean delivery and childhood leukaemia [43] may be influenced by intrauterine factors such as fetal growth [44] but also maternal diet, smoking, parental genetics, and/or exposure to pollutants and toxics.

An environmental determinant of adequate neonatal gut colonization and intestinal immune homeostasis is breast milk. Although the full-term infant is developmentally capable of mounting an immune response, the effector immune component requires bacterial stimulation [24]. Recent studies of the milk microbiome in relation to the way babies are born have detected significant changes according to maternal weight gain, the mode of delivery, and the timing of the operation [20, 23]. Milk samples from obese mothers tend to contain a different and less diverse bacterial community, compared to milk from normal-weight mothers [20]. Milk samples from mothers who had elective but not emergency caesarean section contain a different bacterial community than the milk samples from women giving birth by vaginal delivery. Infants born by elective caesarean delivery have a particularly low bacterial richness and diversity [23]. These data suggest that it is not the operation per se but rather the absence of physiological stress or hormonal signals that could influence the microbial transmission process to milk. Because bacteria present in breast milk are among the very first microbes entering the human body, these data also highlight the need to better understand the biological role that the milk microbiota could potentially play for human health and disease. Interestingly, there are also important differences between prelabour and in-labour factors that can potentially influence the bacterial communities inhabiting human milk. In general, low microbiota diversity can be pathogenic from birth and, for example, colicky babies also present with a low microbiota diversity [45, 46]; thus, theoretically colic should be more common in children born by caesarean section than in those born vaginally; however, there is no evidence supporting this association so far.

Vertical transmission of the microbiome

Evidence for microbial maternal vertical transmission during pregnancy or childbirth is increasingly widespread across different animal species [9]. This collective knowledge compels a paradigm shift, that is, one in which maternal transmission of microbes advances from a taxonomically specialized phenomenon to a universal one in animals. The microbiome has suddenly appeared important to the evolution of animals and plants. All animals and plants establish symbiotic relationships with microorganisms; often, the combined genetic information of the diverse microbiota exceeds that of the host [47]. The 'hologenome' theory of evolution refers to a sum of information that may be transmitted from generation to generation. It demonstrates that changes in environmental parameters, for example, diet, can cause rapid changes in the diverse microbiota, which not only can benefit the holobiont (host plus all of its associated microorganisms) in the short term (adaptation, survival, development, growth, and reproduction) but also can be transmitted to offspring and lead to long-lasting cooperation. The total genetic information transmitted includes the cell's DNA, the cell's mitochondria, and the microbiome [47, 48]. The indigenous microflora has co-evolved with humans for millions of years, and humans have preserved the inherited microbiomes through consumption of fermented foods and interactions with environmental microbes [49]. Through modernization, traditional foods were abandoned, native food starters were substituted with industrial products, vaccines and antibiotics were used, extreme hygiene measures were taken, the rate of caesarean section increased, and breastfeeding changed into feeding with formula.

Pro/prebiotic effects

The gut microbiome can rapidly respond to altered diet, potentially facilitating the diversity of human dietary lifestyles [13]. Effective manipulation of the gut microbiota through diets (both long-term and short-term diet patterns), probiotics (ingested microorganisms that are associated with a beneficial for the microbiome), and/or prebiotics (chemicals that induce the growth and/or activity of the normal gut flora) could have the potential to prevent metabolic disorders such as obesity.

Dietary regulation exerts influences on microbial metabolism and host immune functions through several pathways, which may include selectively bacterial fermentation of nutrients, a lowering of intestinal barrier function, overexpression of genes associated with disorders, and disruptions to both innate and adaptive immunity. In a recent study, mothers with infants at high risk for allergy were randomized to receive either a probiotic mixture or placebo during the last month of pregnancy; then, their infants received it from birth until age six months. Interestingly, the results from this study showed that protection against subsequent childhood allergy was only obtained by the caesarean-born children [29]. There is also limited evidence of a reduction in the rate of gestational diabetes when women are randomized to take probiotics early in pregnancy [50] and thus indirectly of an effect on the colonization of the offspring gut microbiota.

A large number of human intervention studies have been performed that have demonstrated that dietary consumption of certain food products can result in statistically significant changes in the composition of the gut microbiota, in line with the pro/prebiotic concept. Future studies will enable us to understand the link between the maternal microbiome, neonatal transfer of the maternal microbiome at birth, and the pathophysiology of childhood disease and give insights into the rational manipulation of the microbiota with prebiotics, probiotics, or dietary modifications. Thus, identifying specific microbial signatures of mode of delivery, as well as factors that alter microbial populations and gene expression, will lead to the development of new products such as prebiotics, probiotics, antimicrobials and live biotherapeutic products.

Caesarean section and the materno-fetal endocrinology system

Maternal physiological change and fetal development are closely linked throughout pregnancy and are connected via the placental interface, which is in itself an important organ optimizing the intrauterine environment and maternal physiology for the benefit of fetal growth [51]. The placental villous tissue produces two major groups of hormones: steroid hormones, such as progesterone and the oestrogens, and peptide hormones, such as human chorionic gonadotrophin and human placental lactogen. These hormones induce major metabolic changes in all maternal endocrine organs and in particular the thyroid, adrenal, and pituitary glands. Overall, pregnancy is associated with an increase in their size and function with increased circulating levels of the corresponding hormones [52]. The increase in the size of the pituitary gland is quite spectacular (more than a third of its volume, compared to the non-pregnant state). This makes it more susceptible to alteration in blood supply and to peri-partum complications should large maternal blood loss occur.

Oxytocin and pregnancy

Pituitary hormone secretions are significantly affected by pregnancy. The anterior pituitary prolactin level in maternal serum begins to rise from 5 weeks of gestation and by term is ten times higher than at the start of gestation [52]. The principal role of prolactin in pregnancy is to prepare the breast tissue for lactation. Similarly, the level of the posterior pituitary hormone oxytocin increases threefold from the first to the third trimester, and sevenfold at term. During labour, the level of oxytocin rises dramatically to peak in the second stage of labour. The role of oxytocin during and after childbirth has been known for more than a century [53]. Oxytocin is released in large amounts after distension of the cervix and uterus during labour, facilitating birth, maternal bonding, and, after stimulation of the nipples, lactation. Oxytocin is known to exert anxiolytic and antidepressive effects, whereas arginine vasopressin, which is also produced by the posterior part of the pituitary gland, tends to show anxiogenic and depressive actions [54]. A balanced activity of both brain neuropeptide systems is important for appropriate emotional behaviours. Shifting the balance between the neuropeptide systems towards oxytocin, by positive social stimuli and/or psychopharmacotherapy, could help to improve emotional behaviours and reinstate mental health. More recently, it has been found that oxytocin influences many aspects of social behaviour, including recognition, trust, empathy, and other components of the behavioural repertoire of social species; this finding suggests that its effects reach beyond maternal attachment and pair bonds to play a role in affiliative behaviour underlying 'friendships', organization of broad social structures, and maintenance of established social relationships with individuals or groups [55].

Oxytocin and birth

The process of parturition is associated with an intense activation of the oxytocin system (which is not activated in the case of prelabour caesarean section). By contrast, during the first vaginal birth, many women may receive drips of exogenous oxytocin. A recent meta-analysis has shown that, in the case of slow labour, treatment with oxytocin (0.5–4.0 mU/min), as compared with no treatment or delayed oxytocin treatment, did not result in any discernible difference in the rate of caesarean section [56]. Only high-dose regimens of oxytocin ($\geq$4 mU/min) are associated with a reduction in the length of labour and in the rates of caesarean section, and therefore an increase number of vaginal births [57]. Oxytocin is also used routinely during vaginal delivery, during both prelabour and in-labour caesarean section, and also to facilitate placental delivery and prevent post-partum haemorrhage. Thus, the majority of women are exposed to synthetic exogenous oxytocin at some point during labour and/or delivery. Exogenous oxytocin may disrupt the natural physiology of endogenous oxytocin system, possibly influencing maternal stress, mood, and behaviour.

In addition to its peripheral actions during birth, endogenous oxytocin released within the brain is essential for milk ejection (Figure 12.5) and could be a key component in the transition to motherhood, affecting molecular pathways that buffer stress reactivity, support positive moods, and regulate healthy mothering behaviours. Old experiments on animal have shown that, when injected into the third ventricle of lactating rats during suckling, oxytocin increases the basal firing rate of oxytocinergic neurons as well as their activity at the time of each milk-ejection reflex [58]. The oxytocinase enzyme placental leucine aminopeptidase (; P-LAP) is expressed both peripherally and centrally and controls oxytocin degradation. Recent experiments have demonstrated that hypothalamic P-LAP expression and activity increase in lactation in rats and that the prevention of P-LAP activity mimics central oxytocin administration; these findings suggest that P-LAP regulates auto-excitatory oxytocin action during the suckling-induced milk-ejection reflex [59]. The exact effect of oxytocin on the hypothalamus and other brain structures is unclear, and the impact of synthetic oxytocin on P-LAP activity, as well as its secondary effect on the secretion of other neuropeptides, remains unknown.

It has been suggested that the increase in the rates of induced labour and caesarean section could have an epigenetic and neurobiological effect in the deregulation of the oxytocinergic system and thus life-long effects on the development of social behaviours, with a possible link to autism [60]. Recent data from experiments on

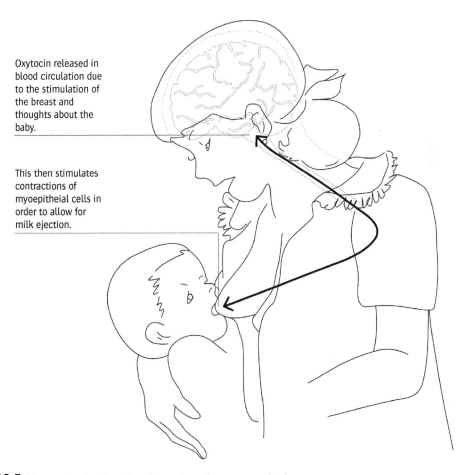

Oxytocin released in blood circulation due to the stimulation of the breast and thoughts about the baby.

This then stimulates contractions of myoepitheial cells in order to allow for milk ejection.

Figure 12.5 Diagram showing the action of oxytocin on the mammary gland.

rats support the conclusion that social stress has transgenerational effects on the social behaviour of the female and male offspring and that these are mediated by changes in the hypothalamic–pituitary–adrenal axis and the hypothalamic–pituitary–gonadal axis [61]. Given evidence that epigenetic states of genes can be modified by experiences, especially those occurring in sensitive periods early in development, it can be hypothesized that the use of oxytocin in modern obstetrics will have an influence on the quality of the oxytocin system in future generations. We use the term 'oxytocin system' to emphasize that we are referring to the capacity to synthesize oxytocin, to secrete it, to use it as a neuromodulator, to store it in the posterior pituitary gland, to release it in

a pulsatile effective way, and to develop receptors. Epigenetic modification of genes involved in oxytocin signalling might be involved in the mechanisms mediating the long-term influence of early adverse experiences on socio-behavioural outcomes, including our reproductive/sexual life, and in all facets of our capacity to love. Furthermore, this system has strong connections with other vital physiological systems, such as the endorphin system, the prolactin system, and the dopamine system.

Should we anticipate a super-brainy *Homo* with a reduced ability to give birth vaginally, breastfeed, and empathize, and with weakened sexual functions [62–64]? Could a super-brainy *Homo sapiens* be endowed with a strong 'emotional intelligence'?

Other emerging issues associated with caesarean delivery

A combination of technical advances has made caesarean births so easy and so safe that we have reached a stage where it is has become acceptable to offer most pregnant women the option of giving birth that way (e.g. see http://www.nice.org.uk/guidance/CG132). In such a context, the main discussion points concern the timing of the operation: prelabour or in-labour caesarean section? One must keep in mind the option of 'planned in-labour caesarean section' [62]. It simply means that the planned operation is performed as soon as the labour has spontaneously begun. Besides the well-known increased risks of neonatal respiratory problems after prelabour caesarean section, and in addition to the data provided by the bacteriological perspective, new reasons for comparing the side effects of prelabour and in-labour caesarean section are now supported by increasing new scientific data. For example, a recent study has shown that uterine contractions are needed for the expression of mitochondrial uncoupled protein 2 by hippocampal neurons; this finding suggests that there could be a negative effect on the fetus of stress deprivation when the caesarean is performed before the labour starts [65]. Such stress deprivation may have long-term effects on individual behaviour and

personality traits. In order to underline the great variety of perspectives that offer reasons for avoiding prelabour caesareans, we can also mention the low adiponectin levels in cord blood after prelabour caesareans. This fact suggests that prelabour caesarean may carry a risk of obesity, independently of other risk factors [66].

The point is that, until now, we have only taken into account the conventional short-term criteria to evaluate the practice of obstetrics (perinatal mortality/morbidity and maternal mortality/morbidity). The list of criteria should increase in the near future, since concomitant scientific advances are pressuring us to think long term and to think in terms of civilization. In spite of spectacular technical advances on the one hand, scientific advances, on the other hand, provide reasons to improve our understanding of the physiological processes in order to disturb them as little as possible. The root of the problem is a cultural lack of understanding of the basic needs of labouring women, and this lack of understanding has been dramatically amplified since the middle of the twentieth century. Is it possible, thanks to the power of modern physiology, to reverse thousands of years of cultural conditioning?

Key learning points

1. EQ (for encephalization quotient) evaluates the relative size of the brain defined by the ratio of the actual to the predicted brain mass for a given animal according to its body weight; *Homo sapiens* has an extremely high EQ compared to other species.

2. Caesarean delivery has allowed bigger babies with higher EQs to survive birth than vaginal delivery could have; thus, we may be at the start of a self-perpetuating evolutionary process, with an increased need for caesarean section being induced by increasing rates of caesarean section.

3. Microbial colonization in the human body begins shortly after birth and, on average, an adult body carries ten times more microbial cells than human cells.

4. The perinatal period is critical as an initial phase of interaction between the newborn host and its developing microbiome and is critical for immune programming.

5. Microbiota disruption around birth (caesarean delivery) and during early development (bottle-feeding) could result in an increased risk of childhood asthma, allergic diseases, syndromes of metabolic dysfunction such as type 2 diabetes and autoimmune disorders.

6. Breast milk samples from obese mothers and mothers who underwent prelabour caesarean section contain different and less diverse bacterial microbiota, compared to those from normal-weight mothers who gave birth vaginally or underwent emergency caesarean sections.

7. The pituitary hormone oxytocin is released in large amounts after distension of the cervix and uterus during labour, facilitating birth, maternal bonding, and, after stimulation of the nipples, lactation.

8. Oxytocin influences many aspects of social behaviour, including recognition, trust, empathy, and other components of the behavioural repertoire of social species.

9. The majority of women are exposed to synthetic exogenous oxytocin, which may disrupt the endogenous oxytocin system and thus influence maternal stress, mood, and behaviour.

10. We hypothesize that modern obstetrics practices and, in particular, the increased number of planned caesarean sections will have an impact on the evolution in humans of the EQ, the microbiome, and the materno-fetal endocrinology system.

References

1. Dahlke JD, Huxley J. Evolution: The Modern Synthesis. London: Allen & Unwin, 1942.

2. Ursell LK, Metcalf JL, Parfrey LW, Knight R. Defining the human microbiome. Nutr Rev 2012; 70(Suppl 1): S38–44.

3. Kruska D. The effect of domestication on brain size and composition in the mink. J Zool London 1996; 239(4): 645–61.

4. Gokhman D, Lavi E, Prufer K, Fraga MF, Riancho JA, Kelso J, et al. Reconstructing the DNA methylation maps of the Neandertal and the Denisovan. Science 2014; 344(6183): 523–7.

5. Wells JC, DeSilva JM, Stock JT. The obstetric dilemma: An ancient game of Russion roulette, or a variable dilemma sensitive to ecology. Am J Phys Anthopol 2012; 149(S55): 40–71.

6. Jones ML, Ganopolsky JG, Martoni CJ, Labbé A, Prakash S. Emerging science of the human microbiome. Gut Microbes 2014; 5(4): 446–57.

7. Walker A. Intestinal colonization and programming of the intestinal immune response. J Clin Gastroenterol 2014; 48 (Suppl 1): S8–S11.

8. Makino H, Kushiro A, Ishikawa E, et al. Mother-to-infant transmission of intestinal bifidobacterial strains has an impact on the early development of vaginally delivered infant's microbiota. PLoS One 2013; 8(11): e78331.

9. Funkhouser LJ, Bordenstein SR. Mom knows best: The universality of maternal microbial transmission. PLoS Biol 2013; 11(8): e1001631.

10. Romano-Keeler J, Weitkamp JH. Maternal influences on fetal microbial colonization and immune development. Pediatr Res 2015; 77(1–2): 189–95.

11. Groer MW, Luciano AA, Dishaw LJ, Ashmeade TL, Miller E, Gilbert JA. Development of the preterm infant gut microbiome: A research priority. Microbiome 2014; 2(1):38.

12. Sherman MP, Zaghouani H, Niklas V. Gut microbiota, the immune system, and diet influence the neonatal gut–brain axis. Pediatr Res 2015; 77(1–2): 127–35.

13. David LA, Maurice CF, Carmody RN, Gootenberg DB, Button JE, Wolfe BE, et al. Diet rapidly and reproducibly alters the human gut microbiome. Nature 2014; 505(7484): 559–63.

14. Hu J, Nomura Y, Bashir A, Fernandez-Hernandez H, Itzkowitz S, Pei Z, et al. Diversified microbiota of meconium is affected by maternal diabetes status. PLoS One 2013; 8(11): e78257.

15. Le Chatelier E, Nielsen T, Qin J, Prifti E, Hildebrand F, Falony G, et al. Richness of human gut microbiome correlates with metabolic markers. Nature 2013; 500(7464): 541–6.

16. Mueller NT, Whyatt R, Hoepner L, Oberfield S, Dominguez-Bello MG, Widen EM, et al. Prenatal exposure to antibiotics, cesarean section, and risk of childhood obesity. Int J Obes (Lond) 2015; 39(4): 665–70.

17. Cabrera-Rubio R, Collado MC, Laitinen K, Salminen S, Isolauri E, Mira A. The human milk microbiome changes over lactation and is shaped by maternal weight and mode of delivery. Am J Clin Nutr 2012; 96(3): 544–51.

18. Gronlund MM, Lehtonen OP, Eerola E, Kero P. Fecal microflora in healthy infants born by different methods of delivery: Permanent changes in intestinal flora after cesarean delivery. J Pediatr Gastroenterol Nutr 1999; 28(1): 19–25.

19. Lif Holgerson P, Harnevik L, Hernell O, Tanner AC, Johansson I. Mode of birth delivery affects oral microbiota in infants. J Dent Res 2011; 90(10): 1183–8.

20. Azad MB, Konya T, Maughan H, Guttman DS, Field CJ, Chari RS, et al. Gut microbiota of healthy Canadian infants: Profiles by mode of delivery and infant diet at 4 months. CMAJ 2013; 185(5): 385–94.

21. Jakobsson HE, Abrahamsson TR, Jenmalm MC, Harris K, Quince C, Jernberg C, et al. Decreased gut microbiota diversity, delayed Bacteroidetes colonisation and reduced Th1 responses in infants delivered by caesarean section. Gut 2014; 63(4): 559–66.

22. Khodayar-Pardo P, Mira-Pascual L, Collado MC, Martínez-Costa C. Impact of lactation stage, gestational age and mode of delivery on breast milk microbiota. J Perinatol 2014; 34(8): 599–605.

23. Cabrera-Rubio R, Collado MC, Laitinen K, Salminen S, Isolauri E, Mira A. The human milk microbiome changes over lactation and is shaped by maternal weight and mode of delivery. Am J Clin Nutr 2012; 96(3): 544–51.

24. Walker WA, Iyengar RS. Breast milk, microbiota, and intestinal immune homeostasis. Pediatr Res 2015; 77(1–2): 220–8.

25. Pistiner M, Gold DR, Abdulkerim H, Hoffman E, Celedon JC. Birth by cesarean section, allergic rhinitis, and allergic sensitization among children with a parental history of atopy. J Allergy Clin Immunol 2008; 122(2): 274–9.

26. Bager P, Wohlfahrt J, Westergaard T. Caesarean delivery and risk of atopy and allergic disease: Meta-analyses. Clin Exp Allergy 2008; 38(4): 634–42.

27. Xu B, Pekkanen J, Hartikainen AL, Järvelin MR. Caesarean section and risk of asthma and allergy in adulthood. J Allergy Clin Immunol 2001; 107(4): 732–3.

28. Roduit C, Scholtens S, de Jongste JC, Wijga AH, Gerritsen J, Postma DS, et al. Asthma at 8 years of age in children born by caesarean section. Thorax 2009; 64(2): 107–13.

29. Kuitunen M, Kukkonen K, Juntunen-Backman K, Korpela R, Poussa T, Tuure T, et al. Probiotics prevent IgE-associated allergy until age 5 years in cesarean-delivered children but not in the total cohort. J Allergy Clin Immunol 2009; 123(2): 335–41.

30. Stensballe LG, Simonsen J, Jensen SM, Bønnelykke K, Bisgaard H. Use of antibiotics during pregnancy increases the risk of asthma in early childhood. J Pediatr 2013; 162(4): 832–8.

31. Jedrychowski W, Gałaś A, Whyatt R, Perera F. The prenatal use of antibiotics and the development of allergic disease in one year old infants. A preliminary study. Int J Occup Med Environ Health 2006; 19(1): 70–6.

32. Glasgow TS, Young PC, Wallin J, Kwok C, Stoddard G, Firth S, et al. Association of intrapartum antibiotic exposure and late-onset serious bacterial infections in infants. Pediatrics 2005; 116(3): 696–702.

33. Bruce A, Black M, Bhattacharya S. Mode of delivery and risk of inflammatory bowel disease in the offspring: Systematic review and meta-analysis of observational studies. Inflamm Bowel Dis 2014; 20(7): 1217–26.

34. McKinney PA, Parslow R, Gurney KA, Law GR, Bodansky HJ, Williams R. Perinatal and neonatal determinants of childhood type 1 diabetes. A case-control study in Yorkshire, UK. Diabetes Care 1999; 22(6): 928–32.

35. Cardwell CR, Stene LC, Joner G, Cinek O, Svensson J, Goldacre MJ, et al. Caesarean section is associated with an increased risk of childhood-onset type 1 diabetes mellitus: A meta-analysis of observational studies. Diabetologia 2008; 51(5): 726–35.

36. Huh SY, Rifas-Shiman SL, Zera CA, Edwards JW, Oken E, Weiss ST, et al. Delivery by caesarean section and risk of obesity in preschool age children: A prospective cohort study. Arch Dis Child 2012; 97(7): 610–16.

37. Blustein J, Attina T, Liu M, Ryan AM, Cox LM, Blaser MJ, Trasande L. Association of caesarean delivery with child adiposity from age 6 weeks to 15 years. Int J Obes (Lond) 2013; 37(7): 900–6.

38. Mesquita DN, Barbieri MA, Goldani HA, Cardoso VC, Goldani MZ, Kac G, et al. Cesarean section is associated with increased peripheral and central adiposite in young adulthood: Cohort study. PLoS One 2013; 8(6): e66827.

39. Blustein J, Attina T, Liu M, Ryan AM, Cox LM, Blaser MJ, et al. Association of caesarean delivery with child adiposity from age 6 weeks to 15 years. Int J Obes (Lond) 2013; 37(7): 900–6.

40. Li H, Ye R, Pei L, Ren A, Zheng X, Liu J. Caesarean delivery, caesarean delivery on maternal request and childhood overweight: A Chinese birth cohort study of 181 380 children. Pediatr Obes 2014; 9(1): 10–16.

41. Turnbaugh PJ, Ley RE, Mahowald MA, Magrini V, Mardis ER, Gordon GI. An obesity-associated gut microbiome with increased capacity for energy harvest. Nature 2006; 444(7122): 1027–31.

42. Larsen N, Vogensen FK, Van der Berg FWJ, Nielsen DS, Andreasen AS, Pedersen BK, et al. Gut microbiota in human adults with type 2 diabetes differs from non-diabetic adults. PLoS One 2010; 5(2): e9085.

43. Francis SS, Selvin S, Metayer C, Wallace AD, Crouse V, Moore TB, et al. Mode of delivery and risk of childhood leukemia. Cancer Epidemiol Biomarkers Prev 2014; 23(5): 876–81.

44. Caughey RW, Michels KB. Birth weight and childhood leukemia: A meta-analysis and review of the current evidence. Int J Cancer 2009; 124(11): 2658–70.

45. de Weerth C, Fuentes S, de Vos WM. Crying in infants: On the possible role of intestinal microbiota in the development of colic. Gut Microbes 2013; 4(5): 416–21.

46. de Weerth C, Fuentes S, Puylaert P, de Vos WM. Intestinal microbiota of infants with colic: development and specific signatures. Pediatrics 2013; 131(2): e550–8.

47. Rosenberg E, Zilber-Rosenberg I. Sybiosis and development: The hologenome concept. Birth Defects Res C Embro Today 2011; 93(1): 55–66.

48. Brucker RM, Bordenstein SR. The capacious hologenome. Zoology (Jena) 2013; 116(5): 260–1.

49. Barzegari A, Saeedi N, Saei AA. Shrinkage of the human core microbiome and a proposal for launching microbiome biobanks. Future Microbiol 2014; 9(5): 639–56.

50. Barrett HL, Dekker Nitert M, Conwell LS, Callaway LK. Probiotics for preventing gestational diabetes. Cochrane Database Syst Rev 2014; 2: CD009951.

51. Burton GJ, Sibley CP, Jauniaux E. Placental anatomy and physiology. In: Gabbe SG, Niebyl JR, Simpson JL, Galan H, Goetzl L, Landon M, Jauniaux E, eds. Obstetrics: Normal and Problem Pregnancies. Philadelphia, PA: Elsevier, 2012; 3–22.

52. Gordon MC. Maternal physiology. In: Gabbe SG, Niebyl JR, Simpson JL, Galan H, Goetzl L, Landon M, Jauniaux E, eds. Obstetrics: Normal and Problem Pregnancies. Philadelphia, PA: Elsevier, 2012; 42–65.

53. Dale HH. On some physiological actions of ergot. J Physiol (Lond) 1906; 34(2): 163–206.

54. Neumann ID, Landgraf R. Balance of brain oxytocin and vasopressin: Implications for anxiety, depression, and social behaviors. Trends Neurosci 2012; 35(11): 649–59.

55. Anaker AM, Beery AK. Life in groups: The roles of oxytocin in mammalian society. Front Behav Neurosci 2013; 7: 185.

56. Bugg GJ, Siddiqui F, Thornton JG. Oxytocin versus no treatment or delayed treatment for slow progress in the first stage of spontaneous labour. Cochrane Database Syst Rev 2013; 6: CD007123.

57. Kenyon S, Tokumasu H, Dowswell T, Pledge D, Mori R. High-dose versus low-dose oxytocin for augmentation of delayed labour. Cochrane Database Syst Rev 2013; 7: CD007201.

58. Freund-Mercier MJ, Moos F, Poulain DA, Richard P, Rodriguez F, Theodosis DT, et al. Role of central oxytocin in the control of the milk ejection reflex. Brain Res Bull 1988; 20(6): 737–41.

59. Tobin VA, Arechaga G, Brunton PJ, Russell JA, Leng G, Ludwig M, et al. Oxytocinase in the female rat hypothalamus: A novel mechanism controlling oxytocin neurones during lactation. J Neuroendocrinol 2014; 26(4): 205–16.

60. Gialloreti L, Benvenuto A, Benassi F, Curatolo P. Are caesarean sections, induced labor and oxytocin regulation linked to Autism Spectrum Disorders? Med Hypotheses 2014; 82(6):713–18.

61. Babb JA, Carini LM, Spears SL, Nephew BC. Transgenerational effects of social stress on social behavior, corticosterone, oxytocin, and prolactin in rats. Horm Behav 2014; 65(4): 386–93.

62. Odent M. Childbirth and the Future of *Homo sapiens*. London: Pinter & Martin, 2013.

63. Odent M. The Caesarean. London: Free Association Books, 2004.

64. Odent M. What about the future of *Homo sapiens*? Hum Evol 2014; 29: 229–30.

65. Simon-Areces J, Dietrich MO, Hermes G, Garcia-Segura LM, Arevalo MA, Horvath TL. UCP2 induced by natural birth regulates neuronal differentiation of the hippocampus and related adult behavior. PLoS One 2012; 7(8): e42911.

66. Hermansson H, Hoppu U, Isolauri E. Elective caesarean section is associated with low adiponectin levels in cord blood. Neonatology 2014; 105(3): 172–4.

CHAPTER 13
Caesarean section: A global perspective

James Walker

Introduction

As described in Chapter 3, there has been a steady rise in caesarean section rates throughout the world. However, these rates vary widely both between countries and within countries [1, 2]. There are many factors that influence this variation, ranging from the levels of skill and training of healthcare providers to the access to obstetric services. There are also cultural and social pressures, which can both inhibit or encourage the uptake of caesarean section.

Although there were isolated cases of caesarean delivery described in early times (see Chapter 1), the procedure was rarely performed except in cases after the mother had died (see Figure 13.1) [3]. The increasing knowledge of anatomy helped those who carried out the procedure to proceed with some confidence, but the maternal mortality rate still reached 75%. It was not until the latter part of the nineteenth century that caesarean delivery became established as a potential alternative management in cases of obstructed labour, following the pioneering work in Glasgow of Murdoch Cameron [4], who carried out 12 caesarean deliveries with no loss of life in women suffering from rickets (Figure 13.2). This improvement in safety corresponded with the development of anaesthesia [5] and anaesthetic machines. The understanding of sepsis, bacterial infection, and

aseptic techniques developed by Lister [6], with whom Cameron had worked, helped encourage operative intervention by increasing the likelihood of survival for the mother and the baby. These advances resulted in an increase in the number of doctors trained in the procedure, promoting a further increase in practice and the development of better techniques. In the 1920s, advanced procedures were developed by Munro Kerr, who popularized the low transverse incisions of the uterus and the abdomen, techniques which improved healing and recovery [7]. Other technological and environmental improvements also contributed making caesarean delivery safer and easier to do than it had been before [8], further reducing the overall mortality rate to less than 10%.

A further impetus for change occurred during and following the Second World War, which brought improved surgical techniques, operating theatres with appropriate lighting, improved operating instruments, and more anaesthetic support than had been available before. But it was the development of blood transfusion and antibiotic therapy by Florey [9] that reduced the chances of the two main causes of maternal mortality. Further developments led first to the use of intubation during general anaesthesia, to reduce the risk of aspiration,

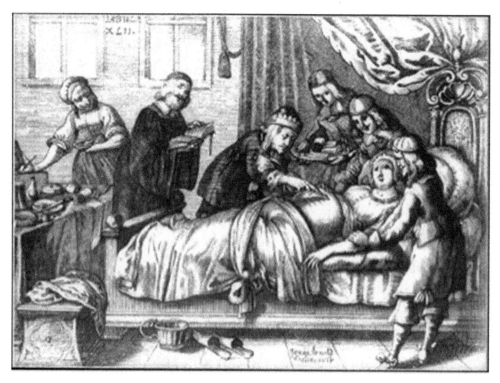

Figure 13.1 A picture from the 1600s depicting a caesarean section with a priest present.

and then to regional anaesthesia, which has helped to make the caesarean section procedure even safer than before (Box 13.1).

These changes did not change the fundamental reasons for caesarean section but changed the balance of risks and benefits of the procedure itself.

Caesarean section has moved from being an operation of the last resort to one that can be done *just in case* [10]. This development has led to the rise in the rate of the procedure in the developed world, with rates of over 50% in parts of countries like China [1, 11, 12].

The global view of caesarean section

These developments in caesarean section and the corresponding steady rise in caesarean section rates are largely developed-world phenomena. However, the rates in the low- or middle-income regions in the world vary markedly, ranging from less than 2% in parts of rural sub-Saharan Africa to over 60% in private practice in Brazil [1]. This variability is not because of differences in need but more to do with the variation in training, facilities available, and social factors.

The World Health Organization has proposed a list of resources that are required to provide a safe caesarean section service (Box 13.2). The World Health Organization has also stated that a minimum caesarean section rate of 10% is required to fulfil basic obstetric needs (Table 13.1) [1]. Conversely, it has been suggested that rates above 20% are not clearly improving maternal or perinatal health, but more data are needed to assess the numerous modern confounding factors associated with rising

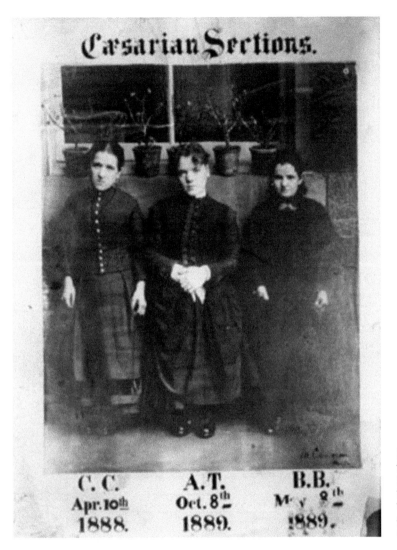

Figure 13.2 A picture of the women from the first three caesarean sections performed by Murdoch Cameron in 1888; they were followed by 14 successful cases with no mortality.

from Glasgow Caledonian University Archives: Heatherbank Social Work Collection

---

Box 13.1 **Factors contributing to the reduction in maternal mortality from caesarean section**

From 1888–1940

- Anaesthesia
- Aseptic techniques
- Suturing of the uterus

Influence of the Second World War

- Safer anaesthesia than before

- Antimicrobials
- Blood transfusion
- Surgical skills and techniques

From 1950 onwards

- Intubation
- Epidural

Box 13.2 **The requirements for developing caesarean section services**

Training
- Operators
- Anaesthetists
- Scrub nurses/assistants
- Theatre support staff
- Recovery staff

Development
- Theatre facilities

- Sterilization equipment
- Maintenance of equipment and supplies
- Blood transfusion services
- Pharmacy services

Planning
- Transport services
- Post-partum contraception
- Management of labour with previous caesarean section

Table 13.1 **World Health Organization assessment of national caesarean section rates. This table shows the percentages of the world's caesarean sections and deliveries in countries classified by national caesarean section rate. Nearly 75% of the world's caesarean sections are carried out in only one-third of the world's countries. In contrast, the majority of deliveries occur in countries which, according to the World Health Organization, have insufficient utilization of caesarean section.**

Countries classified by national caesarean section rate	World Health Organization classification of caesarean section use	Percentage of world's caesarean sections (%)	Percentage of world's deliveries (%)
Countries in which <10% of deliveries are via caesarean section	Underuse of caesarean section	24.7	60.0
Counties in which 10%–15% of deliveries are via caesarean section	Adequate use of caesarean section	2.2	2.5
Countries in which >15% of deliveries are via caesarean section	Overuse of caesarean section	73.1	37.5

Betran AP, Merialdi M, Lauer JA, et al., Rates of caesarean section: analysis of global, regional and national estimates., 2007, Wiley

caesarean section rates and their short- and long-term impacts on maternal and child health.

As the risk of caesarean section to the mother falls, it becomes increasingly justifiable to carry out a caesarean section at a given level of perinatal risk. The occurrence of a fetus with a term breech presentation is a good example of this concept. Based on the short-term results of a randomized trial [13], there appeared to be benefit to the baby from caesarean delivery. This conclusion was buttressed by existing prejudices and fear of litigation and led to a

dramatic change in clinical practice. Following this trial, follow-up studies challenged these results and the subsequent recommendations and changes in practice [14, 15]. However, the die had already been cast, and practice had changed permanently.

Therefore, it is not possible to quote a 'correct' caesarean section rate in any given situation, since it is so dependent on local environment, risks, culture, and perception. However, the frequent following of Western practices has led to an increase in caesarean section in other parts of the world where the risk of caesarean section and its sequelae may not be as low (see Chapter 6, 7, and 8) and the risks of litigation as high as it is in developed countries. Evidence and advice needs to be tailored to the environment where the practice will occur.

The necessity for caesarean section

Unlike other primates, humans walk upright, an activity that ultimately changed the shape of the pelvis, and have a large brain (see Chapter 12). Most other primates deliver their babies in the direct occipital position, whereas humans usually deliver the baby in the direct anterior position after rotation of the fetal head. This approach requires a delivery process that is more complicated than that for most other primates, leading to an increased likelihood of obstructed labour and its attendant risks (e.g. fistula formation, the death of the mother and/or fetus). Obstructed labour or 'failure to progress in labour' with or without fetal distress is the main indication for emergency caesarean section around the world. The two main causes of obstructed labour are cephalo-pelvic disproportion and dystocia (inadequate uterine contraction). Causes of active phase disorders are often combined in cases of fetal macrosomia, fibroids of the lower segment, placenta praevia, and multiple gestation pregnancy, thus increasing the surgical risks and poor outcome for both mother and her baby (or babies). In under-resourced or low-income countries (LICs), up to 9% of maternal death and morbidity is associated with obstructed labour (Figure 13.3) [16].

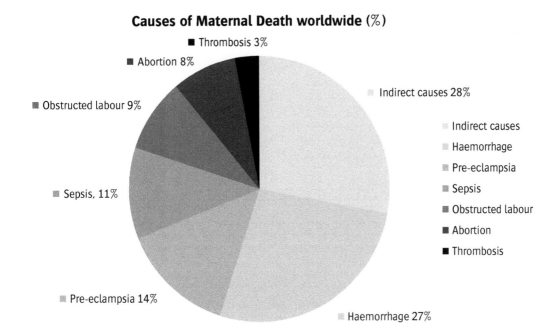

Causes of Maternal Death worldwide (%)

- Thrombosis 3%
- Abortion 8%
- Obstructed labour 9%
- Sepsis, 11%
- Pre-eclampsia 14%
- Haemorrhage 27%
- Indirect causes 28%

Legend:
- Indirect causes
- Haemorrhage
- Pre-eclampsia
- Sepsis
- Obstructed labour
- Abortion
- Thrombosis

Figure 13.3 Global causes of maternal death.

Reprinted from The Lancet Global health, 2, Say L, Chou D, Gemmill A, Tuncalp O, Moller AB, Daniels J, et al., Global causes of maternal death: a WHO systematic analysis., 323–33, Copyright (2014) with permission from Elsevier

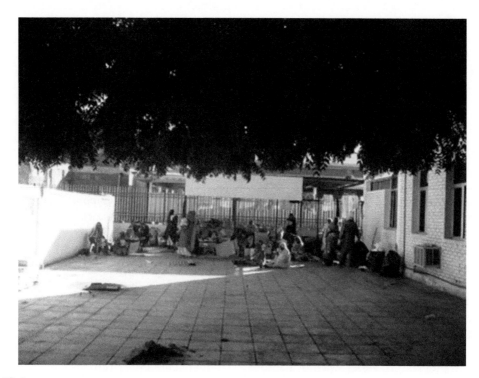

Figure 13.4 Women sitting outside a fistula unit in Khartoum, waiting to be seen and operated on. Many had walked hundreds of miles to get there after being expelled from the family home.

Obstetric fistulae are also a direct consequence of prolonged obstructed labour, with the pressure from impacted fetal presentation leading to the destruction of the vesicovaginal/rectovaginal septum, with consequent loss of urinary and/or faecal control [17,18]. Although obstetric fistula has become a rare complication of delivery in advanced industrialized nations, it remains a major public health problem in many LICs, affecting several million women (Figure 13.4).

Antenatal screening for causes of obstructed labour should be considered as a priority in LICs. Ultrasound imaging can be used to identify a series of prenatal findings clearly associated with increased risk in labour, such as placenta praevia and twins. It can help local healthcare workers to screen their prenatal populations for obstetric and neonatal risks and therefore has the potential to improve outcomes at delivery by providing institutional delivery at facilities with operating rooms and neonatal intensive care services [19]. Basic obstetric ultrasound training using low-cost, portable ultrasound machines in a rural setting supported remotely is feasible, efficient, and sustainable [19]. The training also empowers local health workers and motivates them to work in rural areas.

The ease and safety of caesarean section

In high-income countries (HICs), it was not until the safety of the procedure was established, with the development of improved surgical techniques and suturing, anaesthesia, and infection control, that the use of caesarean section become commonplace. The improvements in safety were paralleled by the development of support services that are required to maximize the safety of the procedure, such as operating theatres and blood transfusion. These developments did not change the fundamental reasons for caesarean section but changed the risks of the procedure itself. These developments need to be repeated in LICs to achieve the same level of benefit. It is not enough simply to train individuals to carry out caesarean section if the support services are not available (Box 13.2).

Training in caesarean section

In many countries in sub-Saharan Africa, there are few obstetricians to provide operative services; if there is one available for a hospital, he or she may be alone and unable to provide 24-hour cover. Thus, a caesarean section can be carried out only some of the time, while at other times the women either has to wait or be transferred, often for several hours, to the next available centre. Therefore, additional trained operators are required to improve access [20]. However, training alone may not fix the problem as, once trained, doctors may leave less resourced settings [20]. This 'brain drain' is a significant problem in many parts of Africa. One solution to the problem is task shifting, with the midwives or medical officer being trained to carry out caesarean section (see Editorial). Nevertheless, they may lack skills, support, and rescue services, so that the safety of the procedure remains suboptimal. Since the main risks of caesarean section are sepsis and haemorrhage, lack of blood for transfusion and a lack of access to antibiotics means that the mortality remains unacceptably high. Also, since anaesthesia in most LICs tends to be general anaesthesia (see Chapter 7), there are further risks which would be averted with the widespread use of regional blockade.

Therefore, even when training is improved, the development of support services and healthcare pathways is required. The complications of caesarean section, both immediate and long term, need to be considered in the overall planning and development of any operative service.

Development of caesarean section support services

Carrying out a caesarean section requires more than just the operator, and major gaps exist in LICs in terms of the physical and human resources needed to carry out basic life-saving surgical interventions. The latest (2011–2013) Saving Mothers report, the National Committee for Confidential Enquiries into Maternal Deaths in South Africa has highlighted the large number of maternal deaths associated with caesarean section (21). The risk of a woman dying as a result of caesarean section during the past three decades was almost three times that for vaginal delivery. Of all the mothers who died during or after a caesarean delivery, 3.4% died during the procedure and 14.5% from haemorrhage afterwards. Including all cases of death from obstetric haemorrhage where a caesarean section was done, there were 5.5 deaths from haemorrhage for every 10,000 CSs performed.

A caesarean section, whether elective or an emergency procedure, requires a nursing assistant, a surgical assistant (who could be the same person as the nursing assistant), a trained operator in anaesthetics, anaesthetic equipment, and the appropriate surgical instruments (Box 13.2). Operating theatres in LICs or middle-income countries are often built apart from the maternity areas, producing difficulty in transferring women for caesarean section. Simple redesign or the building of concrete ramps to allow the pushing of beds to the theatre would make life easier (Figure 13.5). Also, those operating

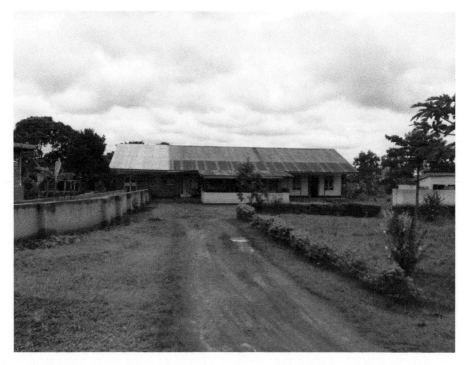

Figure 13.5 An obstetric unit in Uganda. The concrete ramp on the left was built to improve access from the delivery suite to the theatre, which is behind, on the left. On the day the photograph was taken, the man with the key to the theatre was not there, so access to it was not possible.

rooms may not be easily accessed (e.g. they may be locked). Once the operation is over, there needs to be the ability to recover the patient and provide both antibiotic therapy and blood transfusion if required. All these factors need to be considered if caesarean section is going to be a readily available, safe, and reliable procedure in maternity care.

Transferring skills and practice from HICs to LICs needs careful consideration. The immediate risks of caesarean section in modern facilities in HICs are relatively minimal because of the rescue services that are available [22], but the risks at caesarean section are greater in the developing world (Table 13.2) [23–27]. In fact, although caesarean section is used as an intervention to prevent fistula, if those carrying it out are not adequately trained, the procedure can be a cause of fistula itself, in up to 25% of cases [28].

These consequences of caesarean section for the first birth are amplified in any subsequent pregnancy (see Chapter 9). In the United Kingdom, nearly 50% of women requiring a peripartum hysterectomy had a previous caesarean section, with placenta accreta and uterine rupture as the two main causes [22] (Table 13.3). Therefore, developing a caesarean section service in an area that is not equipped to manage women in labour after a previous caesarean section can greatly increase the morbidity of the procedure itself, because of the complications in subsequent pregnancies. There also are other potential late complications of caesarean section, such as subfertility and an increased risk of ectopic pregnancy (see Chapter 9) that can have social consequences as well as impact on immediate maternal morbidity.

Therefore, there is a range of requirements if the benefits of caesarean section are to be brought to an increased number of patients without reducing maternal and perinatal morbidity and mortality in itself (Box 13.2). The experience in Gambia reveals the challenges in developing a programme with these resources. Investigators, in collaboration with

Table 13.2 **Maternal mortality associated with caesarean section. Although Western techniques are available, the mortality rate in sub-Saharan Africa is still significantly higher than that in the United Kingdom. There are multiple reasons for this fact, including pre-existing morbidity and a lack of facilities for blood transfusion and for treating sepsis.**

Years	Location	Rate/1000
1966–74	Lagos, Nigeria [1]	11.0
1979–84	Enugu, Nigeria [2]	8.0
1988–90	United Kingdom [3]	0.2
1998–2000	Malawi [4]	10.5
2010–11	Sub-Saharan Africa [5]	5.0

1. Oyegunle AO. Caesarean section and maternal mortality at the Lagos University Teaching Hospital. Niger Med J 1976; 6(2): 201–5.
2. Megafu U. Maternal mortality from emergency caesarean section in booked hospital patients at the University of Nigeria Teaching Hospital Enugu. Trop J Obstet Gynaecol 1988; 1(1): 29–31.
3. Hall MH. Variation in caesarean section rate. Maternal mortality higher after caesarean section. BMJ 1994; 308: 654–5.
4. Fenton PM, Whitty CJ, Reynolds F. Caesarean section in Malawi: Prospective study of early maternal and perinatal mortality. BMJ 2003; 327: 587.
5. Chu K, Cortier H, Maldonado F, Mashant T, Ford N, Trelles M. Cesarean section rates and indications in sub-Saharan Africa: A multi-country study from Medecins sans Frontieres. PloS One 2012; 7(9): e44484.

Table 13.3 **Women requiring peripartum hysterectomy, and the associated causes in the United Kingdom between 2005 and 2006 (n = 20). Two women died, giving a case fatality rate of 0.6%. (The total adds up to more than 100% because there were some cases with multiple causes.)**

Cause	%
Uterine atony	53
Placenta accreta/increta/percreta	39
Extension of the uterine incision/scar	9
Uterine rupture	8
Uterine infection	5
Fibroids	3
Genital tract laceration	3
Other (including placenta praevia, clotting abnormalities, and placental abruption)	14

Knight M. Peripartum hysterectomy in the UK: Management and outcomes of the associated haemorrhage. BJOG 2007; 114(11): 1380–7.

the Ministry of Health, developed an 'emergency chain of care' for mothers and babies. Multilevel training and infrastructure developments were put in place that produced a framework to allow triage, transport, and access to caesarean section [29]. Nevertheless, major problems remained with low morale, attrition of physicians to the private sector, and difficulty in employing adequate numbers of medical staff. The importance of partnership with the local healthcare providers must be emphasized if a sustainable programme is to be achieved [29]. Also, the economic outlays are not insubstantial. It has been calculated that, in Nigeria alone, it would cost over $68 million dollars a year to institute a comprehensive obstetric care programme, with lesser amounts required in other LICs [2].

References

1. Betrán AP, Merialdi M, Lauer JA, Bing-Shun W, Thomas J, Van Look P, et al. Rates of caesarean section: Analysis of global, regional and national estimates. Paedia Perinat Epidemiol 2007; 21(2): 98–113.

2. Gibbons L, Belizán JM, Lauer JA, Betrán AP, Merialdi M, Althabe F. The Global Numbers and Costs of Additionally Needed and Unnecessary Caesarean Sections Performed per Year: Overuse as a Barrier to Universal Coverage. World Health Report 30. 2010. http://www.who.int/healthsystems/topics/financing/healthreport/30C-sectioncosts.pdf.

3. Boley JP. The history of caesarean section. CMAJ 1935; 32(5): 557–9.

4. Obituary. Murdoch Cameron, M.D., C.M., Ll.D. Br Med J 1930; 1: 930.

5. Dunn PM. Sir James Young Simpson (1811–1870) and obstetric anaesthesia. Arch Dis Child Fetal Neonatal Ed 2002; 86(3): F207–209.

6. Jessney B. Joseph Lister (1827–1912): A pioneer of antiseptic surgery remembered a century after his death. J Med Biogr 2012; 20(3): 107–10.

7. Dunn PM. Professor Munro Kerr (1868–1960) of Glasgow and caesarean delivery. Arch Dis Child Fetal Neonatal Ed 2008; 93(2): F167–169.

8. Basden MM. Caesarean section in infected cases: A series of forty-five caesarean sections in infected or potentially infected cases, with no maternal mortality. Br Med J 1936; 1: 358–60.

9. Florey HW. Penicillin; Its development for medical uses. Proc R Inst G B 1946; 33(150 Pt 1): 23–30.

10. Leitch CR, Walker JJ. The rise in caesarean section rate: The same indications but a lower threshold. BJOG 1998; 105(6): 621–6.

11. Lumbiganon P, Laopaiboon M, Gulmezoglu AM, Souza JP, Taneepanichskul S, Ruyan P, et al. Method of delivery and pregnancy outcomes in Asia: The WHO global survey on maternal and perinatal health 2007–08. Lancet 2010; 375(9713): 490–9.

12. Hannah ME. Planned elective cesarean section: A reasonable choice for some women? CMAJ 2004; 170(5): 813–14.

13. Hannah ME, Hannah WJ, Hewson SA, Hodnett ED, Saigal S, Willan AR. Planned caesarean section versus planned vaginal birth for breech presentation at term: A randomised multicentre trial. Term Breech Trial Collaborative Group. Lancet 2000; 356(9239): 1375–83.

14. Glezerman M. Five years to the Term Breech Trial: The rise and fall of a randomized controlled trial. Am J Obstet Gynecol 2006; 194(1): 20–5.

15. Lawson GW. The Term Breech Trial ten years on: Primum non nocere? Birth 2012; 39(1): 3–9.

16. Say L, Chou D, Gemmill A, Tuncalp O, Moller AB, Daniels J, et al. Global causes of maternal death: A WHO systematic analysis. Lanc Glob Health 2014; 2(6): e323–333.

17. Tebeu PM, Fomulu JN, Khaddaj S, de Bernis L, Delvaux T, Rochat CH. Risk factors for obstetric fistula: A clinical review. Internat Urogynecol J 2012; 23(4): 387–94.

18. Gebresilase YT. A qualitative study of the experience of obstetric fistula survivors in Addis Ababa, Ethiopia. Int J Womens Health 2014; 6: 1033–43.

19. Greenwold N, Wallace S, Prost A, Jauniaux E. Implementing an obstetric ultrasound training program in rural Africa. Int J Gynaecol Obstet 2014; 124(3): 274–7.

20. Kasper J, Bajunirwe F. Brain drain in sub-Saharan Africa: Contributing factors, potential remedies and the role of academic medical centres. Arch Dis Child 2012; 97(11): 973–9.

21. Gebhardt GS, Fawcus S, Moodley J, Farina Z, National Committee for Confidential Enquiries into Maternal Deaths in South Africa. Maternal death and caesarean section in South Africa: Results from the 2011–2013 Saving Mothers Report of the National Committee for Confidential Enquiries into Maternal Deaths. S Afr Med J 2015; 115(4): 287–91.

22. Knight M. Peripartum hysterectomy in the UK: Management and outcomes of the associated haemorrhage. BJOG 2007; 114(11): 1380–7.

23. Oyegunle AO. Caesarean section and maternal mortality at the Lagos University Teaching Hospital. Niger Med J 1976; 6(2): 201–5.

24. Megafu U. Maternal mortality from emergency caesarean section in booked hospital patients at the University of Nigeria Teaching Hospital Enugu. Trop J Obstet Gynaecol 1988; 1(1): 29–31.

25. Hall MH. Variation in caesarean section rate. Maternal mortality higher after caesarean section. BMJ 1994; 308: 654–5.

26. Fenton PM, Whitty CJ, Reynolds F. Caesarean section in Malawi: Prospective study of early maternal and perinatal mortality. BMJ 2003; 327: 587.

27. Chu K, Cortier H, Maldonado F, Mashant T, Ford N, Trelles M. Cesarean section rates and indications in sub-Saharan Africa: A multi-country study from Medecins sans Frontieres. PloS One 2012; 7(9): e44484.

28. Barageine JK, Tumwesigye NM, Byamugisha JK, Almroth L, Faxelid E. Risk factors for obstetric fistula in Western Uganda: A case control study. PloS One 2014; 9(11): e112299.

29. Cole-Ceesay R, Cherian M, Sonko A, et al. Strengthening the emergency healthcare system for mothers and children in The Gambia. Reprod Health 2010; 7: 21.

Index